Marketplace, Power, Prestige

# Medizin,
# Gesellschaft und Geschichte

Jahrbuch
des Instituts für Geschichte der Medizin
der Robert Bosch Stiftung

herausgegeben von
Robert Jütte

Beiheft 70

# Marketplace, Power, Prestige

The Healthcare Professions' Struggle
for Recognition (19th–20th Century)

Edited by Pierre Pfütsch

Franz Steiner Verlag Stuttgart
2019

Gedruckt mit freundlicher Unterstützung der Robert Bosch Stiftung GmbH

Coverabbildung:
„Geherbad" aus dem Robert Bosch Krankenhaus, Stuttgart, 1940.
Quelle: IGM-Archiv

Bibliografische Information der Deutschen Nationalbibliothek:
Die Deutsche Nationalbibliothek verzeichnet diese Publikation in der Deutschen
Nationalbibliografie; detaillierte bibliografische Daten sind im Internet über
<http://dnb.d-nb.de> abrufbar.

© Franz Steiner Verlag, Stuttgart 2019
Druck: Laupp & Göbel GmbH, Gomaringen
Gedruckt auf säurefreiem, alterungsbeständigem Papier.
Printed in Germany
ISBN 978-3-515-12294-8 (Print)
ISBN 978-3-515-12299-3 (E-Book)

# Table of Contents

**Conflicts due to Changes in Social Conditions**

# An Introduction to Conflict Research:
# Illustrative Applications with Healthcare Professions in the 19th and 20th Century

*Pierre Pfütsch*

## Epistemological interest

Currently questions of the best possible care for the population are at the centre of discussion in both the healthcare system and within medicine. While the populations of Western industrial nations are only minimally growing, if at all, there are other factors that push healthcare to its limits. One reason is paradoxically the progress that was made in medicine, hygiene, and nutrition in the past 150 years, which has driven increases in life expectancy. At present, men born in Germany have a life expectancy of 78.18 years and women 83.06 years.[1] In other European countries the situation is similar. In France, life expectancy for men is currently 79.2 years and for women 85.5. In the UK, boys who were born in 2015 will live on average 79.2 years and girls 82.8 years.[2] Model calculation of the Federal Bureau of Statistics in Wiesbaden suggest, however, that boys who were born in 2017 in Germany will on average reach an age of 90 years and girls of 93 years.[3] Since an older age is often accompanied by more diseases and a deteriorating health condition, people above 65 years of age require more medical care and hence have more contact with the healthcare system.[4] In this phase of life cases of multi-morbidity also become more common, which means that consultants with numerous specialities are contacted. Due to the multi-morbidity, the disease patterns are also becoming more complex. Consequently, the healthcare system is frequented more often.

A second reason why the healthcare system is being pushed to its limits is the increasing use of preventative and health-promoting offers on the medical market. Since the 1970s, this development has been linked to the growing significance of health within societal discourse. In the industrial nations, health rose to the position of central leading category of all areas of life. The health scientist Ilona Kickbusch perfectly summarised this development with the term "health society".[5] The reason for using various offers by the healthcare system cannot only be found in the need created by patients, but also in the fact that such offers exist. Until the 1980s, the focus in medicine was foremost to heal diseases. Yet, with the agreement of the Ottawa Charter in 1986, it has increasingly recognised the potential of disease prevention with the term "pre-

---

1    Cf. Statistisches Bundesamt (2016), p. 12.
2    Cf. Eurostat (2017).
3    Cf. Statistisches Bundesamt: Kohortensterbetafeln (2017), p. 16.
4    Cf. Barmer GEK (2017), p. 57.
5    Hartung/Kickbusch (2014).

vention" not only referring to maintaining people's health but also the financial potential of prevention as a market segment. The so-called "second health market" that covers health tourism, wellness offers and services that are not covered by the statutory health insurance is steadily growing in Germany and its importance is rising. In the federal state Hesse alone, there are 30,200 people who work in this area producing a turnover of 5.56 billion Euros per year. Between 2009 and 2012 the employment number rose by 8.6 per cent and the turnover by 17 per cent.[6] Providers of health services and the staff hence prefer to focus on this financially attractive market which has consequences, at least indirectly, for the primary healthcare. Due to the different distribution of resources, this imbalance can have a negative outcome regarding staff capacities and services available.

In addition to these developments in society at large there are also tendencies within the medical system that concern questions of medical care for the population. In Germany we have increasing shortages of doctors in rural areas resulting in a worse standard of care than in the cities.[7] Furthermore, the currently pronounced shortage of nurses also contributes to the fact that the care is at risk as the number of people in need of care keeps growing.[8] Facing this difficult development, the people responsible in the healthcare system have been searching for some time for funding options to prevent a lack of care.

In other Western countries this issue was discussed much earlier and hence, action was also taken much earlier. In Canada, already in 1970 the profession of "nurse practitioner" was introduced. Since 1977, this profession has also been in existence in the Netherlands.[9] Since 1989, in Britain there have been "practice nurses". In Canada, the "nurse practitioners" are registered nurses with an academic degree.[10] "Nurse practitioners" are responsible for serving their patients through all phases of the life, perform smaller examinations, interpreting certain diagnostic tests, documenting findings and managing the patient's medication while staying up to date with the latest research. Overall, these members of staff are the first point of contact for the patient, and they have an extensive medical knowledge and free doctors to focus on more urgent tasks. Similarly, the profession of the "physician assistant" that was established in the 1970s in the US serves to relieve doctors from tasks that a person with less comprehensive, yet specified training could do.[11] With the additional training of medical staff as "care assistants in the GP

6   Cf. Gesundheitswirtschaft Rhein-Main e. V. (2014), p. 51.
7   More specifically on the distribution of doctors in Germany: Albrecht/Etgeton/Ochmann (2015).
8   Current news on the shortage of staff in nursing: Maibach-Nagel (2018).
9   In the US there were already first courses on the topic in the 1960s.
10  On the history of nurse practitioners in Canada: Bryant-Lukosius et al. (2010).
11  On the history of the physician assistant in the US see the homepage of the Physician Assistant History Society (https://pahx.org, last accessed: 17/10/2018). Since 2005, Germany has introduced the first university degrees of "physician assistants". This is a three-year bachelor degree course in which the students acquire a broad medical knowledge. This opens up new opportunities for doctors and other healthcare institutions to delegate

practice" ("Versorgungsassistentin in der hausärztlichen Praxis"), in Germany, general practitioners (GPs) now also have the option to delegate certain tasks to specially trained staff. In this context the professionalisation or academisation of nursing plays an increasingly important role.[12] A current example of this process is the new (model) degree programme of "evidence-based care" that was introduced at the Medical School of the Martin Luther University of Halle-Wittenberg. Yet, these are only first attempts to face this issue. With these current topics that focus on issues of delegating or substituting doctor's services to other health professions we can already recognise areas of tension and conflict. Questions of responsibility and authority will be core areas of conflict.

Historians and social scientists like to research conflicts, tensions, and debates because they bear the potential to disclose information on the conflicting parties and the solutions of the conflict but also on the context of the conflict. This allows the analysis of values, opinions, and patterns of behaviour. The significance of the conflicts lies in their effect for social and societal changes. Conflicts reveal different perspectives, promote change, and serve to generate decisions. The political scientist and researcher of conflict Anton Pelinka thus rightfully claims that without understanding conflict we could not understand changes in society.[13] Furthermore, analysing conflicts enables us to predict conflicts in the future and the development of various constellations of conflict. A historical analysis of conflicts is particularly useful as we can better understand, reconstruct, and interpret current developments.

Conflicts can emerge on various levels and in completely different fields. Within the theory of conflicts, a conflict is defined as follows: various agents perceive their respective interests in a particular area as opposing.[14] The large political and sociological theories of conflict often discuss international conflicts and even wars.[15] Yet, research on peace and conflicts is not an independent academic field but an area of research that is multi-, inter- and transdisciplinary. For that reason, it does not only cover large conflicts such as nuclear crises and world wars but also conflicts within families, communities and structures of society.[16]

At the meso- and micro-level disciplines of work repeatedly appear as a rewarding research project within conflict research. Social history and the history of society are especially well suited for the historical analysis of conflicts

---

tasks, which previously could have only been performed by a doctor. For instance, in the accident & emergency department they can take the medical history of the patient and perform a physical examination, and they can also work in the operating room as an assistant.

12   Since the 1990s, the Robert Bosch Stiftung has been promoting academic degrees in nursing and has been scientifically supporting this movement. Robert Bosch Stiftung/ Kommission (1992); Robert Bosch Stiftung (2000).

13   Cf. Pelinka (2016), p. 17.

14   Cf. Ide (2017), p. 9.

15   For instance: Ruf (2010). And: Geis/Wagner (2017).

16   Cf. Ide (2017), p. 8.

in the professional world because in society, work takes a central position. While presumably every profession and professional area have been marked by conflicts and tension, healthcare in particular is a rich area for research and analysis. On the one hand, health and diseases are central to human life. Every person who lives in an industrialised nation encounters the healthcare system during his or her life. People working in this area literally make life and death decisions for patients. The significance of healthcare as an area of work is also reflected in quantitative information. In Germany in 2015, 5.3 million people worked in the healthcare system.[17] These workers went through numerous training programmes with varying hierarchical levels. The professional world of the healthcare system today is the result of long processes of differentiation, elimination and negotiation. The differentiation of non-physician healthcare professions occurred in parallel with the specialisation of medicine and the development of medical technology, and accelerated at the end of the 19th century. At this time, academically trained doctors had already superseded their competitors with fewer qualifications such as barber surgeons.[18] They only had to fight longer battles with the "quacks" – a term made up by the doctors for non-academically trained healers. In 1903, the German Society for the Eradication of Quacks ("Deutsche Gesellschaft zur Bekämpfung des Kurpfuschertums") fought against the "freedom to heal" ("Kurierfreiheit") that had been announced in 1872.[19] With the foundation of medical associations and achieving the professionalisation that went along with it, the physicians had successfully fought for a position that from now on ensured their large influence in the official recognition of new health professions or professions that required new regulation.[20] They exert this influence to this day. For instance, since the introduction of the profession of doctor's assistant in the 1950s, the State Chambers of Physicians are the "responsible authorities" for the training and further education of medical staff, according to the German Vocational Training Act. Similarly, since increasingly women give birth at the hospital rather than in the private sphere of the home, midwives and doctors have also had a charged relationship. The issue is usually one of status and responsibility.[21] Even between physicians and nursing staff there are often conflicts because of their close collaboration. These conflicts very rarely came to light, as the psychologist Leonard Stein described in the 1960s using what he called the "doctor-nurse game". According to him, the collaboration between the (at the time mostly male) doctors and the (often

---

17  Cf. Statistisches Bundesamt: Statistisches Jahrbuch (2017), p. 10.
18  On the development of the position of physicians and their professionalisation, see Huerkamp (1985); Jütte: Geschichte (1997). On the social history of barber surgeons: Sabine Sander (1989).
19  On the debate between physicians and non-academic medicine: Teichler (2002); Jütte (1996).
20  The first medical association was founded in 1865 in Baden. Cf. Jütte: Entwicklung (1997), pp. 39–40.
21  More specifically on the training of midwives in Germany: Fallwell (2013); Schumann (2009).

female) nurses follows particular rules that do not question the authority of the doctor who has a higher rank in the hierarchy.[22] However, with the professionalisation of nursing, the relationship between doctors and nurses has been slowly changing which is why in the 1980s the "doctor-nurse game" no longer functioned as Stein had described it 20 years earlier.[23] This resulted in more conflicts coming to light more often.

The medical profession offers itself for the analysis of conflicts because scientific progress and the change of the social and societal frameworks had a huge impact on the professional landscape. Following the doctors' initiative to reduce the high mortality of mothers, at the end of the 19th century the profession of a childbed nurse was created. After their training, these nurses were supposed to professionally care for women after they had given birth.[24] However, in the second half of the 20th century, this profession disappeared again. Due to technical progress and improvements in hygiene the mothers spent less time at the hospital. Since the mortality of mothers was now very low, the care during the puerperium lost its justification. Substitution processes through other professions also played a role. Hence, midwives and paediatric nurses campaigned for taking on these tasks.[25] The discovery of new diseases could also result in the development of new working areas. The increase of patients with diabetes mellitus created a need for medical guidance below the rank of the doctor. Thus, slowly diabetes counselling emerged.[26] A more current example is the profession of the scrub nurse who has become necessary because of the increasing specialisation and technicalisation of surgeries. Already in the 1960s, the Netherlands introduced the profession of the "Operatie Assistant".[27] Another example is the emergence of the professional clinical coder. In Germany in 2003, only because of the introduction of a flat-rate per case that is based on the Diagnosis Related Groups (DRG), an independent profession at the interface of technology and medicine could be established. Since conflict research is not only interested in analysing a specific example but also wants to shed light on the context in society and the social framework in which the conflicting agents operate[28], conflict research is an excellent method to analyse the most diverse conflicts in medicine also from a historic perspective. Implicitly, professional sociological reflections play a part in all of these issues.

Beginning with these reflections this current volume serves to explain how and why conflicts emerged within medical professions at all. Who was involved, what coalitions were formed, how did the agents present themselves and what goals did they pursue? Furthermore, we are interested in the extent

---

22    Cf. Stein (1967).
23    Cf. Howell/Stein/Watts (1990).
24    Cf. Waller (2017), p. 114.
25    Cf. Waller (2017), p. 134.
26    Cf. Pfaff (2018).
27    Cf. Cerrahoglu et al. (2014), p. 212.
28    Cf. Pelinka (2016), p. 21.

to which such discussions contributed to changes in services on the medical market and what consequences this had on the demand side. Simultaneously, we want to consider the societal, social and scientific frameworks as central determinants of change.

## Market, Power, and Prestige as Areas of Action

The question about the cause of conflicts and tensions plays a central role in all contributions. In recent years, conflict research has illustrated that the cause of conflicts is most often the distribution of scarce resources but can also lie in the demand for recognition.[29] For that reason and because conflicts are always also linked to questions of power[30], market, power and prestige will be analysed as central areas of action during the interaction of conflicting parties. The agents name the most diverse reasons for their actions depending on the context, yet a closer inspection reveals that the issue can always be linked back to the key areas of market, power, and prestige – and thus to the central elements of distribution of resources and recognition.

Hence, our objective is to open up topics of medical historical origin to address larger societal questions, and thus to utilise them for interdisciplinary historical conflict research. Consequently, the topics discussed here touch on historical but also social scientific and ethnological issues. In addition, medical ethics is also interested in questions of conflict research.

## Corpus of research

The medical market and the conflicts occurring here have been the topic of medical historical research for a long time – sometimes more and sometimes less explicit. The Early modern period[31] and the 19th century have been especially well researched in this regard, as important consolidation processes of the medical market took place during these times. The professionalisation of the rank of doctors was accompanied by numerous conflicts with other groups of healers. Mainly natural healers, homoeopaths and alternative practitioners became the doctors' targets as these did not follow scientifically justified medicine.[32] Especially at the turn of the 20th century and during the time of the Weimar Republic doctors repeatedly demanded a statutory prohibition of the so-called "quacks" which fuelled the "quack debate" even more.[33] Other

---

29 Cf. Pelinka (2016), p. 17.
30 Cf. Pelinka (2016), p. 20.
31 Jütte (1991); Stenzel (2005); Ehrlich (2007).
32 On the history of the natural healing movement: Regin (1995). On the relationship of non-academic healers and the doctors see Faltin (2000). On the history of alternative healing methods: Jütte (1996).
33 Cf. Teichler (2002), pp. 27–31.

critical movements of current medical practice, such as the opponents of vaccinations, have also resulted in conflicts with academic medicine.[34] Despite its hegemonic position, academic medicine could never fully eliminate a certain medical pluralism from society.[35]

The 20th century also produced processes of differentiation and extinction within the health professions but the history of medicine has so far only shown little interest. An exception is here the history of nursing that has already discussed the power structures within nursing and also the conflicts between nursing and medicine.[36] The dimensions of gender and culture have been particularly addressed in this regard.[37] With the exception of possibly midwives, other health professions such as medical technical assistants, emergency medical technicians, diabetes counsellors, physiotherapists and/or occupational therapists have been largely neglected. Yet, they are a rewarding research project from a perspective of the history of professions due to their hierarchical position.[38] Since this topic is often addressed in current debates on medical care, as mentioned at the beginning, it illustrates its centrality and significance.

## Structure

The current volume consists of three parts, arranged on the level of the agents. The first and second parts cover inter-professional and intra-professional conflicts, respectively. And since the framework for conflicts is as important as the agents themselves, the third part is reserved for this issue.

The first part focuses on conflicts between various professional groups or professions. In her article on negotiation processes between nurses and doctors, Karen Nolte uses the example of performing anaesthesia in the 1950s in West Germany. She illustrates how a practice that had previously been performed by nurses slowly became the doctor's task. Eileen Thrower discusses the inter-professional collaboration and the conflicts resulting from it. In particular, she draws on midwives, nurses, and doctors in Georgia in a historical perspective. Pierre Pfütsch focuses in his article on the professionalisation of the non-medical emergency services. He shows how the profession of an emergency medical technician emerged from originally a voluntary job and how it changed into a recognised profession in the Federal Republic of

34   Dinges (1996). In particular on the criticism of vaccinations: Thießen (2017).
35   The volume edited by Jütte provides a fine overview over the history of medical pluralism: Jütte (2013). On conflicts in medical subcultures: Mildenberger (2013).
36   D'Antonio (2010); Fish Mooney (2005). From a sociological perspective: Kirsten Sander (2009). In addition: Malleier (2014).
37   With the inclusion of the category of gender: Loos (2006). With the category of culture: Effelsberg (1985).
38   In addition to some articles on special professions in certain countries, I name as an exception: Twohig (2005).

Germany. He illustrates what impact various agents such as the doctors and aid organisations had in this process.

The second part of the volume discusses conflicts that occurred mainly within a professional group or profession. Christoph Schwamm discusses the history of men in nursing. He asks what masculinity actually meant in the West German professional nursing organisations and illustrates what transformations occurred there. With Geertje Boschma we enter history of psychiatry: she traces the negotiation and tensions around electroconvulsive treatment in Dutch psychiatry. Using the concept of generations, she traces conflict lines between different generations of doctors with regard to the use of this therapy. Sylvelyn Hähner-Rombach focuses on paediatric nursing and hence a special field within nursing that was characterised by the strong bond between patients and nurses. She traces the sources of conflicts between paediatric nurses and the patients' mothers. Using the opening up of the children's wards to mothers, she reveals that changes of management structures can controversially impact hierarchical parameters.

The last part of the volume is dedicated to the general framework of medicine and to the conflicts that result from this. Jane Brooks pursues the question what impact the war as a framework had on the professional role of nurses in Britain during the Second World War. She illustrates how the nurses who had been trained in a strongly hierarchical system developed highly cooperative work forms in collaboration with the doctors at a much larger scale than they would have been able to outside this exceptional situation of wartime deployment. The next article is Eyal Katvan's analysis of the regulation of dental care in British Mandate Palestine. Katvan looks at the development of the profession both from a legal and a medical perspective and points to their interconnections. Simultaneously he discloses the development and extinction of various professional groups within dentistry. Aaron Pfaff focuses on diabetes counsellors and thus directs our attention to a relatively unknown medical profession. He describes in the final article of the volume how the growing significance of diabetes mellitus in societal discourse and the development of the new market of medical technology in this area resulted in the creation of a completely new profession that had to adjust to existing structures.

## Outlook

While the current edited volume addresses the most diverse facets, conflicts, agents, and spaces, we are aware of its limits with regard to its content. All of the articles focus on Western industrial nations and thus the distinct kinds of conflict and issues that have been shaped by Western medicine. When discussing the topic from a global historical point of view, Eastern European countries would be the next focus. Yet the countries in South America, Asia, and Africa would also have to be investigated. This could be an area of research in the future.

Another level for the investigation of conflicts in the healthcare system could and should be the transnational-comparative level. Such a perspective would initially compare conflicts, the context of their development, and the possibilities for solutions in the various countries. The central question is here mainly how the structures of care in the healthcare system impact the development of health professions. At this junction, a comparison between centralist and federalist or capitalist and socialist systems seems to have potential. Since the authors in this volume analyse mainly Western industrial nations, their articles here should also be understood as possible ideas for such a subsequent perspective.

## Bibliography

*Literature*

Albrecht, Martin; Etgeton, Stefan; Ochmann, Richard R.: Faktencheck Gesundheit. Regionale Verteilung von Arztsitzen (Ärztedichte). HNO-Ärzte, Nervenärzte, Orthopäden, Psychotherapeuten, Urologen. Gütersloh 2015.
Barmer GEK: Barmer GEK Arztreport 2016. (=Schriften zur Gesundheitsanalyse 37) Siegburg 2017.
Bryant-Lukosius, Denise et al.: A Historical Overview of the Development of Advanced Practice Nursing Roles in Canada. In: Nursing Leadership 23 (2010), pp. 35–60.
Cerrahoglu, Yahya et al.: Auf den historischen Spuren der OP-Pflege. In: Im OP 4 (2014), pp. 210–214.
D'Antonio, Patricia: American nursing: a history of knowledge, authority, and the meaning of work. Baltimore 2010.
Dinges, Martin (ed.): Medizinkritische Bewegungen im Deutschen Reich (ca. 1870 – ca. 1933). (=Medizin, Gesellschaft und Geschichte, Beiheft 9) Stuttgart 1996.
Effelsberg, Winfried: Interkulturelle Konflikte in der Medizin. Medizinanthropologische Überlegungen. In: Würzburger medizinhistorische Mitteilungen 3 (1985), pp. 29–40.
Ehrlich, Anna: Ärzte, Bader, Scharlatane: die Geschichte der Heilkunst in Österreich. Wien 2007.
Eurostat: Life expectancy at birth, 1980–2015 (years) (2017), available at: http://ec.europa.eu/eurostat/statistics-explained/index.php/File:Life_expectancy_at_birth,_1980-2015_%28years%29_YB17-de.png (last accessed: 17/10/2018).
Fallwell, Lynne: Modern German Midwifery, 1885–1960. (=Studies for the Society for the Social History of Medicine 13) London 2013.
Faltin, Thomas: Heil und Heilung. Geschichte der Laienheilkundigen und Struktur antimodernistischer Weltanschauungen in Kaiserreich und Weimarer Republik am Beispiel von Eugen Wenz (1856–1945). (=Medizin, Gesellschaft und Geschichte, Beiheft 15) Stuttgart 2000.
Fish Mooney, Sharon: Worldviews in conflict: a historical and sociological analysis of the controversy surrounding therapeutic touch in nursing. Ann Arbor 2005.
Geis, Anna; Wagner, Wolfgang: Demokratischer Frieden, Demokratischer Krieg und liberales "peacebuilding". In: Ide, Tobias (ed.): Friedens- und Konfliktforschung. Opladen; Berlin; Toronto 2017, pp. 131–160.
Gesundheitswirtschaft Rhein-Main e. V.: Entwicklungschancen des Zweiten Gesundheitsmarktes in der Rhein-Main-Region und Hessen. Gelsenkirchen 2014.

Hartung, Susanne; Kickbusch, Ilona: Die Gesundheitsgesellschaft: ein Plädoyer für eine gesundheitsförderliche Politik. 2nd ed. Bern 2014.

Howell, Timothy; Stein, Leonard; Watts, David: Sounding Board. The Doctor-Nurse Game Revisited. In: The New England Journal of Medicine 22 (1990), pp. 546–549.

Huerkamp, Claudia: Der Aufstieg der Ärzte im 19. Jahrhundert. Vom gelehrten Stand zum professionellen Experten: Das Beispiel Preußens. (=Kritische Studien zur Geschichtswissenschaft 68) Göttingen 1985.

Ide, Tobias: Einleitung: Konzepte, Themen und Trends der Friedens- und Konfliktforschung. In: Ide, Tobias (ed.): Friedens- und Konfliktforschung. Opladen; Berlin; Toronto 2017, pp. 7–32.

Jütte, Robert: Ärzte, Heiler und Patienten. Medizinischer Alltag in der frühen Neuzeit. München; Zürich 1991.

Jütte, Robert: Geschichte der Alternativen Medizin. Von der Volksmedizin zu den unkonventionellen Therapien von heute. München 1996.

Jütte, Robert (ed.): Geschichte der deutschen Ärzteschaft. Cologne 1997.

Jütte, Robert: Die Entwicklung des ärztlichen Vereinswesens und des organisierten Ärztestandes bis 1871. In: Jütte, Robert (ed.): Geschichte der deutschen Ärzteschaft. Cologne 1997, pp. 15–42.

Jütte, Robert (ed.): Medical Pluralism. Past – Present – Future. (=Medizin, Gesellschaft und Geschichte, Beiheft 46) Stuttgart 2013.

Loos, Martina: Symptom: Konflikte. Was interdisziplinäre Konflikte von Krankenpflegern und Ärztinnen über Konstruktionsprozesse von Geschlecht und Profession erzählen. Frankfurt/Main 2006.

Maibach-Nagel, Egbert: Pflegemangel: Ein wirklich großes Thema. In: Deutsches Ärzteblatt 115 (2018), p. A-505.

Malleier, Elisabeth: Alltag im Krankenhaus – Normen und Konflikte am Beispiel des Wiener "Rothschild-Spitals" um 1900. In: Medizin, Gesellschaft und Geschichte 32 (2014), pp. 51–68.

Mildenberger, Florian: Medikale Subkulturen in der Bundesrepublik Deutschland und ihre Gegner (1950–1990). (=Medizin, Gesellschaft und Geschichte, Beiheft 41) Stuttgart 2013.

Pelinka, Anton: Konfliktforschung. In: Diendorfer, Gertraud et al. (eds.): Friedensforschung, Konfliktforschung, Demokratieforschung. Ein Handbuch. Cologne; Weimar; Vienna 2016, pp. 17–34.

Pfaff, Aaron: "Man darf keine Kenntnisse beim Laien voraussetzen!" Die Genese der Diabetes-Beratungs- und Schulungsberufe. In: Hähner-Rombach, Sylvelyn; Pfütsch, Pierre (eds.): Entwicklungen in der Krankenpflege und in anderen Gesundheitsberufen nach 1945. Ein Lehr- und Studienbuch. Frankfurt/Main 2018, pp. 383–421.

Regin, Cornelia: Selbsthilfe und Gesundheitspolitik. Die Naturheilbewegung im Kaiserreich (1889 bis 1914). (=Medizin, Gesellschaft und Geschichte, Beiheft 4) Stuttgart 1995.

Robert Bosch Stiftung: Pflege neu denken. Zur Zukunft der Pflegeausbildung. Stuttgart 2000.

Robert Bosch Stiftung; Kommission zur Hochschulausbildung für Lehr- und Leitungskräfte in der Pflege: Pflege braucht Eliten. Denkschrift zur Hochschulausbildung für Lehr- und Leitungskräfte in der Pflege. (=Beiträge zur Gesundheitsökonomie 28) Gerlingen 1992.

Ruf, Werner: Islamischer Fundamentalismus. In: Imbusch, Peter; Zoll, Ralf: Friedens- und Konfliktforschung. Vol. 1: Eine Einführung. 5th ed. Wiesbaden 2010, pp. 309–332.

Sander, Kirsten: Profession und Geschlecht im Krankenhaus: soziale Praxis der Zusammenarbeit von Pflege und Medizin. Konstanz 2009.

Sander, Sabine: Handwerkschirurgen. Sozialgeschichte einer verdrängten Berufsgruppe. (=Kritische Studien zur Geschichtswissenschaft 83) Göttingen 1989.

Schumann, Marion: Vom Dienst an Mutter und Kind zum Dienst nach Plan. Hebammen in der Bundesrepublik 1950–1975. (=Frauengesundheit 8) Osnabrück 2009.

Statistisches Bundesamt: Statistisches Jahrbuch 2015. Gesundheit. Personal. Fachserie 12, Reihe 7.3.1. Wiesbaden 2017.

# Interprofessional Conflicts

# The Debate on 'Nurse Anaesthetists' in West Germany during the 1950s and 1960s

*Karen Nolte*

## Introduction

In 1846 the dentists William Green and Horace Wells successfully performed anaesthesia with ether for the first time in Baltimore. A year after the successful use in the US, ether was introduced as an anaesthetic in German operating theatres.[1] In that same year the English obstetrician James Young Simpson successfully used chloroform as an anaesthetic for the first time. Later, it was called "narcose à la reine" because Simpson delivered two of Queen Victoria's babies using chloroform.[2] Soon after, chloroform and ether were used in combination due to the better tolerability. While from the beginning doctors were supposed to perform the anaesthesia, soon inhalation anaesthesia was in the nurses' hands.[3]

In the collective memory initiating and monitoring anaesthesia has always been a doctor's task. However, photographs and textbooks on nursing care from the late 19th century until the middle of the 20th century in Germany reveal a different picture. On these contemporary photographs, the nurse can be seen at the head of the operating table where she independently initiated the inhalation anaesthesia and monitored the condition of the patient under anaesthesia. Nonetheless, today she has disappeared from collective memory. The same is true for the material objects of anaesthesia. The implicit knowledge inherent to objects such as the Schimmelbusch mask, drip bottles for chloroform and ether, and anaesthesia apparatuses that were used by nurses for inhalation anaesthesia has yet to be uncovered. These objects have been preserved in medical historical collections or in museums as items of medical practice and, ironically, this might be precisely the reason why they were collected in the first place. "Nursing items" by contrast are hardly to be found in medical historical collections.[4]

The forgetting of nurse anaesthetists is closely linked to the portrayal of the history of anaesthesia, which has usually been written by doctors and in particular anaesthetists.[5] If nurse anaesthetists are mentioned at all in histori-

---

1    Cf. Dieffenbach (1847); on the first uses in the German-speaking countries cf. Petermann/Nemes (2003), pp. 6–14. In Germany, the surgeon Johann F. Heyfelder (1798–1869) from Erlangen was the first who performed anaesthesia using ether on 24 January 1847.
2    Cf. Petermann/Nemes (2003), pp. 14–16.
3    Goerig/Schulte am Esch (2003), pp. 56–57.
4    Cf. on the preservation of nursing items: Atzl (2017).
5    One example is the "Festschrift" of anaesthesiology in Heidelberg. Here nurse anaesthetists are mentioned in connection with an anaesthesia that was both backwards and

cal overviews, they are merely female representatives of the "old-fashioned" method of inhalation anaesthesia. This method, the reviews seem to say, were happily overturned through the establishment of the specialist for anaesthesia and the mechanisation of anaesthesia in 1953.[6]

In the following I would like to present more than the specialisation – and simultaneous de-specialisation – of nurses. Rather I am interested in the gender-specific connotations and the act of giving anaesthesia, meaning the handling of the objects of anaesthesia well into the 1950s.

This article draws on research on the history of nursing practices and everyday life in nursing after 1945 and especially on pivotal studies that Susanne Kreutzer has produced on the topic.[7] Recently, additional studies have been published on the daily routines in nursing after 1945 and also on health professions beyond the job of the doctor.[8] Furthermore, this article contributes to the innovative and hardly explored research area of the history of material culture within nursing – the "nursing objects".[9]

The source material consists partially of nursing handbooks produced between the 1940s and 1960s, furthermore of nursing journals such as *Die Schwester* (The Nurse), the *Deutsche Schwesternzeitung* (German Nurses Journal), *Die Agnes Karll-Schwester* (The Agnes Karll Nurse), medical journals such as *Der Anaesthesist* (The Anaesthetist) and *Der Chirurg* (The Surgeon), and finally, of manufacturers' catalogues for nursing and hospital supplies.

## History of the professionalisation of nursing in West Germany

In an international comparison, the historical development of nursing in Germany as a profession happened with a strong delay. In Britain, for instance, because of the earlier professionalisation of nursing, initiating and monitoring anaesthesia became a doctor's task already after the First World War.[10] By contrast, in the US anaesthesia also remained a task of the nurses until the middle of the 20th century because the doctors only then became interested in this area.[11] In Germany, the Christian concept of nursing as a labour of

---

unprofessional, cf. Klinik für Anaesthesiologie Universitätsklinikum Heidelberg (2007), p. 24.

6   In the "Festschrift" of the German Society of Anaesthesiology and Intensive Care Medicine ("Deutsche Gesellschaft für Anästhesiologie und Intensivmedizin"), celebrating its 50th anniversary the history of nurses, performing anaesthesia is at least briefly mentioned by characterising it as a brief episode of "collaboration with staff". However, the period of nurses performing anaesthesia in German history is approximately 100 years longer than the existence of medical anaesthesiology that is conducted by doctors, cf. Schüttler (2003), pp. 98–99.

7   Cf. Kreutzer (2005); Kreutzer (2014).

8   Cf. Hähner-Rombach/Pfütsch (2018).

9   Cf. Artner et al. (2017); Atzl (2011).

10  Cf. Nolte/Hallett (2019).

11  Cf. Bankert (1989).

love that the nurses performed for their neighbour shaped the professional concepts and the working conditions of nurses until well into the second half of the 20th century. In 1957, the Nursing Act determined the length of nursing training to be two years with a subsequent work placement of one year. In Heidelberg, already in 1953 a nursing school had been founded with the aid of the Rockefeller Foundation that offered three years of training including 1,200 hours of theoretical instruction. It wanted to set up standards in order to align the German nursing training with international norms. In 1965 these standards were generally introduced in West Germany with the Nursing Act from that year.[12]

Until 1957, the Training Act from 1938 was still effective that required merely 200 hours of theoretical training. In the denominational communities of nurses, the students were largely practically trained on the wards by shadowing experienced nurses. They learned not only important nursing practices but also the Christian work ethos that the older nurses set as an example. The training happened in a community that resembled a family. During the 1960s the concept of the training fundamentally changed and not only because of the significant increase of theoretical instruction: Practical skills were taught at the nursing school and were based on the theoretical knowledge. The increasing specialisation of the departments in the hospital meant that the students could no longer train on just one ward but that they rotated through different wards to get to know a broad spectrum of nursing skills.[13] The changes of the nursing training also reflected the changes of the nursing routines and the development of nursing as a profession. Since the nursing training had not been very specialised until the end of the 1950s, it had also created areas of freedom for the nurses: The students could learn from experienced nurses how to work with X-ray, assist during surgery or become nurse anaesthetists and work quite independently in these areas as I will subsequently show using the example of nurse anaesthetists.

## The historical development of nurse anaesthesia in Germany

Paul Rupprecht (1846–1920)[14], a doctor from Dresden, emphasised in his 1898 textbook for nurses how "responsible" the work of "chloroforming" is and it further states that it can only be learned through "lots of practice under the supervision of a doctor"[15]. This brief statement offers three insights: 1) nurses at this time were supposed to perform anaesthesia using chloroform,

12   Cf. Hähner-Rombach (2018).
13   Kreutzer (2014), pp. 158–168.
14   Paul Rupprecht had been consultant ("Oberarzt") for surgery since 1882 at the Deaconess Hospital in Dresden, in 1897 he became leading surgeon major ("Oberstabsarzt"), in 1898 general senior consultant ("Generaloberarzt") à la suite of the ambulance corps and lecturer of surgery in military medical training courses in Dresden, cf. Pagel (1901), col. 1451–1452.
15   Rupprecht (1890), p. 252.

2) they were to receive long-lasting training in its administration and 3) a physician was always supposed to supervise. In other words, initiating anaesthesia
was understood as assisting the doctor while he performed the surgery. Similarly, the objects that have been preserved point to a female user of anaesthesia instruments. The Medical Historical Collections in Würzburg hold a
chloroform flask from around 1850 that was designed like a perfume bottle
with a drip mechanism that was designed like a tea pot with a small opening.

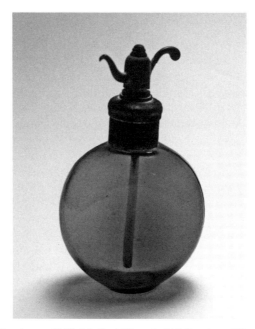

Fig. 1: Chloroform bottle, ca. 1850, Medical Historical Collections, Würzburg,
Photograph: Karen Nolte

Despite the depiction of anaesthesia as an assistant job, the descriptions of
the tasks of an anaesthesia nurse in textbooks for nurses between 1900–1954
show the large responsibility with which a nurse anaesthetist was entrusted
during surgery. She constantly had to monitor the breathing and vital signs
of the patient and also control the blink reflex through regular touches of the
eyelid to evaluate the depth of anaesthesia. This served to decide when the
chloroform mask had to be taken away and when it had to be attached again.
The nurse anaesthetist was supposed to tell the doctor when she observed a
deterioration in the condition of the patient. In case of emergency the nurse
used the mouth-gag by Heister to clear the airways and then initiated decisive
preparations for further life-saving measures such as artificial respiration performed by the doctor. In the "Lehrbuch der Chirurgischen Krankenpflege für
Pflegerinnen und Operationsschwestern" ("Manual for Surgical Health Care
for Nurses and Theatre Nurses") from 1922 the important position of the

nurse anaesthetist in the theatre is emphasised in a number of instances. It is first clarified, however, that this nursing task, while requiring a high level of responsibility in the operation theatre, served to support the doctor:

> For all assisting nurses there should be the rule that they only do what they have been asked to do and that they perform this task with the utmost attention. It happens too often that the nurse has not fully absorbed the necessity of this rule. The surgeon who has to be the master in the operating theatre has given her a specific task.[16]

Over the years the nurse anaesthetist at the head of the bed became part of the familiar image of the operating theatre. In 1940, the "Manual and Textbook of Nursing" by Fischer, Groß and Venzmer had the following to say on the tasks of a nurse anaesthetist:

> Putting a patient under anaesthesia, which requires a lot of practice, experience, concentration, calmness, cold-bloodedness at a moment of danger, and comprehensive knowledge, is an art, albeit one that can be learned. In other words, just as it is with the doctors, the personality that also characterises a good nurse in general, is the crucial element because success does not only depend on technical ability but also on psychological factors, such as a relationship of mutual trust between the nurse and the patient, who, with the beginning of the anaesthesia, entrusted his life for better or worse to the nurse. The nurse must always be aware of that![17]

Not only was it expected that the anaesthesia would be provided and monitored by female nursing staff but there was also the demand that the nurse anaesthetist should have particular human qualities to ensure trust, comfort and safety – all supposedly female qualities. There were both the demand and assumption that nurses particularly embodied these female traits. Accomplished techniques and the feeling of the nurse of how to handle the patient correctly and the operating surgeon appropriately were to become a unit. The significance of emotional qualities while dealing with technology, i.e., especially the technical tools, and the patients was also emphasised for nurses performing X-rays, as the Swiss historian Monika Dommann has shown in her study on the history of X-rays.[18]

The surgeon had to be able to focus exclusively on the procedure. He relied on the fact that the nurse anaesthetist was able to strictly monitor and evaluate the progress of the anaesthesia. She had to observe the "reflexes, breathing, circulation, and after these observations [she had to] set up the amount of the narcotic which [had to] be administered".[19] Furthermore, in the "Manual and Textbook of Nursing" the independent actions of the nurse anaesthetist are emphasised. "Upon request of the surgeon she must be able to immediately count the pulse, and share her observation of its nature, the look of the patient, his or her breathing etc. Without extra prompting she reports every disorder in a loud voice."[20] It was imperative that the physician could

16  Janssen (1922), p. 157. Cf. also Heller (1948).
17  Fischer/Groß/Venzmer (1940), p. 280.
18  Dommann (2003), pp. 139–192.
19  Fischer/Groß/Venzmer (1940), p. 356.
20  Fischer/Groß/Venzmer (1940), p. 356.

rely on the nurse anaesthetist to act calmly and responsibly. Practical inhalation anaesthesia is described in detail in the handbook: At the beginning the methyl trichloride had to be combined with Eau de Cologne to cover up the unpleasant smell of the narcotic to ensure the patient's compliance. To avoid the feeling of choking, the choloroform mask had to be moved slowly towards the face and then carefully placed over mouth and nose. The textbook continues that it was popular to let the patient count but the continuous counting contained the risk that the patient did not breathe deeply enough. The nurse anaesthetist dripped the methyl trichloride continuously on the mask until the so-called "excitation stage" had been overcome and the patient could be put into narcotic sleep – usually this was supposed to happen after approximately 100 drops. Now the nurse had to hold the mask with her left hand while checking the pulse with her right hand. After the "excitation stage" another 60 to 100 ether drops were dripped onto the mask. During the deep sleep, the drip had to be continued at a consistent rate. When the operator gave a sign, the mask was removed and thus the wake-up phase initiated. It was accelerated by administering carbonic acid into the nostrils for three to four breaths. Numerous handbooks for nurses contain instructions for what to do before, during and after anaesthesia, which suggests that this task was a common and also widely respected practice.[21] In 1949, a theatre nurse described how nursing students were instructed on performing anaesthesia during their training segment in the operating theatre.

> Towards the end of her training in the operating theatre the student learns the tasks of a nurse anaesthetist. In theory the young nurse often already knows everything that she needs to know about the types of anaesthesia and possible problems. Perhaps she has experienced one or the other incident herself and realised what large responsibility the nurse anaesthetist has and that, in addition to talent, thorough training and experience are necessary before one can become a really good nurse anaesthetist. The student is allowed to do two or three chloroethyl anaesthesias under supervision so that she can help out in case of emergency. Afterwards she may perform one or two ether drips if a suitable patient must undergo surgery during her time here.[22]

This theatre nurse continued that often experienced nurse anaesthetists would have too little time to teach the students the technique of anaesthesia and to monitor them while they practised. However, it becomes evident that learning the techniques of anaesthesia was already part of nursing training. Furthermore, experienced nurses took on the training of nurse anaesthetist and not the doctors as we can read in the nursing handbooks.

21  Janssen (1922), pp. 173–178; Lindemann (1928), pp. 158–160; Fischer et al. (1949), pp. 438–440.
22  Molterer (1949), p. 15.

## Origin of the consultant anaesthesist in West Germany

Most surgeons were happy with "nurse anaesthesia" because they regarded the initiation and monitoring of inhalation anaesthesia as an assistant job that they directed. Simultaneously however from the end of the 19th century onwards there was a trend in a group of surgeons who regarded anaesthesia as a skill for doctors and who wanted to establish it as a distinct field in addition to surgery. During the 1940s surgeons hardly felt the need to change anything in the established constellation of operator and nurse anaesthetist. Yet, in the post-war years the small group of doctors that had specialised in anaesthesiology gained momentum. Because West German universities were overcrowded the German Council of Science and Humanities aimed at expanding them and funded "small specialist areas" by creating tenured professorships.[23]

Previously, in 1953 the German Medical Assembly ("Deutscher Ärztetag") had decided to include the "consultant anaesthesist" in the consultant regulations. To establish the new speciality, in the same year the German Association for Anaesthesia ("Deutsche Gesellschaft für Anaesthesie") and in 1961 the Professional Organisation of German Anaesthetists ("Berufsverband Deutscher Anästhesisten") were founded. The efforts to establish the young discipline of anaesthesiology as a sub-field of medicine next to surgery looked promising even though the surgeons initially had problems with the new consultants. While the hierarchy and division of labour in the operating theatre had been clear before with nurse anaesthesia, the collaboration between surgeon and consultant anaesthesist had to be newly defined and negotiated. The surgeons had the point of view that they bore the responsibility for the entire operation and that they were therefore in charge and give out directions that the anaesthetists had to follow.[24] For the surgeons who had been used to nurse anaesthetists it was natural to be the only and unquestioned authority in the operating theatre. The new anaesthetists had to underline their greater knowledge relative to nurses and also had to convince the surgeons of the necessity of anaesthesia as an independent medical field.

A female doctor from the US, Jean Emily Henley (1910–1994), who had completed her training in anaesthesia in New York, became a protagonist of the new speciality in West Germany. She brought the important objects needed for intubation anaesthesia with her and worked as an anaesthetist at the university hospital Gießen, the American military hospital, and the university hospital for surgery in Heidelberg where she familiarised her German colleagues with the new anaesthetic machines.[25] She also wrote the decisive handbook on intubation anaesthesia with controlled respiration.[26] The newly emerging speciality of anaesthesia offered opportunities for women to make a career as a consultant even in the German-speaking countries. The "Directory

23  Cf. Petermann/Schwarz (2003), pp. 301–307.
24  Cf. Weißauer (2003), p. 68.
25  Cf. Klinik für Anaesthesiologie Universitätsklinikum Heidelberg (2007), p. 32.
26  Henley (1950).

of Consultant Anaesthesists" ("Verzeichnis der Fachärzte für Anästhesiologie") that listed all male and female consultant anaesthesists in Germany, Austria, and Switzerland for the year 1966 shows that approximately one third of the consultants in this field were women.[27] Nonetheless the argumentation for replacing nurse anaesthesia was heated because of the gender-specific issues as I will show in the following.

Finally, with the recognition of their speciality the anaesthetists reached an important milestone in their conflict with the surgeons: in 1965 they clarified in their "Guidelines on the position of the leading anaesthetist" ("Richtlinien für die Stellung des leitenden Anästhesisten") that the anaesthetist had the full legal responsibility for his speciality and that for that reason he was entitled to "the same independence as consultants of other specialities" in performing his job.[28] Yet, as we will see it took a few more years before anaesthesia was established as a task of a doctor with a specific qualification.

### "Who is allowed to administer anaesthesia?"

At the end of the 1950s the separation of the act of surgery as the doctor's domain and anaesthesia as the nurse's domain, which had been a given until then, was subject to negotiation. At the end the so-called "nurse anaesthesia" was controversially discussed among medics. For instance, Prof. Dr. Fischer, Professor of Surgery from Kiel, emphasised in 1959 in the journal *Der Chirurg* that "experienced nurse anaesthetists were highly regarded due to their good anaesthesia"[29] and that a leading consultant would rather ask an experienced nurse to provide the anaesthesia than an inexperienced licensed doctor. Yet, he also quickly adds that anaesthesia always has to be performed under the supervision of the surgeon. He demanded that nurses working as anaesthetists were to be trained following the American and Swedish model as "nurse anaesthetists". Surgeons like Fischer could not get used to the idea to share the operating theatre with another expert. Hence, they thought nurse anaesthesia could be expanded. In contrast, doctors who had begun to qualify as consultant anaesthesists from the beginning of the 1950s had for obvious reasons a negative view towards a narcosis that had been initiated and monitored by a nurse. The anaesthetist Dr. Hügin from Basel emphasised for example in 1959 that anaesthesia was as important a treatment as the surgical procedure itself. Interestingly, the transition of anaesthesia from being the task of a nurse to being the task of a doctor with special qualification was justified on the one hand with the new technology used to perform anaesthesia and with handling of "complicated apparatuses" and on the other hand with the intubation for endotracheal anaesthesia. He continued that anaesthesia requires in-depth

27  Frey/Kronschwitz (1966).
28  Richtlinien für die Stellung des leitenden Anästhesisten, cited from Weißauer (2003), p. 73.
29  Fischer (1959), p. 535.

knowledge of physiology and pharmacology. Even though a nurse would "admittedly" master the "simple technique" of puncturing a vein, she would be unable to understand the effects of the administered medication. Hence the old simple technique of the inhalation anaesthesia with chloroform and ether could be performed by nurses but, according to the doctor, the nurses lacked the expertise to perform the more complicated endotracheal intubation anaesthesia.[30] Fischer responded to Hügin, explaining that due to the current deficits in consultant anaesthesists one could not spare the experienced nurse anaesthetists. He suggested that while a doctor should perform the intubation the nurses could monitor the anaesthesia after the tube was in place.[31]

As long as monitoring anaesthesia happened without the respective technology it was one of the key areas of nursing. Observing the patients in a precise and professional manner and communicating these observations to the doctor had been part of the nurses' training. While the professional observation and assessment of the patient was far more complex than the technical process of initiating anaesthesia, doctors emphasised that the latter required the skill set of a doctor and had to be part of their area of responsibility.

The dramatic shortage of nurses since the middle of the 1950s due to a lack of newly trained staff finally played into the hands of the anaesthetists in their efforts for professionalisation. As Marianne Schmidbauer[32] and Susanne Kreutzer[33] have shown, in Germany during the 1960s a profound change happened in nursing. The traditional concept of nursing as a Christian service of love for the patient was no longer attractive for women. The deficit of nursing students and the expansion of healthcare following the increasing prosperity in West Germany resulted in a dramatic shortage of nurses.

Ruth Elster (1913–2002), the Principal of the Association of German Nurses ("Deutsche Schwesterngemeinschaft"), emphasised in 1958 that "it was not a nurse's task to provide inhalation anaesthesia, tracheal anaesthesia, intravenous anaesthesia and in short any anaesthesia that requires operating machines."[34] According to her these new types of anaesthesia fell into the doctor's domain of expertise. Pointing to the scarcity of nurses, the suggestion of the physicians who were in favour of nurse anaesthesia to continue to have the nurses oversee anaesthesia and to introduce a 5-year training programme in anaesthesia care was decisively rejected. It is remarkable that the nursing organisation adopted the argument of anaesthetists that now the technology had become too complicated for nurse anaesthetists. This argument is clearly gender biased and ignores the fact that the responsible task of monitoring the patient during anaesthesia, which was a key task of trained nurses, was essential to a successful anaesthesia.

30  Hügin (1960).
31  Fischer (1959).
32  Cf. Schmidbauer (2002).
33  Cf. Kreutzer (2005).
34  Elster (1958), p. 1213.

Now the nurses' task in the operating theatre was supposed to be restricted to preparing the anaesthesia. The task of the nurse anaesthetist focused now on the area of psychologically and physically preparing the patient
and assisting during anaesthesia. While some years before nurses were still
entrusted with calculating the dose of narcotics for the inhalation anaesthesia
now they only had to provide an exact measurement of the body weight. All
instruments and objects that were immediately related to initiating anaesthesia became now doctors' instruments and were subsequently regarded as male
objects. The important task of creating an atmosphere of trust before and
during initiating anaesthesia continued however to have female connotations
so female nurses remained in charge of this aspect of nursing.

It is remarkable that the associations of nurses did not only happily leave
this area of expertise to the doctors but also rejected suggestions by surgeons
to introduce nursing qualifications in anaesthesia following Swedish or British examples. While the hardly standardised nursing training that had taken
place until 1957 (when the Nursing Act took effect) opened up opportunities
to the nurses to become experts in certain specialities such as anaesthesia,
the nurse anaesthetists had no formal training that officially confirmed their
expertise. Following the traditional nursing ethos, the nurses did not define
themselves through their specialist knowledge as e.g. initiating and monitoring anaesthesia but through serving the patients as a labour of love. Elster argues in this sense in the context of staff shortages that nurses would be needed
in this key area of nursing.

The replacement of nurse anaesthesia took longer though than the anaesthetists desired: The handbooks on nursing of this time contain however also
numerous sections that point out the framework that delayed the complete
move of anaesthesia into the doctors' domain of expertise. For example, in the
textbook "Die Pflege des kranken Menschen" ("Nursing the Sick") from 1958
we find a description of how the nurse has to initiate a "deep anaesthesia"
using chloroform and ether upon the doctor's request. In contrast the nurse's
task during intubation anaesthesia was limited to its preparation and handing
the doctor the instruments. Monitoring the patients remained the nurse's task
in the operating theatre which she had to document in an anaesthesia report.
It would be interesting to investigate for how long in smaller hospitals nurses
continued to independently administer anaesthesia with chloroform and ether
since in many places there were no consultant anaesthesists. Fischer and Groß
described the situation in 1957 in their "Handbook of Nursing" ("Hand- und
Lehrbuch der Krankenpflege") as follows:

> Since […] it is impossible in smaller and medium-sized surgical departments to hire an
> anaesthetist in Germany, in the future performing anaesthesia will continue to be one
> of the nurse's tasks. Certain procedures of anaesthesia must not be performed by the
> nurse.[35]

---

35   Fischer/Groß (1957), p. 426.

For that reason the textbook did not continue to discuss those procedures, though explaining the various types of inhalation anaesthesia in detail. The "Little Book on Anaesthesia" ("Kleines Narkosebuch") by the leading consultant of the department of surgery at the community hospital ("Bürgerspital") in Saarbrücken, Fritz Hesse, also emphasises "that general anaesthesia is mainly in the hands of the doctor's assistants" which is why there was the need for the "literary aid" that he provided with his book.[36] The textbooks of the late 1950s suggest that in the hospitals at the periphery nurse anaesthesia remained as it had been before. In 1959, in the "Discussion" section of the *Deutsche Schwesternzeitung* under the headline "Who is allowed to administer anaesthesia?" the board of the German Hospital Federation ("Deutsche Krankenhausgesellschaft") published a statement on the issue of "including assisting staff during operations". It emphasised that the "doctor performing the surgery [...] has the responsibility for the whole operation including anaesthesia and the tasks associated with it, as long it is not administered by a consultant anaesthesist – which would be desirable."[37] Yet an exception was "types of anaesthesia other than intravenous" or "anaesthesia with a strong dampening of the metabolism or with the use of curare" – in other words, the exception was inhalation anaesthesia. The statement continued that doctors could ask nurses "who have the required skill because of their training, experience, and personality" to perform this if they were ready to administer the anaesthesia. In this case – and this was emphasised – the doctor was only responsible for choosing the right "qualified assistants". These nurse anaesthetists who were deemed to be "assistants" would then be responsible for the "technically and objectively excellent performance of the tasks they had been given". This recommendation, however, caused alarm in the communities of nurses who were not willing at all to perform anaesthesia under these conditions.[38] Part of the professionalisation strategy of the anaesthetists was to downgrade nurse anaesthetists to be mere assistants even though they had for nearly 100 years worked alongside the surgeons and carved out their own area of expertise and action despite the doctors' rhetoric. The idea was to deny them the expertise to perform professional anaesthesia. The anaesthetists were quite successful with this strategy as the reaction of the Association of German Nurses showed. Simultaneously, the doctors were confronted with the lack of suitable consultants in most hospitals and small clinics. During the time of transferring anaesthesia from the realm of the nurses to the doctors, the nurses' position was weakened and their expertise was unclear. Yet at the same time they

---

36  Hesse (1950), p. III.

37  *Deutsche Schwesternzeitung* 12 (1959), p. 407.

38  *Deutsche Schwesternzeitung* 12 (1959), p. 407. Cf. also Dörpinghaus (1960), p. 216. Hilde Dörpinghaus emphasised that assisting during surgery was not a task for nurses. She also criticised the recommendation of the German Hospital Federation that ascribed too much responsibility to the nurses. Even monitoring patients during the wake-up period could be only done by a "very thorough nurse".

were ascribed whole responsibility for anaesthesia. It is not surprising that the nurses rejected this responsibility under these circumstances.

## Development of the new profession of nurse anaesthetist

In 1969 the "Deutsche Gesellschaft für Anaesthesie und Wiederbelebung" (German Association for Anaesthesia and Resuscitation) demanded an additional training programme to train nurses as anaesthetists that was to last at least one year. At this point Switzerland had already introduced a two-year additional training programme for anaesthesia nursing.[39]

The anaesthetists had already before thought about the new role the nurse anaesthetist should take on. She was supposed to aid the anaesthetist during complex anaesthesias with curare and intubation and be always at his side. Furthermore, the idea was that she should "psychologically prepare" the patient, "clean the mouth and pharynx including the upper airways [for intubation], arrange the extensive number of instruments on a mobile accessory cart". The nurse anaesthetist was now also supposed to closely monitor the blood circulation of the anaesthetised patient and to document these observations in an anaesthesia protocol. She was also supposed to be responsible for monitoring the patient during the wake-up phase.[40]

Yet the anaesthetists were still aware that there were not enough of them available at that point so doctors remained in charge of the anaesthesia in many places. Even at the University Hospital in Heidelberg, its requirement that each anaesthesia had to be administered by an anaesthetist could not be fully implemented until far into the 1960s because there were not enough consultants available.[41] For that reason the professional association made amends in its guidelines on the training of nurse anaesthetists: "In cases of emergency, nurses can be brought in to administer an ether drip or mask anaesthesia under the sole and expressed responsibility of the doctor."[42] This "exception" was justified by emphasising the doctor's responsibility. Actually, their goal was to transform nurses once and for all into assistants of anaesthetists. Yet, they were supposed to be capable to step in "in case of emergency" and fulfil the task until a doctor arrived. They were expected to bring a "high level of critical observation, fast decision-making and personal responsibility". Yet in the statement of the Physicians' Association on the training of anaesthesia nurses they quickly added: "It is not the anaesthesia nurse's task to conduct an anaesthesia independently nor is it the goal of their training because anaesthesia in its essence and because of its risks is the task of a doctor."[43]

39   Deutsche Gesellschaft für Anaesthesie und Wiederbelebung (1969).
40   Leimbach (1953).
41   Klinik für Anaesthesiologie Universitätsklinikum Heidelberg (2007), p. 41.
42   Bark/Frey (1960), p. 343.
43   Deutsche Gesellschaft für Anaesthesie und Wiederbelebung (1969), p. 230.

The doctors seem to have been well aware of the fine line between the independent work of nurses in anaesthesia care and the doctor's activities in performing anaesthesia. The further development of the specialist training in anaesthesia in the 1970s, when a sufficient number of consultant anaesthesists were available, is a topic for further detailed historical investigation.

## Closing remarks

Since the 1860s nursing anaesthesia had been part of the broadly structured nursing training. The nursing handbooks of the time described inhalation anaesthesia in detail and experienced theatre or anaesthesia nurses taught how to perform and monitor chloroethyl anaesthesias. Only in the late 1950s was this long-ingrained practice questioned. While some surgeons highly respected their nurse anaesthetists, efforts were made to establish the new profession of consultant anaesthesist. The old handbooks on nursing had emphasised specific female qualities as an important condition to perform anaesthesia. By contrast in the 1950s the argument was that nurses were unable to operate the "complicated machines". Initiating inhalation anaesthesias and handling the Schimmelbusch mask or drip bottle were characterised as "simple" techniques. It is remarkable that in the debate about anaesthesia the focus was put on the administration but not on monitoring anaesthesia which was still a task nurses were entrusted and trusted with.

New technology made it possible to justify that anaesthesia became a task of the doctors and was no longer a job for nurses. However, since the "consultant anaesthesist" had been introduced in Germany only in 1953, there was a shortage of qualified doctors until well into the 1960s who could have taken over the nurses' jobs. Hence nurse anaesthetists continued to initiate anaesthesias and thoroughly monitored the patients and the doctors had to emphasise that this was merely an assistant job that could only be done under strict supervision of the doctors. Simultaneously, from the end of the 1950s surgeons rejected the legal responsibility of anaesthesia. Since neither the skills nor the responsibilities were clearly defined for nurse anaesthetists, it seemed only natural that the nurses also declined to be legally in charge of anaesthesia. The unequivocal dissociation of nursing associations from nurse anaesthesia can also be understood in the context of standardisation of the nursing training that took effect with the Nursing Act in 1957 that also defined more clearly which specific tasks were part of nursing care. Finally, the lack of nurses was also a decisive factor for the willingness to give up nursing anaesthesia as a part of the nurses' responsibility.

# Bibliography

Artner, Lucia et al. (eds.): Pflegedinge: Materialitäten in Pflege und Care. Bielefeld 2017.

Atzl, Isabel (ed.): Who Cares? Geschichte und Alltag der Krankenpflege. Begleitband zur Wanderausstellung "Who cares? Geschichte und Alltag der Krankenpflege". Frankfurt/ Main 2011.

Atzl, Isabel: Das materiale Erbe der Pflege. Historische Pflegedinge in Sammlungen und Museen und ihr Potential für die (pflege-)historische Forschung. In: Artner, Lucia et al. (eds.): Pflegedinge. Materialitäten in Pflege und Care. Bielefeld 2017, pp. 51–86.

Bankert, Marianne: Watchful Care: A History of America's Nurse Anesthetists. New York 1989.

Bark, Jochen; Frey, Rudolf: Sollen deutsche Schwestern zu Anaesthesistinnen ausgebildet werden? In: Die Agnes Karll-Schwester 14 (1960), pp. 343–344.

Deutsche Gesellschaft für Anaesthesie und Wiederbelebung: Stellungnahme zur Ausbildung von Schwestern und Pflegern für den Anaesthesiedienst und Intensivpflege. In: Der Anaesthesist 18 (1969), pp. 229–231.

Dieffenbach, Johann Friedrich: Der Aether gegen den Schmerz. Berlin 1847.

Dörpinghaus, Hilde: Die Eigenständigkeit des Berufes der Krankenschwester. In: Die Agnes Karll-Schwester 14 (1960), pp. 173–217.

Dommann, Monika: Durchsicht, Einsicht, Vorsicht: eine Geschichte der Röntgenstrahlen 1896–1963. Zürich 2003.

Elster, Ruth: Hinweis der Schwesternschaft. In: Ärztliche Mitteilungen 41 (1958), p. 1213.

Fischer, A. W.: Wie weit können Schwestern und Pfleger an Narkosen beteiligt werden? In: Der Chirurg 30 (1959), pp. 535–536.

Fischer, Ludolf; Groß, Fritz (eds.): Hand- und Lehrbuch der Krankenpflege. Vol. II: Praktische Krankenpflege. Stuttgart 1957.

Fischer, Ludolf; Groß, Fritz; Venzmer, Gerhard (eds.): Hand- und Lehrbuch der Krankenpflege. Vol. II: Praktische Krankenpflege. Stuttgart 1940.

Fischer, Ludolf et al. (eds.): Hand- und Lehrbuch der Krankenpflege. Vol. II: Praktische Krankenpflege. Stuttgart 1949.

Frey, Rudolf; Kronschwitz, Helmut (eds.): Verzeichnis der Fachärzte für Anästhesiologie in Deutschland, Österreich und in der Schweiz. Heidelberg; New York 1966.

Goerig, M[ichael]; Schulte am Esch, J[ochen]: Die Anästhesie in der ersten Hälfte des 20. Jahrhunderts. In: Schüttler, Jürgen (ed.): 50 Jahre Deutsche Gesellschaft für Anästhesiologie und Intensivmedizin. Tradition & Innovation. Heidelberg et al. 2003, pp. 27–65.

Hähner-Rombach, Sylvelyn: Aus- und Weiterbildung in der Krankenpflege in der Bundesrepublik Deutschland nach 1945. In: Hähner-Rombach, Sylvelyn; Pfütsch, Pierre (eds.): Entwicklungen in der Krankenpflege und in anderen Gesundheitsberufen nach 1945. Ein Lehr- und Studienbuch. Frankfurt/Main 2018, pp. 146–194.

Hähner-Rombach, Sylvelyn; Pfütsch, Pierre (eds.): Entwicklungen in der Krankenpflege und in anderen Gesundheitsberufen nach 1945. Ein Lehr- und Studienbuch. Frankfurt/Main 2018.

Heller, Ernst: Das Handwerk des chirurgischen Stationsdienstes. Leipzig 1948.

Henley, Jean: Einführung in die Praxis der modernen Inhalationsnarkose. Berlin 1950.

Hesse, Fritz: Kleines Narkosebuch. Eine Anleitung zur Erlernung der Allgemeinnarkose für Schwestern und Heilgehilfen. Leipzig 1950.

Hügin, W.: Wie weit können Schwestern oder Pfleger an Narkosen beteiligt werden? In: Der Chirurg 31 (1960), pp. 200–201.

Janssen, Peter: Lehrbuch der Chirurgischen Krankenpflege für Pflegerinnen und Operationsschwestern. Leipzig 1922.

Klinik für Anaesthesiologie Universitätsklinikum Heidelberg (ed.): Anästhesiegeschichte in Heidelberg. Festschrift anlässlich des 40-jährigen Jubiläums des Ordinariats für Anaesthesiologie an der Ruprecht-Karls-Universität Heidelberg 2007. Heidelberg 2007.

Kreutzer, Susanne: Vom "Liebesdienst" zum modernen Frauenberuf: die Reform der Krankenpflege nach 1945. Frankfurt/Main; New York 2005.

Kreutzer, Susanne: Arbeits- und Lebensalltag evangelischer Krankenpflege: Organisation, soziale Praxis und biographische Erfahrungen 1945–1980. Göttingen 2014.

Leimbach, Günther: Die Mitarbeit der Schwester bei der Intratracheal-Curare-Narkose. In: Deutsche Schwesternschaft 6 (1953), pp. 123–127.

Lindemann, Walter: Schwestern-Lehrbuch für Schwestern und Krankenpfleger. München 1928.

Molterer, Marianne: Operationsschwester und Schülerin. In: Deutsche Schwesternzeitung 1 (1949), pp. 13–15.

Nolte, Karen; Hallett, Christine: Crossing the Boundaries: Nursing, Materiality and Anaesthetic Practice in Germany and Britain, 1846–1945. In: European Journal for Nursing History and Ethics 1 (2019), pp. 40–66. DOI: 10.25974/enhe2019-4en.

Pagel, Julius Leopold: Biographisches Lexikon hervorragender Ärzte des neunzehnten Jahrhunderts. Berlin; Wien 1901.

Petermann, Heike; Nemes, C.: Die Entdeckung und Entwicklung der Anästhesie im 19. Jahrhundert. In: Schüttler, Jürgen (ed.): 50 Jahre Deutsche Gesellschaft für Anästhesiologie und Intensivmedizin. Tradition & Innovation. Heidelberg et al. 2003, pp. 2–26.

Petermann, Heike; Schwarz, W[olfgang]: Die Spezialisierung an den Universitäten unter dem Blickwinkel der Anästhesie. In: Schüttler, Jürgen (ed.): 50 Jahre Deutsche Gesellschaft für Anästhesiologie und Intensivmedizin. Tradition & Innovation. Heidelberg et al. 2003, pp. 298–316.

Rupprecht, Paul: Die Krankenpflege im Frieden und im Kriege zum Gebrauch für Jedermann insbesondere für Pflegerinnen, Pfleger und Ärzte. Leipzig 1890.

Schmidbauer, Marianne: Vom 'Lazaruskreuz' zu 'Pflege aktuell'. Professionalisierungsdiskurse in der deutschen Krankenpflege 1903–2000. Frankfurt/Main 2002.

Schüttler, Jürgen (ed.): 50 Jahre Deutsche Gesellschaft für Anästhesiologie und Intensivmedizin. Tradition & Innovation. Heidelberg et al. 2003.

Weißauer, Walther: Die Entwicklung zum selbständigen Fachgebiet. In: Schüttler, Jürgen (ed.): 50 Jahre Deutsche Gesellschaft für Anästhesiologie und Intensivmedizin. Tradition & Innovation. Heidelberg et al. 2003, pp. 68–78.

# "An Extension of Nursing Practice":
# The Evolution of Midwifery in the United States
# as Evidenced in Georgia, 1970–1989

*Eileen Thrower*

Midwifery in the United States has nearly ceased to be an independent profession but rather, has become part of nursing. Midwifery is currently practiced by nurse-midwives almost exclusively in the US.[1] First trained and registered as nurses, then educated at the master's or doctoral level, nurse-midwives practice a combination of nursing, medicine, and midwifery. The American College of Nurse-Midwives represents certified nurse-midwives and certified midwives with the clear majority being nurse-midwives. The American College of Nurse-Midwives defines the scope of practice for midwives as "health care services for women from adolescence beyond menopause including primary care, gynecologic and family planning services, preconception care, care during pregnancy, childbirth and the postpartum period, care of the normal newborn during the first 28 days of life, and treatment of male partners for sexually transmitted infections."[2] This description exceeds the international definition of midwifery as "the health services and health workforce needed to support and care for women and newborns, including sexual and reproductive health and especially pregnancy, labour and postnatal care."[3] The evolution of midwifery to nurse-midwifery in the United States was brought about through complex and often conflicted relationships among the professions of midwifery, nursing, and medicine in the country.

This paper examines the evolution of midwifery within the United States from an apprentice-based trade providing reproductive care of women and families, to a sub-specialty of the nursing profession requiring advanced degrees and providing primary care of women. Relationships among midwifery, nursing, and medicine are examined to identify their role in this evolution. The state of Georgia offers an exemplar demonstrating how the professions of nursing and medicine interacted resulting in the demise of traditional midwifery and the development of nurse-midwifery. Oral testimonies of nurse-midwives working in clinical and education roles in Georgia during the 1970s and 1980s are examined to identify the impact of other healthcare professions on midwifery in Georgia. I argue that the professions of nursing and

---

1  In 2014, certified nurse-midwives and certified midwives (CNMs/CMs) attended 91.3 percent of all midwife-attended births, 12.1 percent of all vaginal births, and 8.3 percent of total US births as reported by Hamilton et al. (2015).

2  Definition of scope of practice for CNMs/CMs from the American College of Nurse-Midwives (2011).

3  Definition of the scope of practice from The State of the World's Midwifery (SoWMy) (2014).

medicine provided support for midwifery, allowing for professional survival, but demanded compromises that prohibited midwifery from thriving.

Midwives have been part of all cultures throughout history beginning in ancient times. Native American women relied on helping women, now known as midwives, but little documentation exists of these earliest midwives in the Americas. Much, however, has been written about the history of midwives in the United States. Caron, for example, used the state of Rhode Island to demonstrate the "long and arduous" work of midwives to preserve a tradition of woman-centered birth in the face of physicians' efforts to undermine the presence of professional nurse-midwives in the state.[4] Reagan argued a two-pronged campaign was waged against midwives and abortion during the Progressive Era linking midwives and abortion in Chicago as a case study.[5] Using oral history interviews of midwives working in Philadelphia, Pennsylvania during the first half of the 20th century, Walsh demonstrated personal and professional relationships supported the role of midwives in their communities and validated them as successful career women.[6] Dawley examined the development of nurse-midwifery's professional identity throughout the 20th century and described a divide between identifying as an advanced nursing specialty or as the independent profession of midwifery.[7]

Traveling to colonial America from Europe, perhaps on the "Mayflower", midwives played a vital role in childbirth throughout the first two centuries of the United States. Childbirth during colonial times was a social experience. A woman in labor would be attended by a midwife and her female friends and family members who would stay for a two to four-week "lying-in" period. Colonial midwives reflected British traditions, receiving no formal training and performing a service considered to be outside the medical profession, social and quasi-religious in nature. Midwives were required to be licensed in some of the colonies, such as New York and Virginia, and held positions of authority regarding women's health. Foreign-trained immigrant midwives were held in high esteem during the early colonial period, provided with housing and a salary in some cases. Midwives in the southern colonies were more typically slaves on large plantations attending other slaves as well as plantation owners' wives and farmers' wives during childbirth.

Knowledge of the quality and outcomes of care given by midwives in the colonial period is limited. Midwives immigrating to the United States came with varying levels of preparation. Some midwives were trained in folklore, while others had received formal midwifery education in Europe. African midwives arrived aboard slave ships prepared with traditions and practices passed down from female relatives. Formal education and regulation of midwifery were rare in colonial America. In 1762, the physician William Ship-

---

4    Cf. Caron (2014).
5    Cf. Reagan (1995).
6    Cf. Walsh (1994).
7    Cf. Dawley (2005).

pen Jr. established a series of lectures on midwifery.[8] Initially training both female midwives and male physicians, his lectures were limited to male students
when Shippen was elected to the medical department of the newly founded
College of Philadelphia in 1765. For a time, midwives remained the primary
maternity care providers in the Colonies, managing simple and complicated
births, and meeting the obstetric needs of their communities. By the late
18th century, however, physicians began to expand their practices to include
attendance of childbirth.

The introduction of the obstetric forceps ushered in great changes in childbirth in the 19th century which would have a major impact on midwives. Developed by the British surgeon Peter Chamberlain, forceps could be a lifesav-
ing intervention for the common problem of labor dystocia. Chamberlain and
his family kept the forceps secret for nearly a century, but physicians gradually
began to purchase forceps from the Chamberlains or made their own.[9] Midwives could seldom afford to buy the instruments and were denied training in
the use of them. Most women in the United States in the 1800s could not afford doctors and continued to employ midwives. However, upper-class women
in urban settings began to call on physicians to attend them in hopes of easier
and safer births. The women in Philadelphia's affluent Drinker family were
attended by Shippen in childbirth, expecting they would receive better care
from a male physician than from traditional female midwives.[10]

Physicians trained in Great Britain were educated in women's anatomy
and the process of parturition. While most American physicians were not
formally trained prior to the 20th century, they enjoyed the elevated status
afforded the male gender and the image of scientific education. Protestant-
ism, with its Puritan prohibition of magic associated with birth, helped to
facilitate a movement away from traditional birth practices and toward an
increased trust in science.[11] Childbirth remained a social event for women in
the 19th century, but the management of it began to be assumed by men in
medicine.

Throughout the 19th century in America, women steadily disappeared
from the practice of midwifery. Four medical schools were founded, but none
admitted female students. Women interested in midwifery education had to
rely on private sources and were encouraged to attend only normal births.
The first American midwifery education program opened in 1848 in Boston.
The school closed in 1874 due to financial difficulties and criticism from the
Boston Medical Society.[12] A few proprietary midwifery schools opened in the
Northeast and Midwest United States in the last half of the 19th century. The
quality of these programs was called into question by Abraham Flexner in his

8   Cf. Leavitt (1986).
9   Cf. Litoff (1978).
10   Cf. Drinker (1937).
11   Cf. Wertz/Wertz (1977).
12   Cf. Donegan (1978).

1910 report on medical education in the United States and Canada.[13] The first formal school of midwifery granting diplomas to women in the United States opened in New York City in 1883. The College of Midwifery closed two years later, after falling into disrepute over student recruitment techniques.[14] Formal education was unavailable to midwives in the United States throughout the 19th century, and they failed to stay current with medical discoveries of the era.

The men attending births in the 19th century were referred to as "man-midwives." They were often informally trained interventionists and frequently caused more harm to women than did traditional midwives. Additionally, the dismantling of home-based midwife care led to a marked increase in obstetric interventions and puerperal fever or sepsis. Maternal and infant mortality rates in the United States increased under the care of the man-midwives, often reaching epidemic proportions. Throughout the second half of the 19th century man-midwives, who began to be referred to as obstetricians, viewed traditional midwives as competition, attacking them publicly. By the end of the century, midwifery began to disappear among middle-class women who were turning to physicians in a belief that science would make childbirth safer and painless.

As scientific study increased the knowledge of reproductive anatomy and physiology, the reliance on folklore and morality decreased. The shift to physician-assisted births brought with it a change in the view of birth reflecting a medical focus on illness and complicated cases. This empirical approach encouraged a view of childbirth as an illness, requiring intervention. An increasing reliance on science moved control of childbirth away from the parturient, her female friends and family, and her midwife, into the male-dominated medical arena.[15]

By 1900, approximately 50 percent of births were attended by midwives in the US.[16] While a similar percentage of births were attended by midwives in the United Kingdom at the turn of the 20th century, the rate rose following the passage of the Midwives Act of 1902 allowing for regulation of English midwives.[17] In contrast, midwifery remained unregulated and most midwives in the United States at the turn of the 20th century were European or Mexican immigrants or African Americans. European midwives were likely to have been formally trained, being better educated than the man-midwives at the time, while African and Mexican American midwives were typically apprentice-trained. These midwives attended women in their communities who were also either immigrants or rural African Americans. Midwifery care was pro-

---

13  Cf. Flexner (1910).
14  Cf. Manley (1884).
15  Cf. McCool/McCool (1989).
16  Cf. Darlington (1911); Abbott (1915).
17  Cf. Donnison (1977).

vided by immigrants and the descendants of slaves and began to be considered inferior to physician care by middle-class women in the United States.[18]

The beginning of the 20th century ushered in the movement of childbirth away from home into hospitals. Growing numbers of hospitals and newly developed automobiles provided increased accessibility to hospital births. Marketing campaigns were undertaken by hospitals to attract paying patients, claiming modern sterility techniques could make the hospital cleaner than the home. Analgesics, anesthetics, labor-inducing drugs, forceps, and episiotomies began to be considered necessary for childbirth. Women endorsed the belief that hospitals offered a safer environment for birth as well as the convenience of a scheduled, painless labor. Additionally, traditional female support networks had become unavailable to many urban women, making the assistance of hospital births the best alternative.

The movement of childbirth to the hospital was accompanied by increasing rates of maternal and infant mortality. Nearly half of maternal deaths at the beginning of the 20th century were due to puerperal fever or sepsis.[19] Midwives were blamed for the increasing rates of puerperal fever. However, women giving birth in the hospital attended by doctors were more likely to contract and die from puerperal fever than women attended by midwives at home.[20] Cities in the northeastern United States, such as Newark and Philadelphia, reported maternal mortality rates for midwife-attended births to be only 15 to 25 percent of the physician-attended births.[21] Despite the poorer outcomes, more than one-third of births took place in the hospital by 1935, with only 15 percent of childbearing women attended by midwives. Nearly 90 percent of white, middle-class women gave birth in hospitals attended by a physician by the end of the 1930s.

Health care reformers in the Progressive Era were alarmed by high maternal and infant mortality rates in the US and particularly in the South. In response to the controversy surrounding midwives in the early 20th century, Frederick Taussig introduced the idea of the nurse-midwife. In a presentation to the National Organization for Public Health Nursing in 1914, this St. Louis physician suggested nurse-midwifery as a solution to the midwife question. He argued for establishing schools of nurse-midwifery so that graduate nurses could be trained in midwifery. In an article for the *Public Health Nurse Quarterly* he wrote, "The nurse-midwife will, I believe, prove to be the most sympathetic, the most economical, and the most efficient agent in the care of normal confinements."[22]

The concept of nurse-midwifery grew as the Federal Children's Bureau, established in 1912 to investigate morbidity and mortality of mothers, infants, and children, identified a need for public health nurses to provide care

18   Cf. Ettinger (2006).
19   Cf. Meigs (1917).
20   Cf. Levy (1923).
21   Cf. Devitt (1979).
22   Taussig (1914), p. 91.

and advice to pregnant women. Leaders of the Children's Bureau suggested prenatal care provided by trained nurses could lower maternal and infant mortality rates. After achieving full enfranchisement, women's organizations successfully worked to enact legislation addressing the poor outcomes affecting women and infants. The Sheppard-Towner Maternity and Infancy Protection Act, passed in 1921, provided financial support for the development of nurse-midwifery as part of states' plans to improve maternal and child health by educating, registering, and supervising midwives.

Public health nurses created a vision of combining nursing with midwifery to create a new specialty: nurse-midwifery. To achieve this vision, nurses joined physicians in a campaign to eliminate traditional midwifery which had become a source of competition for the developing medical specialty of obstetrics.[23] Medical, nursing, and public health professions used racial and gender-biased campaigns to eliminate traditional midwives. Midwives were portrayed as ignorant, illiterate, and dirty, stigmatizing midwifery as unsafe and inferior.[24] Funding provided by the Sheppard-Towner Act resulted in legislation leading to the education and regulation of midwives across the country. In 1923, the director of Maternal and Infant Hygiene of the Children's Bureau reported funds from the Sheppard-Towner Act had enabled 31 states to address "the midwife problem" by providing training and supervision.[25] In the northeast, public health leaders began to call for formal training of midwives and suggested training nurses in midwifery.[26]

With support for nurse-midwifery from physicians and nurses, attempts were made to establish the profession during the mid-1920s. In 1925, the Manhattan Midwifery School opened to train nurses in midwifery. Offering a six-month course in midwifery for graduate nurses, the school graduated at least 18 students who went on to work primarily as missionaries outside the US or in public health settings in the US. The school existed for six years, before closing due to insufficient numbers of patients to train both nurse-midwives and medical students and is little-known today. In 1923, the Bellevue School for Midwives made an agreement with New York City's Maternity Center Association (MCA) to allow nurses to receive training in midwifery. Nurses, working out of thirty centers set up by MCA throughout the city, were providing prenatal care and assisting women giving birth at home. In 1939, Hemschemeyer reported outstanding outcomes of care provided at MCA. Only four maternal deaths occurred in a series of 10,740 deliveries attended by Bellevue midwives, one of which was from pneumonia: "It would seem that their work must have been well done and well supervised. The closing of this school in 1932 was no reflection on the midwives' work nor on the school,

23  Cf. Kobrin (1966).
24  Cf. Crowell (1906/07): an investigation into the conditions of midwifery practice in New York city made under the auspices of the Public Health Committee of the Association of Neighborhood Workers; Abbott (1915).
25  Cf. Rude (1923), p. 987.
26  Cf. Baker (1912); Noyes (1911/12); Van Blarcom (1914).

for coincident with the decrease in this midwife group was a similar increase in hospital facilities for maternity care."[27] The MCA failed when New York City's commissioner of welfare refused to support the project.

The practice of nurse-midwifery was first successfully implemented in the United States in 1925 when Mary Breckinridge established the Frontier Nursing Service (FNS) in Hyden, Kentucky. Breckinridge employed nurse-midwives trained in England, recording remarkable success in decreasing maternal and infant mortality rates. Nurse-midwives provided maternity services, nursing care, and, eventually, family planning services to women in rural Appalachia. They traveled by horseback to attend women in childbirth and other emergencies.[28] Of the first nine thousand women attended by FNS midwives, 98 percent delivered without the use of forceps or cesarean section. At the same time, these interventions were much more common throughout Kentucky.

The nurse-midwives at FNS functioned in an isolated area where few physicians practiced. Writing in support of training nurses in midwifery in 1934, Kosmak referred to the midwives at FNS as proof "that good and effective work can be done by well-trained midwives under the most adverse circumstances."[29] Nearly a century later, Cockerham and Keeling reached a similar conclusion in their synthesis of oral histories gathered through Frontier Nursing University's Pioneer Project. These authors described FNS midwives delivering babies in "primitive and spare mountain cabins", but nonetheless,

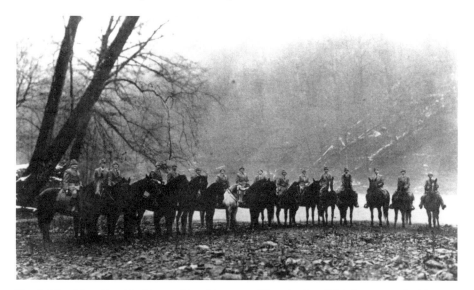

Fig. 1: Mrs. Mary Breckinridge and her Nurses on Horseback – 1931. Image used with permission: Leslie County, Kentucky Photo Gallery

27  Hemschemeyer (1939), p. 1182.
28  Cf. Breckinridge (1952).
29  Kosmak (1934), p. 423.

providing "state-of-the-art obstetrical care."[30] Frontier midwives in the early
20th century cared for low-income women at high medical risk, making their
outcomes even more notable.

The second nurse-midwifery practice in the United States was the MCA
midwifery in New York City in 1931. By the 1940s, nurse-midwives began
to practice in rural areas in North Carolina, South Carolina, Maryland, and
Alabama.[31] In Santa Fe, New Mexico, the Medical Mission Sisters opened the
Catholic Maternity Institute (CMI) in 1944 to serve poor Hispanic families,
offering nurse-midwifery care and training nurse-midwifery students. Women,
primarily of Spanish American descent, were attended by nurse-midwives either in their own homes or at a freestanding birth center called La Casita.
The CMI closed in 1969, succumbing to the financial burden of operating La
Casita as increasing numbers of women opted to deliver at the birth center
rather than at home.[32]

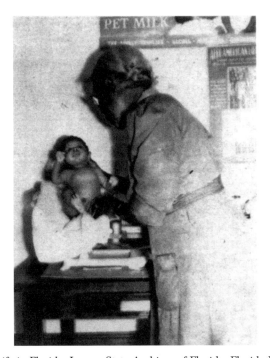

Fig. 2: 1944 Midwife in Florida. Image: State Archives of Florida, Florida Memory

In 1942, the first nurse-midwife led birthing center opened in Rabun County,
Georgia, a county with no practicing midwives. This service expanded in
Georgia to include a home birth service in Thomas County, a hospital-based

30   Cockerham/Keeling (2012), p. 34.
31   Cf. Shoemaker (1947).
32   Cf. Cockerham/Keeling (2010).

service in Walton County, and a second birth center in Lamar County. Counties in which these services functioned experienced a drop in maternal mortality rates, an increase in the average number of prenatal visits, earlier initiation of prenatal care, and increased physician acceptance of nurse-midwives compared to the rest of the state. However, state funding for the projects was discontinued by the early 1960s, leading to their closure.[33]

Despite the success of nurse-midwifery in these regions of the United States, expansion of the profession was slow, and opportunities for clinical practice remained very limited. From its beginning, nurse-midwifery was conceived of as a profession that would serve women outside of the reach of the medical establishment. Early nurse-midwives were faced with the stigma the medical and nursing establishments had created surrounding traditional midwifery. By 1954, there were only three nurse-midwifery practices and schools in the United States: FNS in Kentucky, MCA in New York, and CMI in Santa Fe, New Mexico. Two other schools had opened to educate African American nurse-midwives, one in Tuskegee, Alabama and one in New Orleans, Louisiana. Both schools were short-lived, closing due to issues surrounding.

The movement of childbirth into the hospital provided another obstacle for the development of nurse-midwifery. All three of the existing nurse-midwifery practices had been founded to attend childbirth at home, but by 1950 nearly 90 percent of births took place in the hospital. Nurse-midwives were not welcome in the hospital setting, which was firmly under the control of physicians. A small, 25-bed hospital in Hyden, Kentucky was the only hospital in which nurse-midwives attended births for 30 years. Nurse-midwives began to be welcomed into hospitals after the Second World War due to increasing access to health insurance, growth in hospital construction, rising birth rates, and a shortage of obstetricians.

Hospitals became much safer places for childbirth throughout the 1940s and 1950s. The advent of antibiotics, blood banks, oxytocin, fetal monitoring, and X-ray pelvimetry led to increasing prestige and authority for hospitals and physicians in society. Increasing reliance on hospital services and increasing access to insurance coverage caused a shortage of hospital personnel. Obstetricians began to look to nurse-midwives as a solution to the problem of large numbers of normal deliveries, which left little time to pursue other areas of practice. Nurse-midwifery services were established at Johns Hopkins Hospital in 1953 and Columbia-Presbyterian Hospital in 1954, followed by the MCA practice moving into Downstate Medical Center in 1958. Movement into the hospital created an opportunity for expansion of the profession. It also required nurse-midwives to relinquish control of their practice, to incorporate previously unused interventions, and to function under the authority of physicians.

Changes in women's attitudes regarding childbirth following World War II led to the natural childbirth movement. During the 1940s, most women were given a combination of morphine, scopolamine, and chloroform, known as

33    Cf. Melber (1987).

twilight sleep, which relieved the pain of childbirth, but also caused amnesia of the event. By the end of the decade, public and professional opinion began to move away from twilight sleep due to concerns about its effects on mothers and newborns. Childbirth had become safer than at any time in history, leaving women and providers of maternity care the freedom to focus on the psychological aspects of birth. Nurse-midwives at MCA and Yale University were instrumental in implementing family-centered care, childbirth education, rooming-in, and support for natural childbirth nation-wide. This brought national recognition to the profession and led to a period of expansion and development.

By 1940, nurse-midwifery leaders began to recognize the need for a professional organization to establish standards guiding practice and education.[34] The first American nurse-midwifery association was established in 1929 as the Kentucky State Association of Midwives. The purpose of the association was stated as follows:

> The nature of the business proposed to be transacted, promoted, and carried on by this corporation shall be to foster, encourage, and, in the qualifications for its own membership, to maintain a high standard of midwifery with special reference to rugged, difficult and economically poor areas [...]; and thereby to raise the standard of midwives and nurse-midwives, who are or have been or may hereafter be engaged in the active practice of midwifery, to a standard not lower than the official standards required by first class European countries in 1929.[35]

In 1938, there were 44 members, all but one being FNS staff members. Annual meetings were held on the Thanksgiving holiday at Wendover, Kentucky, the headquarters of the FNS. The organization's name was changed to the American Association of Nurse-Midwives in 1940 to allow membership to nurse-midwives outside of Kentucky. By 1942, the organization consisted of 76 midwives, but remained primarily FNS graduates.[36] Dawley and Burst argued the American Association of Nurse-Midwives failed to become the national organization for nurse-midwifery due to its history of racial exclusion, and a failure to set standards for nurse-midwifery practice.[37]

In 1947, a section of the National Organization of Public Health Nurses, an organization open to nurses of color, was organized to represent nurse-midwifery.[38] This section existed until 1952 when the National Organization of Public Health Nurses was dissolved, and the American Nurses Association and the National League of Nursing became the two major national nursing organizations. Both organizations refused to create an autonomous section for nurse-midwifery, expressing concern that nurse-midwives practiced medicine rather than nursing. Sister M. Theophane Shoemaker led a committee on organization, guiding the formation of the American College of

34   Cf. Shoemaker (1947).
35   Kentucky State Association of Midwives, Inc. (1939), p. 19.
36   Cf. Shoemaker (1947).
37   Cf. Dawley/Burst (2005).
38   Cf. Shoemaker (1947).

Nurse-Midwifery in 1955. Hattie Hemschemeyer became president and Sister Theophane Shoemaker became president-elect of the newly formed organization. The American College of Nurse-Midwifery merged with the American Association of Nurse-Midwives in 1969, becoming the American College of Nurse-Midwives, as it is known today.

During the1960s, nurse-midwives were practicing primarily in Kentucky, New Mexico, and New York City, the only three areas which had laws allowing their practice. Nurse-midwifery had disappeared in Georgia following the closure of the state-funded demonstration projects. The institution of Medicaid in 1965 set the stage for nurse-midwives to participate in maternal healthcare programs. Medicaid set limits on the fees which could be charged for services, resulting in physician unwillingness to participate in the fee-capped program. Nurse-midwives stepped in to fill the resulting gap in access to care for low-income women.

Nurse-midwifery developed in the United States to care for women lacking access to physicians, primarily serving poor women in inner-city or rural areas. Private practice, even in 1970, was unheard of due to financial limitations, resistance from the medical establishment, and a long-standing commitment by nurse-midwives to care for underserved populations. Nurse-midwifery's entrance into private practice was facilitated by obstetricians who were so overworked with normal deliveries they had no time to practice gynecology, and by women seeking nontraditional care within the hospital setting.[39]

As nurse-midwifery developed, a union between midwifery and nursing was sealed. As women gained the right to vote and began to participate in the country's workforce, traditional midwives began to disappear, and the medical specialty of obstetrics began to gain economic, political, and social dominance. Supporters of midwifery at the beginning of the 20th century believed midwifery could not stand on its own in the United States as it did in European countries because "the medical profession was too strong, and the takeover of midwifery by physicians was too complete."[40] Midwifery was only allowed as an attachment to nursing and under the direct supervision and control of medicine.

Nurse-midwifery developed as a nursing specialty as a matter of professional survival. However, this position within the nursing profession created confusion regarding professional identity. Ambivalence regarding identity as either advanced practice registered nurses or as midwives has existed since the establishment of the profession. In 1957, Hattie Hemschemeyer, the president of the American College of Nurse-Midwifery, stated, "You and I know that midwifery and nursing are two distinct professions."[41] While just a year later, in 1958, a report from that college identified nurse-midwifery as a nurs-

---

39 Cf. Gatewood/Stewart (1975).
40 Burst (2010), p. 406.
41 Hemschemeyer (1957), p. 53.

ing specialty.[42] A compromise was reached in the College which recognized nurse-midwifery as a separate profession drawing on knowledge from both nursing and medicine and affirmed the American College of Nurse-Midwifery as the professional organization responsible for setting educational and practice standards.

The compromises which allowed for the creation of the nurse-midwifery profession provided legitimacy within the health care system but resulted in a loss of the autonomy which traditional midwives had enjoyed. One nurse-midwifery leader, Helen Varney Burst, suggested "without autonomy and independence then the concepts of team and collaboration may simply mask the reality of continuing a century's worth of supervision and control by both medicine and nursing."[43]

In the state of Georgia, traditional granny midwives persisted into the mid-20th century, much longer than in most of the US, primarily in rural parts of the state. In the 1940s, Georgia's Department of Public Health began requiring midwives be educated, certified, and supervised. The number of midwives decreased significantly following these requirements. Between 1946 and 1951, nurse-midwives were hired to train and supervise the traditional midwives, educate public health nurses in maternity care. Nurse-midwife demonstration projects began between 1947 and 1951 in three Georgia counties. The projects were shown to be effective but were discontinued due to financial constraints and lack of available nurse-midwives.[44]

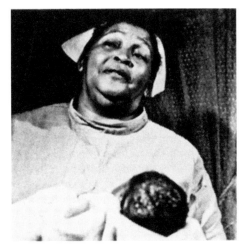

Fig. 3: Mary Francis Hill Coley Holding new Baby. Image: All My Babies, Film Documentary, 1952

42   Burst (2010), p. 406, reported the American College of Nurse-Midwifery's 1958 report on the Work Conference on Nurse-Midwifery: "the group took as a working assumption that nurse-midwifery is a clinical nursing specialty."
43   Burst (2010), p. 409.
44   Cf. Melber (1987); Sharp (1987).

By 1960, midwifery nearly ceased to exist in Georgia; traditional midwives were becoming rare, and no nurse-midwives were practicing in the state. But change was on the horizon. In 1970, nearly 8,000 babies were born at Grady Memorial Hospital. Residents from the Emory School of Medicine were overwhelmed attending this large volume of deliveries. At that time, a Maternal and Infant Project focused on high-risk patients, but there was an increasing need for care of low-risk patients. One of the attending physicians, Dr. Newton Long, had worked with Elizabeth Sharp at Johns Hopkins University. Long, recognizing the value of nurse-midwives in the care of low-risk patients, convinced Sharp to undertake the establishment of a nurse-midwifery service at Grady. Sharp brought students and faculty from Yale University to Grady Memorial Hospital for clinical experiences in the summer of 1971. Permanent midwifery staff were then recruited, and two of the faculty and one student from Yale were employed.[45] In 1971, Elizabeth Sharp was recruited to open a nurse-midwifery service to care for low-risk women, relieving some of the burden on the obstetrical residents. Sharp went on to establish a nurse-midwifery education program at Emory University in 1977.[46] The program remains in operation at the time of this writing and, as of 2015, reported 370 total nurse-midwifery graduates.

After being established at Grady Memorial Hospital, nurse-midwifery spread to other areas of the state where physicians struggled to keep pace with the high volume of births. Obstetricians in one town in rural Georgia sought Sharp's advice as they started the first private-practice nurse-midwifery service in 1973. The same year, nurse-midwives began working in five other rural areas of the state. These nurse-midwifery programs were established primarily to provide maternity care to uninsured and underinsured women. However, insured women began seeking out nurse-midwifery care as it gained a reputation for providing patient safety and patient satisfaction. In 1983 the first private nurse-midwifery practice in Atlanta was established, and soon, the profession spread to physician's offices and private hospitals throughout the city.

Relationships among nurse-midwifery and other health care professions, particularly the relationships with nursing and medicine, played a key role as nurse-midwives worked to establish the profession in Georgia. A nurse-midwifery service was established at Grady Memorial Hospital in Atlanta, Georgia in 1971. This service represented the first hospital-based practice in the state. A nurse-midwife on staff at the Grady service from 1974 to 1976 stated, "Sharp had great support from the OB [Obstetrics] chief, and she had great support from nursing."[47] The inter-professional relationships Sharp built with physicians and nurses were instrumental in the success of the nurse-midwifery service at Grady.

---

45   Cf. Sharp (1987).
46   Cf. Thrower (2016).
47   Thrower (2016), p. 125. From a 2016 interview with Ellen Martin, CNM, conducted by the author.

Another nurse-midwife at Grady Memorial Hospital from 1976 to 2016, described nurse-midwifery as an extension of nursing. She recalled choosing to work with Sharp at Grady Memorial Hospital, rather than staying in New York with Dorothea Lang at the MCA, because of Sharp's midwifery paradigm. She stated, "Liz's view was that we were nurse-midwives, not midwives. We came from a nursing perspective."[48] Sharp's view of nurse-midwifery as an expansion of nursing was confirmed in her 1996 interview. Sharp stated,

> Nurse-midwifery, the midwifery part, was an extension of nursing practice, so that while you were doing your nursing care, it just made sense, if you were listening to the baby's heartbeat, your hands were on the abdomen, why not, figure out where the baby was lying, how it was lying, or measure the fundal height, so that if you were taking care of the patient in labor, you would gather more information and add more management decisions. Now, she did say at the time of birth, if you were doing the hand maneuvers, and doing all the things that you do there, you would need a nurse to help with that, but you did have to focus on that; you couldn't do everything at once […] Nurse-midwifery as an expansion of nursing, and because I really was very into nursing, this did not seem like I was leaving nursing […] to go to something else. It was just a natural expansion of the nursing practice. And, that's how I have always seen it.[49]

A nurse-midwife who provided home birth services starting in 1976, expressed similar sentiments regarding nursing when she stated, "We depend on nursing. I know there's a thought that too bad it isn't just midwifery programs like they have in England. But we evolved differently."[50]

Other narrators emphasized a distinction between the professions of nurse-midwifery and nursing. One midwife recalled, "The midwives who were at Grady before us were older, sort of seasoned, a little set in their ways, and a little bit more nursey than we were. We were willing to … to assert ourselves, just sort of change the flow of the practice. I think we'd matured it from a real nursey kind of program to something that really reflected more midwifery."[51] Sharp discussed the complicated nature of nurse-midwifery's relationship to nursing saying, "It wasn't until I got back into nurse-midwifery down at Grady and beginning to recruit nurse-midwives that I began to realize that some of the nurse-midwives went into nurse-midwifery to get away from nursing […] and saw it very separate and hearing about how we weren't nurses and how […] we were midwives."[52]

Despite differing opinions about the position of nurse-midwifery within nursing, the narrators voiced a dependence on the support of nurses and the nursing profession. One midwife expressed this as she described the process used for hiring nurses to work at West Paces Ferry Hospital:

---

48   Thrower (2016), p. 125. From a 2016 interview with Denise McLaughlin, CNM, conducted by the author.
49   Sharp, oral history interview 1996.
50   Thrower (2016), p. 126. From a 2016 interview with Linda Segal, CNM, conducted by the author.
51   Thrower (2016), p. 126. From a 2016 interview with Ellen Martin, CNM, conducted by the author.
52   Sharp, oral history interview 1996.

She hired the nursing staff by saying, "We're going to have a brand-new unit here. It's all new; it's fresh; it's beautiful and we're going to have midwives. And so how do you feel about working with midwives?" And if the nurse that was the interviewee said, "I don't want to, I don't believe in that," she didn't get the job.[53]

Similarly, another midwife described the importance of the nursing staff to the labor, delivery, and recovery unit at Grady Memorial Hospital: "The other wonderful thing at the beginning was that the nurses that we had were recruited specifically for this unit, and most of them went on to be nurse-midwives […] I think that made, you know, we were such a little hardworking, coherent unit. I mean, I look back on that period as the heyday of midwifery at Grady."[54]

Narrators also emphasized the role medicine played in establishing nurse-midwifery, and the inter-dependence between the two professions. According to a nurse-midwife from the Grady service:

When Liz started the practice, she was asked to come for three reasons … One was to model continuity of care; one was to develop an interdisciplinary approach to OB; and one was to take the load off the residents. When they started here in 1970, they only had six residents per year […] and they just didn't have enough residents. So, in 1973, July, they doubled their residency program, but they still needed the midwives, so that's really where it came from.[55]

Recounting her career at Associates in Obstetrics and Gynecology (OB/GYN) in Dalton, another midwife recalled the mutual respect and reliance she shared with the physicians:

Dr. Gregory, I worked with him for […] 25 years and I'd say […] he had a sixth sense for obstetrics and helped me […] so much. I always knew I could count on him. If I called him, he was there for me. He was […] a wonderful mentor. [The physicians] […] could see what we were saying, and they understood that we were bringing in money, and they couldn't do it without us.[56]

One midwife recalled the support she received from the physicians who helped convince the medical director at Crawford Long Hospital to grant her hospital privileges. She also described the support of these two physicians as they promoted nurse-midwifery to patients:

I mean when, when Jeff and Michael were there, […] they would say, you know, […] "If everything is normal, you're going to get much better care from the nurse-midwives than you're going to get from me, 'cause they'll spend more time with you, and they'll understand what's going on with you," you know, "emotionally and physically."[57]

53  Thrower (2016), p. 127. From a 2016 interview with Elaine Moore, CNM, conducted by the author.
54  Thrower (2016), p. 127. From a 2016 interview with Mickey Gillmor, CNM, conducted by the author.
55  Thrower (2016), p. 127. From a 2016 interview with Denise McLaughlin, CNM, conducted by the author.
56  Thrower (2016), p. 127. From a 2016 interview with Sanna Wagner, CNM, conducted by the author.
57  Thrower (2016), p. 128. From a 2016 interview with Maureen Kelly, CNM, conducted by the author.

Sharp credited physician Newton Long with bringing nurse-midwives to Grady Memorial Hospital. She recalled Long agreeing to accept a faculty position with the Emory University School of Medicine that had been offered to him by John Thompson saying, "If you can promise me that at some point we'll have nurse-midwives."[58]

The narrators described struggling to keep their services in operation within a health care system which could be unsupportive of nurse-midwifery. Many of the difficulties were related to competing for patients and financial stresses. The director of the faculty practice at the Emory University Clinic described the closing of the clinic using the phrase "mission versus margin" to represent the challenges of providing midwifery care to women while remaining financial sustainable. She recalled:

> They figured that we weren't making [...] we weren't paying for ourselves, because they didn't count any of the patients that came in as ours, necessarily, unless they declared themselves, um, wanting to see a midwife [...] when they first came in [...] Right. And so there [...] were some who were [...] actually a number of years where Marla Salmon, our dean, was paying part of our salaries because she believed in the model. There was a year that she got the Woodruff fund to pay for our salaries and so the OB/GYN department, you know, got away with not paying for what we were doing there for a number of years, four or five years. And finally, the dean said, you know, "I can't do this, and I can't continue to do this. And if they're gonna sort of stack the deck against you," um, "if they're not willing to support midwifery [...]" and I was in this terrible meeting with some administrators from Crawford Long, and an OB/GYN from Crawford Long, and they said, "Maureen, we're just gonna, you know, it's just not gonna work. We're not going to be able to do it."[59]

Nurse-midwives in the 1970s and 1980s were often viewed as competition by physicians in their communities. A nurse-midwife from Athens, Georgia recalled the physicians "really trashed us, in a lot of ways ... because we, we probably took some of their patients."[60] The physicians she worked with viewed the nurse-midwives as competition and attempted to limit them to seeing women who were uninsured or indigent. Eventually, an uninsured student from the University of Georgia filed a successful lawsuit against the hospital, winning entrance into the nurse-midwifery service. The midwife recalled: "The judge ruled ... They either settled it – I mean, it wasn't for money or anything, it was admission into the program ... I can't remember the whole thing; it's been so long ago. We ended up getting them. We ended up getting the students."[61]

A midwife from Savannah, Georgia recalled the birth center in Savannah being viewed as competition despite delivering small numbers of babies:

58   Sharp, oral history interview 1996.
59   Thrower (2016), p. 138. From a 2016 interview with Maureen Kelly, CNM, conducted by the author.
60   Thrower (2016), p. 140. From a 2016 interview with Angela Best, CNM, conducted by the author.
61   Thrower (2016), p. 140. From a 2016 interview with Angela Best, CNM, conducted by the author.

"I think that physicians, at least in Savannah, I can't speak for the rest of them, have always seen us as competition. I mean, we're only, even at the biggest year, we've done two-hundred and seventy births. That's not competition for OB/GYN, really."[62]

A nurse-midwife from the Emory University nurse-midwifery education program articulated the relationship between physicians and nurse-midwives saying:

> At first when nurse-midwives took hold … in different places and different institutions, I think we were always relegated to […] taking care of poor women. And we provided a big service for the institution, but then when middle-class women and people who had insurance decided they would like to take advantage of nurse-midwives, I think that's when there was tension with some of the doctors 'cause they saw it as taking their patients away.[63]

Finding physicians willing to provide consultation, collaboration, and emergency transfer services was a challenge for the narrators, particularly those who were self-employed, or worked for hospitals. A male nurse-midwife described the physicians at Cobb Hospital rotating to provide backup services to the nurse-midwives. He recalled one physician group refusing to provide coverage for the nurse-midwives after being "accused of fraud for billing for all the deliveries the midwives were doing."[64]

The director of the birth center in Savannah, Georgia recounted the difficulty she had finding a collaborating physician due to misconceptions associated with nurse-midwifery. She stated:

> That's always been the hardest part, getting a backup physician because their peers are so against us […] but [it] was just basically ignorance to start with, and then once they could've educated themselves, they didn't. And then once they could've looked at our record, they didn't. And I think, also […] they thought we were so counterculture, I don't think they wanted to understand.[65]

When asked about obstacles she faced in the 1980s, a nurse-midwife faculty member from Emory University responded:

> Education of the public about nurse-midwives because, in Georgia, in particular, midwives were delivering babies for a long time but they were, granny midwives. There was […] educating women about the services, and educating doctors […] There was such a misconception about who we were, and what we did, and why would somebody have a midwife when they could have a doctor.[66]

---

62  Thrower (2016), p. 141. From a 2016 interview with Nancy Belin, CNM, conducted by the author.
63  Thrower (2016), p. 141. From a 2016 interview with Marianne Scharbo DeHaan, CNM, conducted by the author.
64  Thrower (2016), p. 141. From a 2016 interview with Michael McCann, CNM, conducted by the author.
65  Thrower (2016), p. 141. From a 2016 interview with Nancy Belin, CNM, conducted by the author.
66  Thrower (2016), p. 142. From a 2016 interview with Marianne Scharbo DeHaan, CNM, conducted by the author.

Obtaining hospital privileges was often difficult for the narrators. Gatewood and Stewart[67] described the considerable effort required to open the first private nurse-midwifery practice in the state, particularly related to credentialing the nurse-midwives to work at the Sumter County Hospital. These physicians struggled for five months to gain approval from the medical staff hospital authority for nurse-midwives to obtain hospital privileges. A nurse-midwife from Dalton, Georgia reported resistance from the medical staff as she sought to obtain hospital privileges saying, "they had to get me approved through the medical staff, and there were a lot of docs who were resistant."[68] Another midwife recalled being denied privileges at Piedmont Hospital despite having the support of staff physicians. The birth center midwife stated: "So finally, [...] we got it [...] Every year, we applied and the first year they said, 'We don't have any pieces of paper for you to fill out.' So [...] they had a committee studying it, that whole dragging their feet nonsense."[69]

Relationships and connections weighed very heavily in the narrators' accounts of the establishment of nurse-midwifery in Georgia. Support received from physicians, nurses, administrators, communities, and peers sustained the pioneer nurse-midwives and the profession. Connections between the narrators and their communities played a key role in the development of many nurse-midwifery practices in the state. Relationships built with physicians, nurses, and administrators facilitated expansion of nurse-midwifery into the arena of private obstetrical practice, and into Emory University's Nell Hodgson Woodruff School of Nursing. Relationships with mentors and fellow nurse-midwives sustained the narrators as they dealt with the responsibilities inherent in care of women during childbirth. A home birth midwife stated, "What we do is a really big thing," as she described one of her mentors helping her find the courage she needed for nurse-midwifery.[70]

The sole male nurse-midwife interviewed described a hierarchical relationship with medicine saying:

> There's a certain level in midwifery where in the [...] hierarchy, you're always never going to be top dog. And you've got to kind of come to grips with that. Is that, there's always going to [be] this person with an MD behind their name that can sort of supersede you [...] and change plans and, and ultimately, at this point in time has a, has authority that until healthcare systems change, they'll all supersede you, and so [...] you got to be comfortable with the fact that you can be superseded, especially if you need their service.[71]

---

67   Cf. Gatewood/Stewart (1975).
68   Thrower (2016), p. 142. From a 2016 interview with Ellen Martin, CNM, conducted by the author.
69   Thrower (2016), p. 142. From a 2016 interview with Nancy Belin, CNM, conducted by the author.
70   Thrower (2016), p. 152. From a 2016 interview with Linda Segal, CNM, conducted by the author.
71   Thrower (2016), p. 153. From a 2016 interview with Michael McCann, CNM, conducted by the author.

While many physicians provided sustaining support for nurse-midwifery, others raised considerable opposition. Physicians blocked access to hospital privileges for nurse-midwives, placed limits on the types of insurance nurse-midwives could accept, wrote letters to local newspapers maligning nurse-midwives, and refused to collaborate with nurse-midwives in Georgia during the 1970s and 1980s.

In conclusion, complex relationships existed among midwifery, nursing, and medicine in the 1970s and 1980s as nurse-midwifery was established and developed in Georgia. One midwife summarized the position of nurse-midwifery at the time as "halfway between a doctor and a nurse."[72] Compromises were made with nursing and medicine which ushered nurse-midwifery into the 21st century. These compromises allowed for the survival of the profession but placed limitations on the autonomous practice of midwifery. Relationships with nurses and physicians played key roles in establishing nurse-midwifery in Georgia and developing the profession throughout the state. However, opposition from the more powerful medical profession constrained the growth of the profession. Ultimately, an interdisciplinary symbiosis developed among nurse-midwives, nurses, and physicians which was foundational for the profession of nurse-midwifery in Georgia in the 1970s and 1980s.

## Bibliography

*Oral history interview (Author's private collection)*

Sharp, Elizabeth S., oral history interview by Kay Johnson in February 1996

*Literature*

Abbott, Grace: The Midwife in Chicago. In: American Journal of Sociology 20 (1915), pp. 684–699.
American College of Nurse-Midwives: Definition of midwifery and scope of practice of certified nurse-midwives and certified midwives (2011), available at: http://www.midwife.org/ACNM/files/ACNMLibraryData/UPLOADFILENAME/000000000266/Definition%20of%20Midwifery%20and%20Scope%20of%20Practice%20of%20CNMs%20and%20CMs%20Dec%202011.pdf (last accessed: 24/10/2018).
Baker, S. Josephine: Schools for midwives. Read before the Annual Meeting of the Association for the Study and Prevention of Infant Mortality held in Chicago, IL, November 1911. New York 1912.
Breckinridge, Mary: Wide neighborhoods: A story of the Frontier Nursing Service. Lexington, KY 1952.
Burst, Helen Varney: Nurse-Midwifery, Self-Identification and Autonomy. In: Journal of Midwifery and Women's Health 55 (2010), no. 5, pp. 406–410.

---

72 Thrower (2016), p. 155. From a 2016 interview with Ellen Martin, CNM, conducted by the author.

Caron, Simone M.: "It's Been a Long Road to Acceptance": Midwives in Rhode Island, 1970–2000. In: Nursing History Review 22 (2014), pp. 61–94.

Cockerham, Anne Z.; Keeling, Arlene W.: Finance and faith at the Catholic Maternity Institute, Santa Fe, New Mexico, 1944–1969. In: Nursing History Review 18 (2010), pp. 151–166.

Cockerham, Anne Z.; Keeling, Arlene W.: Rooted in the mountains, Reaching to the World: Stories of Nursing and Midwifery at Kentucky's Frontier School, 1939–1989. Louisville, KY 2012.

Crowell, F. Elisabeth: The Midwives of New York. A report submitted on December 20, 1906, at a special meeting of the Committee of the Association of Neighborhood Workers held at the New York Academy of Medicine. In: Charities and the Commons 17 (1906/07), pp. 667–677.

Darlington, Thomas: The Present Status of the Midwife. In: American Journal of Obstetrics and Diseases of Women and Children 63 (1911), pp. 870–876.

Dawley, Katy: American Nurse-Midwifery: A Hyphenated Profession with a Conflicted Identity. In: Nursing History Review 13 (2005), pp. 147–170.

Dawley, Katy; Burst, Helen Varney: The American College of Nurse-Midwives and its Antecedents: A Historic Time Line. In: Journal of Midwifery and Women's Health 50 (2005), pp. 16–22.

Devitt, Neal: The Statistical Case for Elimination of the Midwife: Fact Versus Prejudice, 1890–1935 (Part 2). In: Women & Health 4 (1979), no. 2, pp. 169–186.

Donegan, Jane B.: Women & Men midwives: Medicine, Morality, and Misogyny in Early America. Westport, CT 1978.

Donnison, Jean: Midwives and Medical Men: A History of Inter-Professional Rivalries and Women's Rights. New York 1977.

Drinker, Cecil K.: Not So Long Ago: A Chronicle of Medicine and Doctors in Colonial Philadelphia. New York 1937.

Ettinger, Laura E.: Nurse-Midwifery: The Birth of a New American Profession. Columbus, OH 2006.

Flexner, Abraham: Medical Education in the United States and Canada: A Report to the Carnegie Foundation for the Advancement of Teaching. (=Carnegie Foundation Bulletin 4) New York 1910.

Gatewood, Thomas Schley; Stewart, Richard B.: Obstetricians and Nurse-Midwives: The Team Approach in Private Practice. In: American Journal of Obstetrics and Gynecology 123 (1975), no. 1, pp. 35–38.

Hamilton, Brady E. et al.: Births: Final Data for 2014. In: National Vital Statistics Reports 64 (2015), no. 12, pp. 1–64.

Hemschemeyer, Hattie: Midwifery in the United States. In: The American Journal of Nursing 39 (1939), no. 11, pp. 1181–1187.

Hemschemeyer, Hattie: Maternity Care Within the Framework of the Public Health Service. Presented before the International Confederation of Midwives 11th International Congress, Stockholm, June 24, 1957. In: Bulletin of the American College of Nurse-Midwifery 2 (1957), no. 3, pp. 49–56.

Kentucky State Association of Midwives, Inc. In: The Quarterly Bulletin of the Frontier Nursing Service, Inc. 16 (1939), no. 4, p. 19.

Kobrin, Frances E.: The American Midwife Controversy: A Crisis of Professionalization. In: Bulletin of the History of Medicine 40 (1966), no. 4, pp. 350–363.

Kosmak, George W.: The Trained Nurse and the Midwife. In: The American Journal of Nursing 34 (1934), no. 5, pp. 421–423.

Leavitt, Judith Walzer: Brought to Bed: Child-Bearing in America, 1750–1950. New York 1986.

Levy, Julius: Maternal Mortality and Mortality in the First Month of Life in Relation to Attendant at Birth. Read before the Child Hygiene Section of the American Public Health

Association at the 51st Annual Meeting, Cleveland, OH, October 18, 1922. In: American Journal of Public Health 13 (1923), no. 2, pp. 88–95.

Litoff, Judy Barrett: American Midwives: 1860 to the Present. Westport, CT 1978.

Manley, Thomas H.: Women as Midwives. Read November 19, 1884 [at a meeting of the New York State Medical Association]. In: Transactions of the New York State Medical Association 1 (1885), pp. 370–375.

McCool, William F.; McCool, Sandi J.: Feminism and Nurse-Midwifery: Historical Overview and Current Issues. In: Journal of Nurse-Midwifery 34 (1989), no. 6, pp. 323–334.

Meigs, Grace L.: Maternal Mortality from all Conditions Connected with Childbirth in the United States and certain other countries. (=US Children's Bureau, Pub. 19) Washington, D.C. 1917.

Melber, Ruth B.: Georgia Midwifery from Granny to Nurse: An Overview of the Development of Nurse-Midwifery in Georgia (1987, May). Commissioned by the Georgia Department of Human Resources, Division of Public Health [Manuscript, author's private collection].

Noyes, Clara D.: Training Schools for Midwives at Bellevue and Allied Hospitals. In: The American Journal of Nursing 12 (1911/12), no. 5, pp. 417–422.

Reagan, Leslie J.: Linking Midwives and Abortion in the Progressive Era. In: Bulletin of the History of Medicine 69 (1995), no. 4, pp. 569–598.

Rude, Anna E.: The Midwife Problem in the United States. In: Journal of the American Medical Association 81 (1923), no. 12, pp. 987–992.

Sharp, Elizabeth S.: CNMs in Georgia, 1946–1987. In: Current News for Nurse-Midwives 1 (1987), no. 1, pp. 1–6 [Author's Private Collection].

Shoemaker, Mary Theophane: History of Nurse-Midwifery in the United States. Master's Thesis. Washington, D.C. 1947.

The State of the World's Midwifery (SoWMy) 2014: A Universal Pathway. A Woman's Right to Health, available at: https://www.unfpa.org/sites/default/files/pub-pdf/EN_SoWMy2014_complete.pdf (last accessed: 24/10/2018).

Taussig, Fred J.: The Nurse-Midwife. In: Public Health Nurse Quarterly 6 (Oct. 1914), pp. 66–91.

Thrower, Eileen J.B.: Blazing trails for midwifery care: Oral histories of Georgia's pioneer nurse-midwives [Doctoral Dissertation]. Mercer Univ. 2016, available from ProQuest Dissertations and Theses database, UMI No. 10302242.

Van Blarcom, Carolyn Conant: Midwives in America. In: American Journal of Public Health 4 (1914), no. 3, pp. 197–207.

Walsh, Linda V.: Midwives as Wives and Mothers: Urban Midwives in the Early Twentieth Century. In: Nursing History Review 2 (1994), pp. 51–65.

Wertz, Richard W.; Wertz, Dorothy C.: Lying-In: A History of Childbirth in America. New Haven, CT 1977.

# Emergency Medical Services in Germany: The Conflictual Development of a Professional Field

*Pierre Pfütsch*

## Introduction

The emergency medical services in Germany today are a highly complex and efficient system for the fast and professional aid of people who have fallen ill or are hurt.[1] Thus throughout the entire country there is a tight net of rescue coordination centres that coordinate the emergency services.[2] The ambulance and emergency vehicles conform to state-of-the-art technology and are thus largely independent treatment units.[3] Approximately 51,000 full-time Emergency Medical Technicians (EMTs) are working for the emergency services in Germany providing round-the-clock[4] pre-clinical professional emergency care[5]. Both "pre-clinical" and "professional" are two key attributes here that were not part of emergency care from the beginning but began to evolve during the 1960s as we will subsequently show.

In addition, the current emergency services involve many different kinds of agents who are responsible for their functioning. Foremost these are emergency staff and emergency doctors. Furthermore, there are the employees in the call centres of the rescue coordination centres and the doctors in the emergency departments of the hospitals. Finally, there are the patients with their families, their treating general practitioners (GPs) and consultants. Well-functioning teamwork of all these agents is crucial in this area as the smallest error can decide over life and death. The paramedic plays a particular role in this area of interaction because he is in contact with most of the other agents and this forms the central interface between everyone. Thus, it was not an accident that in the restatement of the German legal framework for EMTs in 2014 the ability for teamwork as an express goal of training was explicitly included in the wording of the law:

---

1    In 2012/2013 alone, there were 8,553,311 emergency service responses in Germany (excluding the normal ambulance service). Cf. Gesundheitsberichterstattung des Bundes: Einsatzfahrtaufkommen (2018).
2    Already in 2000 there were 270 rescue coordination centres and more than 1,830 ambulance stations. Cf. Gesundheitsberichterstattung des Bundes: Rettungswachen (2018).
3    On the equipment and the structure of an ambulance vehicle: Cf. Bundesstadt Bonn (2016).
4    Cf. Statistisches Bundesamt (2017), p. 11.
5    Cf. Wiedenfeld (2013), p. 26.

> In accordance with the commonly accepted norms of emergency, medical and other scientific insights, the training of Emergency Medical Technicians must include expert, personal, social and methodological competencies to perform emergency care and transport of patients either independently or as part of a team.[6]

To register such skills in writing in norms and laws can be read as an indication that previously there must have been issues between EMTs and members of other professions.

The complex emergency services system with its numerous interfaces offers also the potential for conflict. Yet, as mentioned above, the emergency services of today are the result of a long development that began in the German Federal Republic in the 1960s and went through numerous tumultuous phases of dispute.

## Epistemological interest

These disputes will be at the centre of this subsequent analysis. My first question is which kinds of conflict had existed in the emergency services and which groups had been involved in them. How did the various agents argue during the disputes? Which effects did the outer framework have on the development of conflicts? Did they result in changes in if so, what kind? In addition, I am foremost interested in the reasons that led to conflicts. Were the issues mainly specific to the emergency service or were they rather issues of teamwork? When we consider that the shift of competencies and opportunities for action in the area of medicine has resulted in a number of problems we must address the question what effect the market, power and prestige as motivations for action for the individuals had on these issues. Were they central catalysts for the conflicting parties or were there additional other factors?

To answer these questions, I want to address first why it is worthwhile to analyse conflicts within the health care system from a historical perspective. Subsequently I will examine two conflicts from the emergency services in Germany as examples. One of the conflicts deals with the voluntary elements within the groups of EMTs, i.e., the professional and voluntary emergency aid workers. The other concerns disputes between doctors and EMTs and the tasks the professional EMTs were "allowed" to do. This selection brings two different kinds of conflict into focus. One is a conflict between hierarchically distinct groups and the other is an example of conflicts between agents who are hierarchically in a similar position. Before analysing these conflicts, it is necessary to briefly summarise the development of the German emergency services.

---

6   Gesetz über den Beruf der Notfallsanitäterin und des Notfallsanitäters (2014), Article 4. For the practice policy in England cf. College of Paramedics (2017).

## Conflicts as a category of analysis

What is a conflict? A conflict is determined by a particular behaviour of conflicting parties that points to the conflict. In addition, there is a contradiction between the goals of conflicting parties as well as their attitudes and positions.[7] The analysis of conflicts through theories of conflict enables us to provide prognoses of conflicts in the future and the development of various constellations of conflict. In addition to the conflicting parties the subject of conflict, the source and progress of a conflict and the function of conflicts are interesting. But why are historians even paying any attention to conflicts? If conflicts occur, then these are exactly the situations, in which something "happens", in which something deviates from the norm and is thereby special. This means, that conflicts can both form the launch pads for changes and act as catalysts. At the same time, they give us an insight into processes of social change. In my opinion therefore, with regard to the healthcare professions, conflicts can represent an analytical probe to find out more about the history of specific professions, their frameworks and negotiation processes. The view of conflicts is also interesting, because they are created on multiple levels: sometimes they occur simultaneously, or they can work against each other. A structured analysis may help to understand certain processes of change better.

As mentioned above, the emergency services are virtually predestined for numerous conflicts due to the many people involved, its importance for healthcare, and the large impact on all agents when it does not function smoothly. Let us just think of the conflicts between emergency doctors and emergency staff or between the rescue coordination centres and the EMTs. Yet there can also be conflicts between the EMTs as employees and the aid organisations as their employers. Furthermore, the patient and his or her environment can also contribute to conflicts, e.g., when family members interfere with the initial emergency care or the patient does not want to cooperate. In all of these cases solutions must be found so that the emergency service remains functional. If the service does not function properly from the first minute of care there can be fatal consequences for the patients.

During the analysis of the conflicts mentioned here we must differentiate between two levels. On the micro-level we discuss disputes between individual subjects. These are for instance discussions between a particular EMT and an emergency doctor or between a patient and an EMT. The solutions are here of particular interest because in a concrete case, quick action is vital. The other group are conflicts that also take place within emergency care but between groups of organisational units. These include unions, professional organisations, employer organisations, expert associations and similar institutions. Methodologically this is called the meso-level. The most important agents in the emergency services are specifically the professional association of EMTs ("Berufsverband der Rettungssanitäter", BVRS), the German Medical Association ("Bundesärztekammer", BÄK) and aid organisations such as

---

7    More specifically on this: Imbusch/Zoll (2005). And: Galtung (2007).

the German Red Cross ("Deutsches Rotes Kreuz", DRK). We cannot analyse both levels independently from one another because developments on one level often also caused changes on the other levels. For that reason, it often makes sense to compare the developments on both levels with each other and to put them, if applicable, in juxtaposition to each other. While both levels would be important investigating the conflicts that the emergency services postulate, this article can only focus on the meso-level. Due to the complicated situation of source with merely letters from the public we can only superficially scratch at the micro-level.[8]

## Paramedics or EMTs

Even the correct designation of this profession is not easy. From 1989 to 2013, the workers were officially called "Rettungsassistent" (paramedic assistant). With the restructuring of the training, the name changed to "Notfallsanitäter" (critical care paramedic). However, in general conversation, the term "Rettungssanitäter" (paramedic) that was generally used before 1989 is still common. Yet a comprehensive translation into English is not possible. While US paramedics may be similar to the "Rettungssanitäter", their training and scope of tasks are far more complex. Hence I chose the term "Emergency Medical Technician", even though their training standards fall somewhat below those of a German "Rettungssanitäter".[9]

## Background

For a long period of time, the emergency service was primarily concerned with moving the patient or injured person to a medical facility and not with providing medical care at all. Since the founding of the Federal Republic of Germany, the charitable organisations have slowly emerged as the central supporters of the emergency service. They include the German Red Cross as the leading association, the religious associations of the "Malteser Hilfsdienst" and the "Johanniter-Unfall-Hilfe" as well as the "Arbeiter-Samariter-Bund" (ASB). At the beginning, it was only a question of the correct organisation of transport. In the opinion of all the experts, no special medically-trained personnel was required for this.[10] Barely anything changed until the end of the 1950s. However, with the subsequent numerous social changes the emergency services changed too. For example, the strong increase in the use of motor-

---

8   We plan however, to investigate the micro-level further using interviews with contemporary witnesses.
9   EMTs usually receive training between 120 and 150 hours whilst paramedics are trained for 1,200 to 1,800 hours. In addition, paramedics execute their emergency service completely without the aid of doctors.
10  Cf. Pfütsch (2018), p. 360.

ised vehicles led to a huge increase in the number of accidents. Furthermore, the field of medicine itself made important progress. New forms of treatment made time an increasingly important factor. Examples include use of defibrillators, blood transfusions, or rediscovery of older resuscitation techniques.[11]

In addition, the first scientific studies showed, that in the Federal Republic of Germany, 43.7 per cent of those killed on the roads, died within an hour of the accident.[12] This meant, that it was possible to help more and more people, provided that medical assistance was given in a timely manner. For this reason an idea which had occasionally been discussed among medical experts re-emerged: providing medical assistance directly at the location of an accident. Slowly the so-called "Stay and Play" principle won out over the "Load and Go" principle.[13] With this initiative of some experts in the mid-1960s, there was a slow reorganisation of the emergency service into a medical service. In a comparable way to medical historian Francisca Loetz, Nils Kessel talks of a "medification of the emergency service", meaning that the "reclassification of primitive treatment [was] performed by laypeople outside hospitals with subsequent transport to a medical activity organised under medical conditions."[14] From now on, the emergency service was increasingly considered as an area of medical action. In so doing, the focus was no longer primarily on transport, but on rapid medical treatment. In turn, this meant, that the competencies of the non-medical personnel increasingly became the topic of public discussions.

## Conflict area: voluntary work

During the discussion on the development of the profession of the EMT there were numerous discussions how to deal with the voluntary aspect within emergency care. What kind of tasks should voluntary workers take on and which tasks should be avoided? Among the main agents in this area of conflict are the employed professional and the voluntary EMTs.

The basic problem emerged due to a changed framework. Emergency services had become more than a transport system for people and consisted increasingly of the expert medical care of people in need. At the end of the 1960s and the beginning of the 1970s, i.e., the time when discussions on the role of voluntary work within the emergency services emerged, emergency services were still largely provided by voluntary workers. In 1971, a total of 96 per cent of all emergency care workers who worked for the ASB were volunteers.[15] By contrast, at the DRK the number was only 80 per cent.[16] Some

---

11   Cf. Kessel (2008), p. 63.
12   Cf. Kessel (2008), p. 62.
13   Cf. Nößler (2012).
14   Kessel (2008), p. 74; Loetz (1994).
15   Cf. Hahn (1994), p. 45.
16   Cf. Hahn (1994), p. 45.

of these people also held other jobs and worked for the emergency services in their spare time. The training that these employees had received until that point had been brief and mainly focussed on the transport. The key point was instruction on how to correctly position the patient for safe transport to the hospital. In addition, the volunteers had to be able to operate the radio equipment properly and steer the ambulance in such a way that the patient arrived quickly but without additional injuries that occurred because of the transport. During the training courses of the ASB the volunteers had to learn specific positioning techniques for particular injuries and the lifting up of a patient as well as bring the patient into the lateral recumbent position. The loading and unloading of an ambulance was also part of the curriculum.[17] Medical knowledge was barely taught in these courses: This was limited to a standard first aid course of eight double units, followed by another training course of twelve double units. The EMTs thus had the medical knowledge that anyone could pick up in two weeks.

Table 1: Example of a day during a basic training course of 14 days

| Time | Topic |
| --- | --- |
| 8.00–8.45 am | Breathing difficulties, stopped breathing, resuscitation |
| 9.00–9.45 am | Resuscitation |
| 10.00–10.45 am | Resuscitation with aids (airway and orospirature) |
| 11.00 am–12.00 pm | Technical ventilation (bag resuscitator, resuscitator 63, pulmotor) |
| 2.00–2.45 pm | Aspiration, suction |
| 3.00–3.45 pm | Inhalation |
| 4.15–5.00 pm | Practical resuscitation exercises |
| 5.15–6.00 pm | Continuation of the practical exercises |

Source: BArch, B189/13113, Deutsches Rotes Kreuz, Landesverband Niedersachsen: Programme for a basic training course of 14 days

The new emergency service focussing on a pre-clinical treatment required additional skills and knowledge from the emergency staff – foremost in the medical area. But the increased technisation, specialisation and scientification of medicine made a "rapid introduction" into the medical discipline almost impossible. In the light of the new treatment options through the progress in medicine, the gap between available and theoretically available care became even greater.

In addition, there were a few professional EMTs working full-time. While they were a minority in terms of numbers they were the group that defined the public debates in subsequent years. The professional organisation of EMTs (BVRS) that was founded in 1979 represented the concerns of professional

17   Cf. Arbeiter-Samariter-Bund (n. d.).

EMTs. It demanded that volunteer emergency staff were to be placed hierarchically lower than the professionals.

> While volunteer work was highly regarded by the professional organisation, the person's qualification must match the tasks he or she had to perform. For that reason, the organisation suggested that in the long run volunteers should accompany two professionals in the ambulances. Their role was to be called, for instance, emergency helper. In addition, the organisation imagined roles in ambulances and the call centres that volunteers could continue to fulfil. They would be valuable helpers without taking away necessary jobs.[18]

The professional organisation thus did not only want to introduce a hierarchy supporting the task of the professional EMTs but also to limit the competencies of the volunteers and subsequently their area of work.

On the micro-level professional EMTs increasingly shared their criticism of the equalisation of their profession with volunteers:

> I have been working for the emergency services of the German Red Cross for eight years and I hold the RS [qualification as an EMT]. II. The problem: On weekends, ambulance and emergency services are performed in my area by volunteers. It happens that I have to perform emergency calls with a volunteer who only has had emergency medical training. Furthermore, it is normal that people doing civilian service and who had ambulance training answer emergency calls with the voluntary emergency helpers. [...]

> In the interest of our emergency patients I am no longer willing to accept this situation (each emergency doctor call costs approximately 100.00 DM). I think the patients have a right to well-trained staff.[19]

The argument for the hierarchy in this letter – similar to the meso-level – is the different training. There are no concrete examples of any wrong-doing of a volunteer or that their quality of work was worse. However, the last sentence suggests that there were numerous problems.

The voluntary emergency helpers who had conducted the majority of all emergency services without the aid of any professionals until the beginning of the 1970s felt downgraded and undervalued through the increasing criticism by the professional EMTs. In October 1989, the EMT Reinhard Holzhausen (his letter does not state whether he was a volunteer or a professional) wrote for instance to the journal *Rettungsdienst*:

> As is well known emergency and ambulance services have their roots in voluntary work. Both volunteer fire brigades and voluntary sanitary trains were the first that organised and conducted the transport of sick and injured people in our country. Voluntary, mind you! Without the voluntary commitment the current sufficient emergency services would not have developed the way they did. Emergency services would probably have been run by the state and the "private firms" would have no means of existence.

> Instead of fighting stomach pains you should [...] take off your hat to those people who cancel their holidays in order to train to become an emergency medical technician and who sacrifice their spare time only to help on weekends when they perform their voluntary service.

---

18  BArch, B189/35729, Berufsverband der Rettungssanitäter e. V.: 10 Thesen zur Ausbildungssituation der Rettungssanitäter (10 theses on the training situation of EMTs) (1985).
19  Unknown (1985), p. 594.

> For sure, there are also some bad apples among volunteers who want to attract some
> public attention with their stories from emergency calls. Yet, you will find those among
> the professionals too. I have experienced more than once how a professional "saviour",
> intoxicated from alcohol, entertained the whole pub with stories from emergency opera-
> tions.[20]

The lack of appreciation from the perspective of the volunteers is quite apparent in this letter. The voluntary staff was indeed willing to continue their professional development as can be seen in a letter to the journal by the voluntary
EMT Peter Thienemann. He laments the lack of training opportunities for
voluntary emergency workers which is why he always depended on reading
the journal *Rettungsdienst*.[21] Various sides also argued in favour of the voluntary helpers as 70 per cent of operations were scheduled hospital transports,
with only 30 per cent being proper emergency operations.[22] These hospital
transports could have performed without any problem by voluntary EMTs.

At the meso-level the conflict mainly took place on the level of the federal
government and was influenced by the further development of the emergency
services. In October 1970, the so-called "Bund-/Länder-Ausschuss 'Rettungswesen'" (joint German Federal/Länder Committee "Emergency Services")
was founded, bringing together political representatives of both the German
Länder and the German federal government. It developed into the central
political point of contact for any issues concerning the emergency services.
It developed minimal requirements for people working for the emergency
services. The main focus was the training. Initially the minimal requirement
contained 1,200 hours of training as a basis for work. In general the assumption was that the higher the demands for training the fewer voluntary EMTs
would be willing to perform the training as hardly anyone would be willing
to invest that much time into an unpaid job. The aid organisations who were
the largest employers of EMTs rejected this suggestion by the joint committee
of federal and Länder representatives.[23] Their argument was the importance
of the voluntary element in emergency services and its meaning for society.[24]
Simultaneously, and in their opinion this was an even more important point,
the phasing out of volunteers would have massively increased costs for the aid
organisations as they would have had to use mainly professional EMTs. After
additional negotiations between the committee and the aid organisations they
agreed in 1977 on a compromise, the so-called "520-hour training". This compromise was developed as a temporary solution, but it was used in practice for
twelve years. The 520-hour training included that people working for emergency services, both voluntary and professional EMTs, should have 160 hours
of theory and 160 of practical training in a hospital, followed by an internship
of 160 hours at an ambulance station and a final training course of 40 hours

---

20   Holzhausen (1989), p. 658.
21   Cf. Thienemann (1987), p. 151.
22   Cf. Kessel (2008), p. 103.
23   Cf. Pfütsch (2018), p. 364.
24   Cf. Pfütsch (2018), p. 371.

including an exam.[25] Yet this compromise did not satisfy either of the conflicting parties completely. The voluntary workers regarded the length of the training as exaggerated, the professional EMTs thought it was not enough training. Thus, the compromise could only reduce the conflict but not resolve it. With the progression of the possibilities in the emergency services the conflict inevitably erupted again. Nils Kessel noticed this re-emergence of the conflict through the increasing number of letters on the topic that were published.[26] However, this was merely an indication as the purposeful publication of the letters could have been a strategy of the editors or publishing board at the journal to fuel the conflict. Thus we cannot say for sure whether the readers wrote indeed more letters.

The professional organisation of EMTs massively supported an independent job profile for professional EMTs from at least the beginning of the 1980s. The organisation received support from the German Employees Union ("Deutsche Angestellten-Gewerkschaft", DAG) that wanted to strengthen the position and rights of employees. In contrast, both politicians and the aid organisations supported the idea of maintaining the voluntary aid. Changing parameters influenced the conflict also on this side. Many Länder introduced laws for the emergency services at the end of the 1970s to better organise and regulate them. These laws also prescribed that emergency services were to be available around the clock. The Law on Rescue Services of Baden-Wuerttemberg, effective in 1975, stated for instance: "The rescue coordination centres must be ready to operate 24/7."[27] This fact forced the aid organisations to increasingly employ professional EMTs because they did not have the capacities with merely volunteers to secure the functioning of the emergency services in the morning, afternoon, at night and on weekends. Many volunteers had day jobs after all. Thus the proportion of professional staff automatically increased during the 1980s.[28] For instance in 1974 the ASB had 163 professional EMTs, in 1981 317 and in 1989 488.[29] This fact resulted in the DRK, the largest employer of EMTs, to change its previously negative opinion on an independent job profile for professional EMTs and from 1984 onwards it began to support it.[30] The reason was that the DRK no longer had to fear huge increases in staff costs.[31] The largest hurdle had thus been overcome and the decision for the development of an independent job profile for EMTs had been made. Yet the discussion what this job profile should entail lasted nearly for another five years. In 1989 the "Gesetz über den Beruf der Rettungsassistentin und des Rettungsassistenten (RettAssG)" (Law on the profession of paramedics and EMTs) was passed that was effective until 2013. This provided a two-year

25  Cf. Pfütsch (2018), p. 364.
26  Cf. Kessel (2008), p. 116.
27  Gesetz über den Rettungsdienst (1975), p. 379.
28  Cf. Lüttgen (1980), p. 13.
29  My own calculation based on the annual reports of the ASB.
30  Cf. Schlegelberger (1986), p. 63.
31  Cf. Pfütsch (2018), p. 372.

training for emergency assistants ("Rettungsassistent" – the official term) that included 1,200 hours of theory and a practical period of 1,600 hours at training ambulance centres. Since nobody wanted to give up the voluntary service completely temporary regulations were passed and voluntary aid could still be integrated. EMTs who had completed their 520-hour training or were still going through this training could get the permission to call themselves emergency assistant if they provided evidence of 2,000 hours of work experience within the emergency services. The 520-hour training was also kept to give voluntary workers the opportunity to work within the emergency services. They were not allowed to call themselves emergency assistant after their training and could not do all of the tasks their professional colleagues performed. From the volunteers' perspective this laid down what they had fought against for nearly 20 years: a hierarchy within the emergency services and the loss of the emergency services as an originally voluntary task. Hence it is not surprising that they strongly criticised the law.

Shortly after the RettAssG had been passed the voluntary EMT Gerold Hoopmann wrote a letter to the journal *Rettungsdienst* and shared his displeasure with the new law:

> For us "voluntary emergency medical technicians" a new era has begun. We hope for an interim solution to be put in place very soon so that we do not have to look at an ambulance only from the outside one day.
>
> Will the volunteers only fill in forms in the future or be behind the steering wheel? What about disaster management, ambulance services, all social services that we perform on a daily basis? What use are training courses and practical instructions if we no longer receive the opportunity to gain practical experience and use this theoretical knowledge?

He wrote furthermore:

> A law has been passed. There are high demands on us. It is not that we don't want to do the training – quite the contrary. But when? During our thirty days of holidays or possibly during an educational leave. But what about the family? What about all the volunteer tasks that must be completed? Overloading the volunteers is already inevitable in many aid organisations and the day when this becomes reality is getting closer and closer.[32]

Here he verbalised the basic problem of the emergency services. Even if the volunteers wanted to complete the training they simply did not have the time for it. Despite interim solutions and exceptions for voluntary workers the new RettAssG favoured professional EMTs and the reason for that were probably the overall changes that had taken place in society.

## Conflict area: responsibilities

A second major area of conflict in the emergency services in (West) Germany were the responsibilities of the professional EMTs, and here the conflicting parties were mainly doctors and EMTs. Connected to the question of respon-

---

32  Hoopmann (1989), pp. 752 f.

sibilities were implicit issues such as market, power, and prestige. In a letter
to the journal *Rettungsdienst* one EMT wrote about the general collaboration
with doctors:

> I have experienced it myself that an ambulance was called to take a patient to the hos-
> pital. At the inspection these patients were seriously or acutely ill – but the vehicle had
> been ordered by a specialist. When asking about the details I received in these cases the
> following information (and so did my professional colleagues): "He is not doing so well
> and has to be taken to hospital quickly. You could just give him some oxygen along the
> way." Unfairly, the referral is usually written in such jargon that was common during the
> 1920s so that the "stupid EMT" would not draw the right conclusions and call the rescue
> van with an emergency doctor. The patients in question have been knocked out with
> morphine and Valium so that they can barely answer our questions.[33]

The micro-level thus also reveals some conflicts. From the perspective of the
EMT, the doctor played up his scientific training to show the EMT his higher
position within the hierarchy of medical professions. At the same time, he
was so uncooperative that the EMT had no opportunity to benefit from the
doctor's knowledge. This isolation mechanism simultaneously prevented the
emergence or growth of new competitors in order to secure market, power
and prestige for one's own profession. The doctors' perspective on the collaboration with EMTs was – not surprisingly – different. For instance, in another letter the son of a doctor reported about the collaboration of his dad
with the EMT and adopted the doctor's perspective.

> My father (a GP with over 40 years of professional experience) is called out to an el-
> derly patient on a Sunday morning as part of the standby service. She is complaining
> of pain in the lower part of her body. After an introductory examination, he diagnosed
> "appendicitis" and requested an ambulance, which arrived soon after. The paramedics
> and ambulance staff (highest age 21 or 25 years) stormed into the flat and the following
> discussion unfolded:
>
> <u>Doctor</u>: Good morning gentlemen. This lady must immediately be transported to the
> surgery department of … hospital. I have spoken with the doctor on duty, a bed is avail-
> able, here are the referral and the transport documents.
>
> <u>EMT</u>: (After a brief glance at the referral) So, appendix. So, we've got to carry the old
> lady. Can we put the siren on?
>
> <u>Doctor</u>: I do not see any need for that. I require careful but speedy transport of the
> patient.
>
> <u>EMT</u>: Doctor, are you sure of your diagnosis? I mean if something bursts … (The EMT
> probably means a perforation of the appendix).
>
> <u>Doctor</u>: (Annoyed) Young man, have I been the GP of this lady and have looked after her
> for more than 20 years or have YOU?
>
> This is where the argument ended. The lady was loaded into the ambulance in a grudg-
> ing and disinterested manner and driven away.[34]

In contrast to the previous letter the EMTs were portrayed in a negative light
in this one. They questioned the doctor's instructions without any reason and

33   Wachsmuth (1986), p. 485.
34   Schmidt (1986), p. 485.

thus overstepped the professional boundaries. Simultaneously the letter suggests that the EMTs treated the doctors without respect.

In the following the writer addresses also another problem:

> There are also other instances where the GPs' special knowledge and their experience
> are seriously affected by EMTs (and here in particular volunteers show off) in front of
> the patients. The problem is that voluntary EMTs (whose service I highly respect as they
> are the ones who help their fellow citizens without pay in their spare time) try to achieve
> dubious prestige or respect from their ill fellow citizens through the way they appear
> (white protective clothing, emergency bag, using many abbreviations in their speech)
> and the equipment they carry (radio, siren etc.). Doctors (though not in their presence)
> are degraded in one inconsiderate sentence even though they have been served their
> community for decades by people who do not work in a medical profession but once
> a week or once a month put on a white shirt and white trousers and clip on a beeper.
> Such statements project themselves too easily into the vocabulary/the memory of the pa-
> tient because they, medical laymen themselves, believe the deception: "The gentlemen in
> white from the ambulance must know as that is their day job." That way public opinions
> are easily and unnoticeably formed that each objective EMT should be ashamed of.[35]

The medical layperson can barely distinguish between doctor and EMT and
believes that both are experts. According to the author of the letter it often
happened that EMTs copied the habitus of doctors on purpose. Apart from
deceiving the patients such behaviours could become triggers for conflicts between EMTs and doctors. Doctors might have felt threatened and the struggle
for market, power and prestige could have become public.

The conflicts pointed at on the micro-level similarly occurred on the meso-
level. The conflict between mainly professional EMTs and doctors was very
similar to the one between voluntary and professional EMTs. To be precise,
the conflict culminated in the fundamental question of whether EMTs should
be permitted to intubate, to infuse, and to administer injections. These questions were more often asked when during the 1980s there was a debate about
the professional profile of EMTs. The professional EMTs argued for performing these tasks. In addition, starting in the late 1970s they had become more
professionalised. This enabled EMTs to place their demands at the respective
authorities and be taken more seriously. Thus, for example, the journal *Der
Rettungssanitäter* was published from 1978 onwards. In 1980, it published the
first training manual for EMTs with the title "Der Rettungssanitäter – Ausbildung und Fortbildung". It made a significant contribution to the structuring
and standardisation of EMT tasks. The professional EMTs experienced a further push towards professionalisation in 1979 when the professional organisation BVRS was founded. They organised annual conferences for EMTs.
For example, the first "Bundeskongress für Rettungssanitäter" took place in
Dormagen in 1979.

The main conflicting party was the doctors. Institutionally and organisa-
tionally, doctors were represented in the discussions on the emergency service
by, on the one hand, the German Medical Association and, on the other hand,
various associations for emergency medicine, such as the German Interdisci-

---

35   Schmidt (1986), p. 486.

plinary Association for Intensive and Emergency Medicine ("Deutsche Inter-disziplinäre Vereinigung für Intensiv- und Notfallmedizin e. V.", DIVI).

From their side, the expansion of responsibilities of non-medical emergency service personnel was observed in detail and with critical comments. Both the German Medical Association and the other organisations argued for a regulated occupational profile of the EMTs. They were of the opinion that this was the only way to guarantee a high quality emergency service. According to the doctors, EMTs were supposed to receive the best training possible. One emergency doctor wrote for instance in a letter about the tasks of EMTs:

> Of course, EMTs or emergency assistants should be able and allowed to intubate and set up infusions. The reasons are obvious: First, the EMT is often earlier at the site than the emergency doctor and often it is the EMT who calls the emergency doctor. Second, in traffic accidents for instance in rural areas there is more than one patient who needs to be taken care of. Here the emergency doctor is grateful when she or he can also delegate so-called "doctors' tasks". Since I worked as a voluntary EMT while I was a student I, thirdly, had the experience that many of the doctors (not emergency doctors) whom Herr Knuth [Peter Knuth, anaesthesiologist and medical director of the German Medical Association – P. P.] praises so highly were unable to set up an infusion, let alone intubate. As a committed emergency doctor I want to improve the preclinical care of the emergency patients without considering rank or class. This is only possible with a highly qualified EMT who is legally covered to perform additional medical measures. If Herr Knuth wants to stop this, he harms the emergency patients and leaves the EMT in the lurch who, hopefully, will continue to intubate if he can save life.[36]

There was however also a different perspective:

> An EMT found an 81-year old female patient in a comatose condition. Her blood sugar stick showed a blood sugar level of 40 mg/dl. The EMT established a venous access and administered an infusion of 500 ml glucose 5 % and 20 ml glucose 40 %.

> When she was admitted to the intensive care unit she received another infusion of 500 ml glucose 10 %. At admission the blood sugar level was 168 mg/dl and the patient was still comatose, her breathing shallow and accelerated. Even without a stethoscope one can hear her wheezing whilst breathing.

> Diagnosis at admission: Global heart insufficiency with pulmonary congestion and suspicion of a myocardial infarction.

> Conclusion: The volume administered by the EMT was completely contraindicated and could have resulted in the death of the patient.[37]

This quote at least points to the danger that can emerge when doctors' tasks are delegated to EMTs. The EMT's wrong assessment could endanger a patient's life if the wrong measures are taken. At the same time the quote can be understood as a criticism of the current training of EMTs that would simply not allow EMTs to act independently. Thus an improvement of the training and continuous professional development of EMTs would have been recommended. From the perspective of the medical associations, i. e. on the meso-level, paradoxically we see both: the danger of delegating doctors' tasks but

---

36  Pless (1987), p. A-2773.
37  Katterwe (1988), p. 118.

also the necessity for a better training of EMTs. Yet while the medical associations demanded the best possible training for EMTs this did not mean at all that they favoured EMTs to be granted to use their skills in practice. That would have meant that EMTs would have completed tasks that were expressly the responsibility of doctors. Following the logic of the medical associations this would have meant losing an area of responsibility – or at least facing the danger of such a loss – that had become exclusive for the doctors only during the 1960s. This argument was used with respect to injections, infusions and intubations with the right of practising medicine. According to the Non-Medical Practitioners Act only doctors and non-medical practitioners (alternative practitioners) have this right. Here, it was the German Medical Association in particular that argued to clearly distinguish between the tasks of doctors and of EMTs. It was not trying to prevent the professionalisation of the full-time rescue service staff, but requested that this should occur within clear limits and only up to a certain point. This "certain point" was precisely the spot where the influence of the doctors began.

*Solution of the conflict*

This simmering conflict that had started at the beginning of the sixties and peaked for the first time in the mid-seventies was full-on from the mid-eighties onwards. As the agents' points of views were so far apart and it was impossible to agree on a compromise, the question of the responsibilities was excluded during the drafting of the EMT law. Only after this exclusion it could be passed in 1989. The distinct definition of the EMT as an "assistant to the doctor" by law clearly established the roles of the doctor and the EMT. The EMTs were to follow the instructions of the emergency doctor. The emergency doctors in turn were to delegate tasks to the EMTs. Thus, a suggestion by the German Medical Association prevailed. It had demanded that EMTs should learn to intubate and administer injections and infusions perfectly. Yet it was the doctor who had to announce when the need for these tasks was indicated and he remained in charge. Even though this principle has been repeatedly discussed since its implementation, it still remains the basis for the emergency services in Germany.

   This form of co-operation worked as long as an emergency doctor was present. However, because EMTs and the emergency doctor travel separately to the site of an accident due to the German "rendezvous system", often there is no emergency doctor with the patient and to this day EMTs have been often working alone. In these cases, the *modus vivendi* took hold that the EMT should exchange information through close radio contact with the medical head in the emergency HQ and should, if necessary, receive the permission from them to perform specific measures. While this model of co-operation sounds good in theory it actually contained a range of pitfalls. For instance, it was possible that, in rural regions, radio contact failed or could not even be established. In other cases, the emergency situation required immediate action, leaving no time for agreements. In these cases, the emergency assistant could take specific measures within the framework of so-called emergency competence, which was technically only allowed in an emergency if it could save the life of the patient. Yet, these measures were regularly carried out under unclear legal conditions, as emergency competence from a legal point of view represented an individual decision and thus, theoretically, had to be reviewed frequently. Acting in the sense of emergency competence was subject to the principle of relativity. That principle means that only measures with minimal intervention yet leading to success were to be used. If, for example, breathing with a ventilation bag was effective, then intubation with its greater risks was not permissible.[38]

## Summary

The goal of this article was to present and analyse specific conflicts in the history of healthcare in Germany to question their connection with issues such as market, power and prestige. My aim was to illustrate that the analysis of conflicts offers a good option for tracing and presenting processes of social change.

For my brief analysis, I chose the emergency services because the lengthy debate of about thirty years facilitates the presentation of the points of view and interests of the professional and voluntary EMTs, the non-profit employer organisations, the doctors as the main competing professional group, and the state as a regulator. I could show using the (limited) range of tasks EMTs are permitted to perform and the responsibilities granted to them that not only the well-being of the patient but also a wide range of other influences could be paramount for decision-making. At the same time, I illustrated the impact general social conditions (such as the attitude towards voluntary work) can have on conflicts.

The first conflict was the debate between professional and volunteer EMTs. The volunteer EMTs were primarily concerned with performing voluntary work and thus helping the general populace. They were critical of any type of training regulations and regarded them as an obstacle in exercising their voluntary work. Hardly any volunteer was prepared to invest a lot of time in training courses. Surely, there were certainly volunteers who welcomed the opportunity for further training. Yet according to them these courses should have been at a low level and not particularly time-intensive. By contrast, the professional EMTs who earned a living with this job demanded an occupational profile that was to go hand in hand with high-level training. This was very important to them: Through improved training they hoped to see a broadening of their responsibilities and thus an increase of social rec-

38   Cf. Bundesärztekammer (1992).

ognition of their profession. Naturally, this request was also connected to the desire for better working conditions such as increased salaries.

The second conflict was the debate between the (professional) EMTs and doctors. Here, the main issue was also the question about the responsibilities of EMTs. Should EMTs have been permitted to carry out intubations, injections and infusions, and should these tasks have stayed within the sphere of the doctors? The professional EMTs wanted to expand their training to such a degree that they could have performed tasks that were previously exclusive to doctors. The doctors regarded this ambition for a wider area of responsibilities as an intrusion into their own professional realm and fought against it with all their might.

The healthcare conflicts that took place in the emergency services occurred on various levels, between various agents and at different times. Often, they had to do with financing, training standards, and the competence to act and thus they were linked to the (medical) market, power and prestige. The areas of conflict were frequently closely interconnected. For that reason, an individual analysis is often impossible. Conflicts could be a concrete demand for action but they could also play out on a meta-level. Both types of conflicts could affect each other. With regard to the healthcare system as a whole these conflicts proved to be a fruitful point of access as all kinds of interests collided because of their complexity.

The market, power and prestige were the most important catalysts for these conflicts. Yet, if we do not only regard conflicts as a negative symptom but also see them as innovators for change, then the market, power and prestige are also the central reasons for such change.

## Bibliography

*Archives*

Bundesarchiv Koblenz (BArch)

B189/13113
B189/35729

*Published sources*

Arbeiter-Samariter-Bund e. V., Bundesschule: Lehrplan SIII. Samariterausbildung als Fortsetzung der Helferausbildung. Köln n. d. (ca. 1967–1972).
Bundesärztekammer: Stellungnahme der Bundesärztekammer zur Notkompetenz von Rettungsassistenten und zur Delegation ärztlicher Leistungen im Rettungsdienst (1992), available at: http://www.bundesaerztekammer.de/fileadmin/user_upload/downloads/BAEK_Stellungnahme_Rettungsassistenten.pdf (last accessed: 17/10/2018).

College of Paramedics: Paramedic – Scope of Practice Policy. Bridgwater 2017, available at: https://www.collegeofparamedics.co.uk/downloads/171121_Paramedic_-_Scope_of_Practice_Policy.pdf (last accessed: 17/10/2018).

Gesetz über den Beruf der Notfallsanitäterin und des Notfallsanitäters (Notfallsanitätergesetz – NotSanG) (2014), available at: https://www.gesetze-im-internet.de/notsang/BJNR134810013.html (last accessed: 17/10/2018).

Gesetz über den Rettungsdienst. In: Gesetzblatt für Baden-Württemberg (1975), pp. 379–383.

Holzhausen, Reinhard: Letter to the journal. In: Rettungsdienst 12 (1989), p. 658.

Hoopmann, Gerold: Letter to the journal. In: Rettungsdienst 12 (1989), pp. 752–753.

Katterwe, Rüdiger: Letter to the journal. In: Rettungsdienst 11 (1988), p. 118.

Lüttgen, Roderich: Hauptberufliche und ehrenamtliche Tätigkeit im Rettungsdienst. In: Leben retten (1980), pp. 12–15.

Pless, Harald: Delegieren. In: Deutsches Ärzteblatt 84 (1987), p. A-2773.

Schlegelberger, Hartwig: Rettungsdienst und Ehrenamt. In: Leben retten (1986), pp. 62–66.

Schmidt, Joachim: Letter to the journal. In: Rettungsdienst 9 (1986), pp. 485–486.

Thienemann, Peter: Letter to the journal. In: Rettungsdienst 10 (1987), p. 151.

Unknown: Letter to the journal. In: Rettungsdienst 8 (1985), p. 594.

Wachsmuth, Klaus: Letter to the journal. In: Rettungsdienst 9 (1986), p. 485.

## Literature

Bundesstadt Bonn, Feuerwehr und Rettungsdienst: Medizinisch-technische Ausrüstung und medikamentöse Bestückung. Bonn 2016.

Galtung, Johan: Frieden mit friedlichen Mitteln. Friede und Konflikt, Entwicklung und Kultur. Münster 2007.

Gesundheitsberichterstattung des Bundes: Einsatzfahrtaufkommen im öffentlichen Rettungsdienst (Anzahl). Gliederungsmerkmale: Jahre, Deutschland, Einsatzart, available at: http://www.gbe-bund.de/gbe10/trecherche.prc_them_rech?tk=14501&tk2=16801&p_uid=gast&p_aid=60104562&p_sprache=D&cnt_ut=1&ut=16801 (last accessed: 17/10/2018).

Gesundheitsberichterstattung des Bundes: Rettungswachen, Rettungsleitstellen und Rettungshubschrauber im öffentlichen Rettungsdienst. Gliederungsmerkmale: Jahre, Region, available at: http://www.gbe-bund.de/gbe10/trecherche.prc_them_rech?tk=14501&tk2=16801&p_uid=gast&p_aid=60104562&p_sprache=D&cnt_ut=1&ut=16801 (last accessed: 17/10/2018).

Hahn, Christian: Entwicklung des öffentlichen Rettungswesens in der Bundesrepublik Deutschland unter besonderer Berücksichtigung Schleswig-Holsteins. Mag.-Arb. Univ. Kiel 1994.

Imbusch, Peter; Zoll, Ralf (eds.): Friedens- und Konfliktforschung. Eine Einführung. Lehrbuch. Wiesbaden 2005.

Kessel, Nils: Geschichte des Rettungsdienstes 1945–1990. Vom "Volk von Lebensrettern" zum Berufsbild "Rettungsassistent/in". (=Medizingeschichte im Kontext 13) Frankfurt/Main 2008.

Loetz, Francisca: "Medikalisierung" in Frankreich, Großbritannien und Deutschland, 1750–1850. In: Eckart, Wolfgang Uwe; Jütte, Robert (eds.): Das europäische Gesundheitssystem. Gemeinsamkeiten und Unterschiede in historischer Perspektive. Wiesbaden 1994, pp. 123–161.

Nößler, Denis: Notfallsanitäter. Rettung für den Rettungsdienst. In: Ärzte Zeitung (10/10/2012), available at: https://www.aerztezeitung.de/politik_gesellschaft/article/823546/notfallsanitaeterrettung-rettungsdienst.html (last accessed: 17/10/2018).

Pfütsch, Pierre: Rettungssanitäter – Rettungsassistenten – Notfallsanitäter: Ein Berufsbild im Wandel, 1949–2014. In: Hähner-Rombach, Sylvelyn; Pfütsch, Pierre (eds.): Entwicklungen in der Krankenpflege und in anderen Gesundheitsberufen nach 1945. Frankfurt/Main 2018, pp. 350–382.

Statistisches Bundesamt: Statistisches Jahrbuch 2015. Gesundheit. Personal. Fachserie 12, Reihe 7.3.1. Wiesbaden 2017.

Wiedenfeld, Carsten: Das deutsche Rettungswesen im Spannungsfeld zwischen hoheitlicher Aufgabe und Marktleistung. Der Einfluss des europäischen Vergaberechts auf die Leistungserbringung. Masterarbeit Juristenfakultät der Universität Leipzig. Leipzig 2013.

Conflicts Within a Profession

# Hegemonic Masculinity and the Gender Gap in Caregiving: The Contentious Presence of West German Men in Nursing since around 1970

*Christoph Schwamm*

## Masculinity and professional caregiving in history – a contradiction?

Today some twelve per cent of all nurses in Germany are men.[1] Compared to other Western countries this is a relatively high number, although still small enough to reinforce the stereotypical view of nursing as a woman's profession.[2] Among these, many work in particular areas of focus such as psychiatric units or urology departments.[3] Men are overrepresented in positions that require higher qualifications, whereas the opposite is the case for positions requiring little qualification like nursing auxiliaries or assistants.[4] Some of these aspects have changed over time, while others have remained remarkably stable. Among the latter, perhaps most notable is the fact that contrary to widely-held assumptions, men have worked as caregivers for the sick and elderly throughout history.[5] The presence of men in the profession is not a recent innovation. While Nursing Studies is well aware of male nurses in premodern history, even here similar misunderstandings prevail. Publications about the "feminisation" of nursing suggest that during the heyday of motherhouse nursing in the late 19th and early 20th century, men were basically excluded from providing professional care in hospitals.[6] This was simply not true. Being called "Krankenwärter" ("wardens"), "auxiliaries" or other names, men provided care for patients to an extent not entirely different from today.

Yet even considering this, the statistics depict a situation of inequality prone to gender conflicts. In contrast to family caregiving, professional caregiving has become a gainful means of employment since the latter half of the last century. Working conditions, however, as well as social prestige remain bad and women still predominate in the field. The gender gap in caregiving remains a point of contention between those who advocate for more equal sharing of this burden and those who do not.

In any case, the situation cannot be satisfactorily understood without a more precise analysis of gender relations. Nursing Studies often characterises masculine gender identity as a hindrance to men becoming caregivers. An oft-heard opinion in this regard is that hegemonic or socially desirable masculinity prevents men from entering the nursing profession in the first place.

---

1   Cf. Hähner-Rombach (2018), p. 214. See also Statistisches Bundesamt (2012).
2   Cf. D'Antonio (2010), p. 188; Genua (2005); O'Lynn/Tranbarger (2007), pp. 207–208.
3   Cf. Hähner-Rombach (2018), p. 216.
4   Cf. Hähner-Rombach (2015), p. 124.
5   Cf. Evans (2004); O'Lynn/Tranbarger (2007).
6   Cf. Bischoff (1992).

Even the few who actually become nurses are said to assume positions within the profession removed from actual caregiving. Teaching or management are allegedly preferred by men because they allow for the embodiment of masculine roles in a field that is otherwise deeply feminised.[7] The unequal distribution of carework within society as a whole (men avoid becoming nurses) is mirrored within the nursing profession itself (male nurses avoid activities involving carework). And like the former, the latter engenders intense controversy, only within the much more focused internal discourse of the nursing profession. Feminist commentators tend to criticise this imbalance by blaming masculinity in one way or another for the inequality. When male nurses justify themselves, the result is, as we will see below, that they often find own things at fault with gender relations in nursing, making the debate conflict-prone.

Historiography is often pressed into service to provide evidence for the belief that masculinity and caregiving are mutually exclusive.[8] While only anecdotal evidence can be provided here, it seems that many people believe male caregivers to only be a recent phenomenon. While as mentioned above, Nursing Studies is aware of the centuries-old traditions of volunteer and professional male caregiving, it tends to disregard the fact that the profession was alive and well during the first half of the 20th century. According to the accepted narrative, starting around 1900, the profession gradually became systematically feminised until most of the men had vanished. By the end of the first half of the 20th century, nursing had become *the* prime example of "women's work". This changed at least partially with the so-called nursing desegregation of the 1960s. While men could once again become nurses, it was no coincidence that they quickly entered positions most compatible with their gender identity. Newly technology-related positions appeared in operating rooms and intensive care units (ICUs). New executive nursing positions also sprang up. All of these paid higher than average, particularly the latter.

While there is certainly some truth to these historical interpretations, many questions remained unanswered. For instance, in the case of Germany it is still unclear whether the terms "segregation" and "desegregation" are adequate descriptions for what took place. It is true that more men work or worked as caregivers than did before the 1970s. But at no time did men ever come close to ceasing to work as nurses in Germany.[9] Moreover, many of them were highly organised – but not in the same organisations as female nurses in motherhouses or women-only associations.[10]

So the question remains: To what extent was the alleged admittance of men to nursing anything more than a fusion of formerly gender-separated professional organisations? And how well does the theory of masculinity as a barrier to male caregiving match the facts? If not because of masculinity, then why are women still vastly overrepresented in nursing? Even more in need of

---

7    Cf. Krampe (2013).
8    Cf. Mackintosh (1997); Wetterer (2002).
9    Cf. Hähner-Rombach (2018), p. 214.
10   Cf. Schwamm (2018), p. 37; Bauer (1965), p. 368.

explanation is the current overrepresentation of men in key positions in the profession. All these phenomena can hardly be addressed without taking the reforms of the 1960s and 1970s into account. And masculinity has played a significant role, but, as will be shown in this article, not always the role that it is usually thought to play. All this implies that Nursing Studies views of the profession's past cannot be entirely accurate. But our current understanding of the statistics is still rife with assumptions. In particular, the question remains: To what extent is masculine identity to blame for the unequal distribution of caregiving in society as well as in nursing? These questions cannot be answered through simple deduction from sociological theories. A thorough consideration of the historical evidence will be required.

The topic is far too broad-ranging to cover sufficiently in an article of this scope. But as a start, it deems promising to analyse representations of masculinity in the context of two historical phenomena which have been described as the precursors of the present male nurses' situation. The first is the often quarrelsome professional discourse during the creation of gender-inclusive professional nursing as part of the reforms around 1970. The second was the unexpected success of the alternative civilian service for conscientious objectors, also around 1970, which resulted in hundred of thousands of young German men working as nursing auxiliaries. Regarding the first, relevant discussions took place in the journals or magazines of professional nursing associations and unions. The second phenomenon, the civilian service as an institution, has already been investigated with a multitude of sources by Patrick Bernhard.[11] Bernhard was well aware of the importance of his findings for the history of gender relations. He was not able to put his results systematically into a context of the history and theory of masculinity. Even today, such a framework hardly exists outside of the realm of cultural studies, let alone in 2005 when his work was published. Importantly, some of the contradictions in his findings with regard to Nursing Studies' views of masculinity have still not entered historiography's awareness.

## Hegemonic masculinity in the context of nursing

Before describing the journals and Bernhard's findings more closely a few things must be said about the theory of masculinity. In its critique of unequal distribution of carework, Nursing Studies relies on an understanding of the sociology of the workplace based on theories of power-related social inequality.[12] Nursing is understood as a social field in which both gender-specific behaviour itself and representations of gender-stereotypical behaviour (in the media, for example) reinforce inequality between men and women. A crucial point is that carework is associated with femininity whereas technological

---

11    Cf. Bernhard (2005); Bernhard (2006).
12    Cf. Dressel/Wanger (2008); Notz (2008); Wetterer (2002); Ummel (1997); Heintz (1997); Williams (1993).

skills and leadership are associated with masculinity. In theory this results in men being overproportionally supported when they wish to become highly skilled and paid nurses, head nurses or nursing teachers. Crucial to these theories is an assumption that men emphasise their gender identity, unlike women in "manly" jobs who tend to adapt their habitus to their male environment. According to this assumption, male nurses exhibit particularly "manly" behaviour in contrast to their colleagues which in turn reinforces the mechanisms of inequality.[13]

These models of patriarchal power dynamics conform seamlessly to more recent theories of masculinity. For some years, Australian sociologist Raewyn Connell's concept of "hegemonic masculinity" has been the accepted paradigm for the study of men and masculinity.[14] In accordance with the sociological models just described, Connell assumes that the prevalent binary gender order is constructed. This happens through a process in which people within a society are attributed certain sets of mutually exclusive properties and behaviour. These are retrospectively declared "typically male" or "typically female" and thus naturalised. The groups of males subject to this attribution are represented as naturally dominating and instrumental. Females, however, are designated as subordinate and caring. This endorses an unequal distribution of power. It is clear how such a distribution supports the notion that men would not be effective caregivers. But contrary to the models common in nursing theory, Connell also suggests an explanation. Why exactly is this the case and why do at least some men who end up working in nursing choose not to embody femininity?

The answer implies more than simply the positions these men wish to have in relation to their female colleagues or to women in general. The relationships men have with other men must also be taken into account. According to Connell, all men tend to attempt to embody what she calls "hegemonic masculinity". This dynamic set of properties is the embodiment of all attributes socially desired from men at a given time. Typical men want it and typical women desire the men who have it. Although perceived by Connell as a context-dependent power distributor rather than as an ideal type, research has shown that it indeed has a certain core of properties.[15] These have remained relatively stable for at least 200 years. Of these properties, almost all are incompatible to working as professional caregivers. This starts with hegemonic masculinity limiting men's sexual desire towards women and forbidding them to embody attributes coded as female or to behave accordingly. Men who do so nevertheless, embody what Connell called "subordinate masculinity".[16] For Connell, gay and bisexual men as well as transsexual persons identified by their environment as biological males fall under this category. Working in

13  Cf. Ummel (1997); Wetterer (2002).
14  Cf. Connell (2015), originally published as Connell, R[obert] W.: Masculinities. Berkeley 1995. All quotes are from the 2015 German translation.
15  Cf. Dinges (2005), pp. 8–19.
16  Cf. Connell (2015), p. 132.

a field coded as feminine such as nursing puts male nurses into the direction of subordinate men and – viewed from a socio-psychological perspective – under considerable pressure for two different reasons. Men who desire other men or identify with women though finding opportunities for self-realisation become direct targets for homophobia. In West Germany until 1969 (and beyond) this could well include criminal persecution. For cis-heterosexual male nurses societal misperceptions ("all male nurses are gay") or disregard for their attempts to be desirable partners for women may also cause tensions.[17]

Secondly, a man who embodies hegemonic masculinity has to be sufficiently successful in economic terms to provide an above-average standard of living for his family. This certainly was not the case for caregivers during the period of time investigated here and arguably it is neither today. Hegemonic masculinity is also constituted by emphasising the inadequacy of the men incapable of holding this kind of economic power. When men are accused of not being economically "potent", and react defiantly to these accusations by claiming that they are "real" and desirable men nevertheless, they embody what Connell called "marginalised masculinity".[18] Although male nurses did not belong to the very lowest strata of income distribution, their status until the 1970s was without a doubt associated with marginalisation. There were two reasons for this. Female nurses often received nothing more than an allowance. Their male colleagues did actually receive regular payments but it was not a lot either. Moreover, they were associated with lower social strata because they had to deal primarily with stigmatised patients from mental institutions or hospitals for venereal diseases.[19]

So in comparison to other men – not to their female colleagues – the agency of male nurses can be described as decreased. This loss of agency results in theory in the unwillingness of men to adapt their habitus to their allegedly allochthonous (associated with femininity) working environment. The intensified variant of this behaviour, hypermasculine compensation, causes gender inequality and eventually causes clashes with those unwilling to accept it. Recent masculinity studies along with the sociology of the workplace have to be taken into account when approaching the question of how male nurses could exist in the past at all, how their relation to caregiving was shaped by their masculinity and possibly how contentious their presence was in earlier days in their profession.

As mentioned above, the sources analysed here are journals from professional organisations. These journals functioned as forums for different nursing-related groups to present their work, announce events and to discuss controversial issues. And, coming straight to the point, virtually all articles by or about male nurses belonged to the "controversial" category. It can be safely assumed that male nurses felt a pronounced need to defend their presence in formerly female-only associations. The articles written by male nurses or

17   Cf. Harding (2007).
18   Cf. Connell (2015), p. 173.
19   Cf. Evans (2004), p. 322.

their female allies within the organisations are clearly vindications of the male nurses' right to exist on (at least) equal footing in the new modernised profession. An evaluation of the masculine roles portrayed in these articles is an evaluation of strategical representation, of the way male nurses wanted to be seen, not necessarily of their actual behaviour. These public relation efforts nevertheless shed light on the paradoxes of masculinity in the nursing profession. If nursing was coded as female, then how could men represent themselves as capable of doing the job while continuing to embody masculinity?

### Machine operator or sensitive caregiver?
### Representations of male nurses around 1970

I chose three journals:

– First, *ÖTV-Presse/ÖTV. Sanitätswarte* of the public services union ÖTV.
– Second, the *Agnes-Karll-Schwester* belonging to the largest association of non-motherhouse-nurses, the "Agnes-Karll-Verband" (AKV). The latter's successor, the DBfK ("Deutscher Berufsverband für Pflegeberufe"), is the largest nursing association in Germany to this date.
– The third journal is the *Deutsche Schwesternzeitung*, edited jointly by various nursing-related associations and institutions.

These particular publications were chosen because they were the most relevant for men in nursing at the time. The ÖTV represented nurses employed in public service. Since the regional states ran large psychiatric hospitals, large numbers of male nurses were employed there. Moreover, during the postwar era more and more communities built hospitals where they increasingly employed their own staffs instead of relying on contracts with female-only motherhouses (confessional and other). Thus many male nurses were organised within the ÖTV and ran their own department there.[20] During the extended postwar era, the AKV became the other large organisation to include male nurses.[21] Although it was not a union but a professional organisation, like the union it represented nurses not employed by motherhouses. In contrast to the motherhouses, the AKV was flexible enough to change with the times by admitting male nurses from the mid-1960s onwards.

Most of the mentioned reforms first took place in these two organisations. Between 1950 and 1990 about 35 articles on topics concerning men in nursing were published, most of them between 1965 and 1975. These were the formative years of the modern, gender-inclusive nursing organisations. The "desegregation" was part of a broader process in which nursing was supposed to be restructured as regular employment comparable to other professions. This included among other things regular working hours, career plans and individual accomodation. As mentioned above, the "desegregation" in West

20  Cf. Kreutzer (2005), p. 52.
21  Cf. Elster (1967), p. 223.

Germany was to a large extent institutional, not one that fundamentally began with the access of men to the profession. From 1967 onwards, men could join the hitherto female-exclusive AKV, while the gender-separated departments in the ÖTV union were merged in 1968.[22]

Like other aspects of this modernist agenda, the integration of male caregivers was opposed by a traditionalist fraction which led to considerable clashes. It is not particularly easy to determine the power of this opposition. When men started to join the organisations, a new generation of leaders in the AKV and ÖTV were decidedly in favour of the modernisation.[23] From the mid-1960s onwards the opposing traditionalists apparently had no say in determining the direction in which the organisations were heading. Their outcry could only be heard in the workplace, not in the organisations themselves. But there the resistance was significant. This is clearly reflected by the analysed articles in the journals.[24] Explicit denial of men's ability to become nurses clearly did not sit well with the editors and was given no platform in the journals. There were abundant statements by traditionalists within the hospitals themselves, however, arguing that men were incapable of caregiving. The traditional assumption was implicitly present everywhere within the profession. Thus the modernists fought a culture struggle rather than a power struggle within the associations. Things like job adverts adressing only female nurses ("Krankenschwestern") persisted. A modernist female nurse, in favor of more men in the profession, complained about the following advert for a nursing school: "Nursing – a nice and womanly profession, in which all the dispositions of a young girl are fostered in the best possible way [...] where a woman finds satisfaction even if she remains unmarried." Only at the end of the text could be read in small print: "We also accept men."[25]

Young male trainees were required to read textbooks about the nurses' "natural role" as a substitute mother. This grounded their supposed unsuitability (for the job they were already doing) firmly in biology.[26] Female-only accomodation soon became a real logistical problem, with male nurses complaining about having to rent their own rooms for a lot of money or having to sleep in places like unheated attics or cellars adjacent to the hospital morgue.[27]

While these things were far from being pleasant, the most urgent reason why male nurses relied on access to the associations was another one: by rivalling the motherhouses, the AKV and somewhat later an ÖTV-related institute were the only providers of higher qualification training willing to admit men. Contrary to many female nurses of the time, who dropped out of their jobs rather early to start families, men had to get trained in order not to do

22  Cf. Kreutzer (2005), p. 10.
23  Cf. Elster (1967), p. 223; Elster (1968).
24  The actual extent of these confrontations will have to be investigated separately using other sources like personnel files or interviews with contemporary witnesses.
25  Heyn (1965), p. 348.
26  Cf. Bauer (1959), p. 207; Fricke (1967).
27  Cf. Bauer (1959), p. 207; Krankenpfleger (1971), p. 504.

the same job for the rest of their lives. The higher qualifications were also a means by which male nurses could escape their subordinate and marginalised masculine status. Traditionalists against male nurses working in key positions often associated male nurses with lower-class coarseness. As the following examples will illustrate, this was something of an ironic argument, as the traditionalists themselves were often upper-middle-class women.

Crucial about the perceived association with the lower classes was that it made it possible for traditionalists to portray the men not as real nurses but as something different. The fact that they still overproportionally worked with society's outcasts enabled such a portrayal.[28] Patients in mental asylums and institutions for alcohol addiction were obviously among these. But patients in dermatological or urological clinics, or suffering from venereal diseases are also to be named here. These disciplines were frowned upon to such an extent that even the physicians working there were not entirely free of stigma, let alone the nurses.[29] The prison-like character of these places is also the reason that at the time of deinstitutionalisation male nurses were still often addressed as "Wärter" or warden, drawing a clear line between the duties expected of male and female.[30] This perception of male nurses had undesired effects for them. Male nurses were more likely to be hired if they embodied these stereotypes, as nobody felt it was necessary for male nurses to be skilled in the tasks women were supposedly better at anyhow. As late as 1968 a nurse complained: "Given the physically demanding tasks due in every hospital, one is tempted to turn a blind eye to certain other insufficiencies when chosing male candidates for a job."[31] Even a male nurse and ÖTV unionist had to concede that many of the traditionalists' arguments against men in nursing were not entirely unfounded. "Certainly there were and still are people who chose this profession out of dubious motives. But there are slouches among female nurses too. And who would deny that good male nurses exist?"[32] Concessions like this provided arguments that male nurses should be given access to more training and qualification, not less.

Access to higher qualification was paramount to stopping the traditionalists' ultimately futile attempts at gatekeeping. The gatekeeping was not limited only to aspiring men. Geriatric and assistant nurses were equally excluded by the nursing elite.[33] As one can imagine, the fight against traditionalist upper-middle-class women from which head nurses, motherhouse matrons and academy teachers were recruited was especially bitter within the union. "What are we actually for our bourgeois society?" complained a member of the ÖTV. "Bluntly spoken, they imagine us as a bunch of uneducated ruffians,

28   Cf. Hähner-Rombach (2015); Evans (2004).
29   Cf. Scholz (2013), pp. 90–93; Moll/Schultheiss (2015).
30   Cf. Reimann (1968), p. 3.
31   Reimann (1968), p. 3; also Berron (1970).
32   Bauer (1965), p. 365.
33   Cf. Grabe (2016), p. 52.

whose intelligence barely amounts to enable us to handle some bedpans and maybe inject an enema."[34]

While many male nurses apparently complained about their ongoing marginalisation, the resulting PR offensives used as countermeasures against the proponents of separate gendered spheres were varied. Some men clearly tried to take advantage of the gender injustice prevalent in society in general. These men claimed their position in the nursing associations in a series of articles describing themselves in ways compatible with socially desired masculinity. The most prevalent of the rhetorical strategies was the association of men with technological skills. It envisioned the male nurses as technophile "medical engineers" ("Medizinalingenieur"). This term was one of several proposed to replace the term "Krankenpfleger" with something more prestigious-sounding.[35] The way in which these articles depicted male nurses' masculinity barely concealed denying that women were capable of handling machines in a hospital: "In the course of the mechanisation of our age and the improved advanced education available [now] for male nurses too, the era of the subordinate position of the male nurse will hopefully come to an end."[36] Or as another male nurse put it: "Progress in the field of medicine and the evolution and the development of technology in the hospitals require more and more men in nursing. Today a hospital without highly skilled male nurses has become inconceivable."[37] Similarly, a few articles claimed that male nurses were inevitable because of their dominance and decisiveness. It is hardly surprising that their authors decidedly rejected what they deemed "feminine" as a trait for male nurses:

> The patient population in psychiatry is characterised to quite a high percentage by sub-criminal or even openly criminal elements. A young [male] nurse will soon realise that a psychiatric hospital with its large dimension (e.g. 3,000 beds and more) requires strict order and good discipline on the job, to the point that it is actually comparable to service in a military organisation. [...] It goes without saying that sexual perverts, for example persons with homosexual tendencies, should refrain from working in psychiatry.[38]

A young nurse summarised this position in the following call:

> [Having to do menial, low-prestige labour] demands from male nurses that they supress the very things that in our culture define masculinity: Responsibility, skill, dynamic activity and creativity. [...] All male nurses should to a higher degree appropriate the element in nursing associated with masculinity, i.e. the medical-technical one and unleash their full potential here. Every male nurse has to withdraw from basic care to participate in building new self-esteem within his group.[39]

It can be safely assumed that this construction of what Raewyn Connell named "hegemonic masculinity" by leading male nurses did at least facilitate

---

34   Krett (1965), p. 351.
35   Cf. Winter (1968), p. 9; Berron (1970), p. 236.
36   Krett (1965), p. 351.
37   FDK (1970), p. 238. See also Wollscheid (1968), p. 16.
38   Frinken (1965), p. 348.
39   Pousset (1973), p. 472.

the de-feminisation of the associations. It provided a cultural framework by overcoming the perceived incommensurability of masculinity and caregiving. The unequal distribution of carework prevalent in nursing became a reality. And its ideological origins certainly have important ties to the struggle of male nurses for representation in the nursing associations around 1970. In this respect Nursing Studies' second assumption has been confirmed: that masculinity can function as a cultural agent which prevents men from doing carework. On the other hand this is far from the whole story. It is in fact misleading to limit the role of masculinity to this interrelation. It does not take into account the fact that this kind of identity politics facilitated the entry into carework for many men. For one thing, it made it easier for male nurses to legitimise their career choice when faced with sceptical parents, friends and other associates. The hospital the authors of the articles had envisioned, however, in which men only used machinery and women washed patients and made beds, was never to be realised. Once they had entered the profession, men made beds and washed patients just like everybody else. Assigning hegemonic masculinity the sole role of preventing male carework is a position hardly defensible in empirical terms.

The latter becomes even more clear when taking a look at the consequences of male nurses justifying their nursing abilities with quite the opposite strategy. Many authors were noticeably concerned with their colleagues' representation of hegemonically masculine nurses. They emphasised in their own articles that a) basic caregiving was vital to being a nurse, regardless of whether the person was male or female. According to them, a nurse not doing carework was not a nurse; b) men were perfectly capable of being caring; and c) gender differences should be reduced rather than artificially increased. Men should work as subordinates to women where required. And women in general should be able to operate machinery. A group of 14 young male nurses in training rejected the above-cited call to abstain from basic care in a reply. "It follows neccessarily that there is no menial labour (cleaning urine bottles and making beds etc.) in this profession."[40]

A male nurse working at a dermatological clinic argued similarly. On his ward quite different things were demanded, empathy, for example ("A patient suffering from a skin disease must know that people are not disgusted by them").[41] Concerning possible conflicts between male and female nurses he urged that "in mixed-gender teams it is vital to work hand-in-hand with the female nurses" ending his article as followed: "Which job is better for a man than one where he can help others? And which occupation grants the opportunity to do so? Nursing."[42] Another male nurse emphasised that part of being a nurse meant subordinating to female colleagues if necessary: "The [female]

40   Pousset (1973), p. 468.
41   Fiedler (1965), p. 352.
42   Fiedler (1965), p. 353.

nurse will find it helpful, if [the male nurse] supports her, draws a syringe for her, prepares and cleans tools, in short has an eye for her situation."[43]

One male nurse reporting from an educational trip to Finland stressed that male nurses there were allowed to work in every possible way in the hospitals, even in gynecological wards.[44] While there were indeed many images of male nurses operating machinery at least as many depicted them in unambiguously female-coded situations like carrying babies.[45]

Among the most powerful critics of gendered labour-division in nursing were the men dominating the Association of Male Nurses ("Fachverband Deutscher Krankenpfleger", FDK). This organisation had strong ties to the churches in West Germany. A church-related institution like the FDK might particularly approve of male caregiving, as it exemplified the ideal of charitable service. A member of the organisation's board wrote: "The reason for [the current association of nursing with femininity] is certainly not that men lack the natural gift of caring, affectionate and joyful service." "[Such a claim] is contradicted by the honorable history of male nurses during the first centuries after Christ, let alone by the medieval orders."[46] He criticised a "common drawing of men and women in terms of black and white", emphasising that "one should [also] not deny women at the outset technological skills, like those required in an operating room" and furthermore, that "male nurses are no sidekicks at the sickbeds and that their service for the ill is not limited to being some beast of burden for heavy items or to be a manservant".[47] He expressed understanding for the frustration of his colleagues and acknowledged that there was still a long way to go. "If [the correction of the unfavourable male nurses' image] has not been achieved yet, the reason is not necessarily lack of goodwill of the female nurses."[48]

But just as the portrayal of male nurses in terms of hegemonic masculinity had unintended consequences, so did its opposition. And equally paradoxically, the FDK's ideals of male caregivers in nursing in no way kept men from occupying key positions overproportionally, quite the opposite. In the AKV it paved the way for males to get into key positions in the first place. The FDK had a pioneering role in creating the required training programmes, whose syllabi promoting male charity were at least in vital parts far from advocating hegemonic masculinity.[49] Apparently there is no unequivocal result when evaluating the impact of male nurses publicly portraying themselves and the role of their gender: Claiming they were tough, unambiguously heterosexual and technophile or rather that they were gentle, caring and empathetic did not result in distinguishably different long-term outcomes. For better or

43   Fery (1965), p. 361.
44   Cf. Tschierschke (1967), p. 46.
45   Cf. Wandel (1968), p. 11; Bayerns (1973), p. 506.
46   Schimmelpfennig (1965), p. 344.
47   Schimmelpfennig (1965), p. 344.
48   Schimmelpfennig (1965), p. 344.
49   Cf. Schimmelpfennig (1973).

worse – both strategies facilitated men becoming caregivers and made "desegregation" possible but also enabled the current unequal labour distribution
in nursing. At least in relation to the male nurses' public relations efforts, the
received narrative of patriarchal power dynamics fails to fully explain the precise nature of the relationship between masculinity and carework.

In regard to masculinity, the story of how male nurses became an integral
part of the nursing profession is one of unintended outcomes. At least this can
be said for the "desegregation" of nursing in West Germany during the second half of the 20th century. Both the affirmation of hegemonic masculinity as
well as its wholehearted rejection seem to have provided a somewhat favour-
able climate for the advent of the modernised gender-inclusive profession.
Quantifying this influence in order to establish a correlation with the increase
in the number of male nurses is far more difficult to achieve. The statistics are
notoriously difficult to analyse, given the ever-changing job titles and work
activities assigned to men present in the wards. How should the job of a man
be categorised who carries heavy items all the day, some of which are actual
patients, while being called on every now and then when sensitive tasks like
the intimate care of male patients required his help? It is certain, however, that
since the reforms of the 1960s there has been an increase of male nurses with
(almost) identical education and activities as female nurses.

## Nursing as forced work for conscientious objectors.
## The unintended consequences of gender shaming in West Germany

While in all likelihood the reforms contributed significantly to this increase,
there is another phenomenon whose positive impact on the number of male
nurses is much more likely to be proven in terms of causality: The existence
of an alternative civilian service for men who did not wish to attend the basic
military service, obligatory in West Germany starting in 1956. From the beginning, the civilian service played a significant role in increasing the number
of men doing carework. It is estimated that by the late 1960s around half of
the participants worked in jobs comparable to nursing auxiliaries.[50] Many
of them stayed in the field and became trained nurses after the end of their
service.[51] By the beginning of the 1970s there were about 4,000 young men
doing civilian service in hospitals and nursing homes, a considerable number
given the fact that the overall number of male nurses was estimated to be
about 14,000 at that time.[52]

And like the culture struggle during the "desegregation" of the nursing associations, this was a story of ambiguity and unintended outcomes. Increasing
social justice by increasing the number of men doing carework was not on the
agenda of any of the political groups who designed the civilian service in the

---

50   Cf. Bernhard (2005), pp. 420–422.
51   Cf. Bernhard (2006).
52   Cf. Bernhard (2005), pp. 420–422.

late 1950s, quite the contrary. Officials looked for ways to make it as undesirable as possible because they feared that young men would go to great lengths to avoid military service. "Do you really think we are that stupid, making the alternative service [...] attractive?" asked one official in charge at the Ministry of Defence.[53] While longer service times and other chicaneries were used for discouragement, the most important was without a doubt the shaming of the conscientious objectors. The masculinity of the young men was central to this. Despite the recently lost war, military service remained a central part of contemporary hegemonic masculinity in West Germany. Objectors were widely considered as deeply deplorable people, and the military's will to put as much pressure on them as possible was shared by large parts of the society. In so-called "trials of consciousness" objectors had to prove the sincerity of their plea before a committee. Besides being called back-stabbers and worse, objectors were stigmatised as "sissies", "non-men", "no real guys"[54], and the work they had to do during the service was characterised as "essentially untenable for a man". Gender-shaming of young men unwilling to do military service was far from a mere side issue. Patrick Bernhard comes to the conclusion that it was the single most effective deterrent for young men in the beginning years of the alternate service until after 1968, when it ceased to be effective.[55]

From then onwards more and more young men preferred to object, even if this meant having to do carework, even though the cultural climate remained hostile well into the 1980s. Around 1980, 17,000 young men per year did civilian service in nursing-related jobs; in the mid-1980s, 26,000; in 1990, 45,000; while around the turn of the century the number peaked at 70,000.[56] Consequently ten of thousands of young men first experienced nursing during their civilian service, and many stayed.

Again it becomes clear that strategies representing male caregiving as effeminate with the aim of preventing men from working in nursing-related jobs have unpredictable outcomes. Although propagated again and again, the anti-caregiving faction within the nursing organisations did not realise their vision of a distinct male nursing profession devoid of any activities associated with femininity. Neither was the aggressive gender-shaming of conscientious objectors an effective deterrent in the long run. This paradoxical pattern can be found even within the distinct culture that developed among the young men in civilian service. Just because they were portrayed as effeminate did not mean that they themselves were willing to let go of male privilege.

In the years following 1968, young objectors went to some lengths to affirm publicly that they were not unmasculine. In the spirit of the student protests which increased the influx of men into the service, "sexual liberation"

53  Bernhard (2005), p. 94.
54  Bernhard (2005), pp. 57–58.
55  Cf. Bernhard (2005), p. 55.
56  For the exact numbers in every single year see Bernhard (2005), pp. 420–422. The percentage of all objectors doing nursing-related work in hospitals and nursing homes was consistently about 50 per cent.

was a significant part of the objectors' agenda. This included comparisons of
their virility to that of their peers who had opted for the military: "18 months
of military will make you impotent" or "In order to fuck freely you have to
free yourself from the military. Fuck the Bundeswehr, let's get out and let
the soldiers jerk off alone by themselves." Slogans like this were printed on
leaflets and handed out to potential objectors.[57] Such politically motivated
breaches of taboo were soon to be criticised as sexist by the second wave of
feminism but remained alive and well among young men attaining civilian
service. The desire to embody hegemonic masculinity was also among the
reasons why doing politics rather than caregiving was prioritised by many
of them. Politicising patients and hospital staff in the fight against the soon-
to-be collapsing capitalist establishment was seen as the primary goal. These
men never imagined themselves as caregivers embodying a masculinity more
compatible with gender equality. They rather saw themselves in the role of
workers, leaders, liberators of the opressed, a self-perception often at conflict
with the fact that they had actual work to do and had to accept direction from
superiors.[58] Many of these superiors were women nurses. "The head nurse is
a drill instructor"[59] was a common slogan among the activists. This indicates
that they had some trouble dealing with women who had the authority to
issue directives and represented them as "battle-axes".[60] However the large
majority of men attending civilian service did their job satisfactorily and after
the beginning of the 1970s political protest also became less disruptive.[61] The
civilian service continued to attract more and more men, many of whom
remained in nursing. Those aspects of countercultural masculinity embodied
by the conscientious objectors who embraced male caregiving (if only for one
mandatory year) remained and became exemplary for hundred and thousands of German men.

## Conclusion

Up to now, Nursing Studies' narrative of the role of masculinity can be summarised as follows: Hegemonic masculinity prevents men from doing carework. On the level of society as a whole, it strongly limits the number of men
willing to choose caregiver careers as they are incompatible with received ideals of masculinity. The resulting inequality is an important part of the feminist
critique of gender relations in society as a whole and of the conflicts resulting
from this critique. Within the nursing profession the few existing male nurses
tend to avoid actual carework and end up overrepresented in positions like
management, teaching or technology-related nursing. Here too, masculinity

57  Cf. Bernhard (2005), pp. 131–132.
58  Cf. Bernhard (2005), p. 136.
59  Bernhard (2005), p. 138.
60  Darbyshire/Gordon (2005), p. 69.
61  Cf. Bernhard (2005), pp. 219–224.

is the essential agent. Men in occupations coded as feminine emphasise their gender overproportionally to compensate for their decreased agency. Thus, they recapitulate gender inequality which is prone to conflicts in the workplace as well as in internal professional discourse. However an analysis of how masculinity has functioned in contemporary history in two important fields casts significant doubt on the assumption that representations and behaviour associated with hegemonic masculinity correlate negatively with the number of men entering the nursing profession and on the overall amount of carework they do if they do remain in the field.

The public relations efforts of organised male nurses during the "defeminisation" of nursing does not provide unambiguous evidence for such a link. While re-masculinising efforts were an important part of the campaign, at least as many articles explicitly rejected hegemonic masculinity and actively embraced reduced gender difference and equality at the workplace. Paradoxically, the former strategy has undoubtedly contributed to legitimising the existence of male nurses, while the underlying vision of male nurses not doing carework at all was realised only to a limited extent. Equally paradoxically, the idea of promoting gender equality in nursing was put forward by exactly those institutions which worked to gain access to key positions, thus enabling the eventual gender-care gap within the nursing profession. The thesis of hegemonic masculinity as an anti-caregiving agent comes into question because of the success of the carework-oriented civilian service, despite the gender-shaming used to deter men from enlisting in it. This does not disprove the extensive research done by Nursing Studies showing that gender relations result in an unequal distribution of carework in nursing. It calls, however, for an empirically grounded evaluation of the role masculinity plays in these power dynamics. The history of nursing could contribute further to such an evaluation, analysing the history of everyday hospital life in this regard.

## Bibliography

Bauer, Franz: Steht der Krankenpfleger im Hintergrund? Sorgen wegen des nötigen Berufs-
    nachwuchses. In: ÖTV. Sanitätswarte 11 (1959), p. 207.
Bauer, Franz: Geschichte der Krankenpflege. Kulmbach 1965.
Bayerns erster Kinderkrankenpfleger. In: Deutsche Krankenpflegezeitschrift 26 (1973), p. 506.
Bernhard, Patrick: Zivildienst zwischen Reform und Revolte. Eine bundesdeutsche Institu-
    tion im gesellschaftlichen Wandel 1961–1982. München 2005.
Bernhard, Patrick: Zivis in der Pflege. Zur Geschichte einer besonderen Mitarbeitergruppe
    im bundesdeutschen Sozialsystem, 1961–1990. In: Braunschweig, Sabine (ed.): Pflege –
    Räume, Macht und Alltag. Zürich 2006, pp. 140–151.
Berron, Thomas: Das Image des Krankenpflegers. In: Deutsche Schwesternzeitung 23 (1970),
    pp. 233–237.
Bischoff, Claudia: Frauen in der Krankenpflege. Zur Entwicklung von Frauenrolle und
    Frauenberufstätigkeit im 19. und 20. Jahrhundert. Frankfurt/Main 1992.
Connell, Raewyn: Der gemachte Mann. Konstruktion und Krise von Männlichkeiten. Wies-
    baden 2015.

D'Antonio, Patricia: American Nursing. A History of Knowledge, Authority and the Meaning of Work. Baltimore 2010.

Darbyshire, Philip; Gordon, Suzanne: Of Nurses and Nursing. In: Daly, John et al. (eds.): Professional Nursing: Concepts, Issues, and Challenges. New York 2005, pp. 69–92.

Dinges, Martin: Einleitung. In: Dinges, Martin (ed.): Männer, Macht, Körper. Hegemoniale Männlichkeiten vom Mittelalter bis heute. Frankfurt/Main 2005, pp. 7–34.

Dressel, Kathrin; Wanger, Susanne: Erwerbsarbeit: Zur Situation von Frauen auf dem Arbeitsmarkt. In: Becker, Ruth; Kortendiek, Beate (eds.): Handbuch Frauen- und Geschlechterforschung. Theorie, Methoden, Empirie. 2nd ed. Wiesbaden 2008, pp. 481–491.

Elster, Ruth: Fachverband Deutscher Krankenpfleger im Agnes-Karll-Verband. In: Die Agnes-Karll-Schwester 21 (1967), p. 223.

Elster, Ruth: Das heutige Berufsbild des Krankenpflegers. In: Die Agnes-Karll-Schwester, der Krankenpfleger 22 (1968), pp. 187–188.

Evans, Joan: Men nurses: a historical and feminist perspective. In: Journal of Advanced Nursing 47 (2004), no. 3, pp. 321–328.

FDK: Der Mann in der Krankenpflege. Ein Beitrag zum Tag der Krankenpflege. In: Deutsche Schwesternzeitung 23 (1970), pp. 238–239.

Fery, Rolf: Der Krankenpfleger in der urologischen Abteilung. In: Die Agnes-Karll-Schwester 19 (1965), pp. 358–361.

Fiedler, Martin: Der Krankenpfleger in der Hautklinik. In: Die Agnes-Karll-Schwester 19 (1965), pp. 352–353.

Fricke, Anneliese: Statistisches. In: Die Agnes-Karll-Schwester 21 (1967), pp. 217–220.

Frinken, Walter P.: Der Krankenpfleger in der Psychiatrie. In: Die Agnes-Karll-Schwester 19 (1965), pp. 346–348.

Genua, Jo Anne: The Vision of Male Nurses: Roles, Barriers and Stereotypes. In: InterAction. The Official Publication of the American Assembly for Men In Nursing 23 (2005), no. 4, pp. 4–7.

Grabe, Nina: Altenpflege, ein Beruf nur für Frauen? Die stationäre Versorgung alter Menschen in der Nachkriegszeit (1945–1975). In: Geschichte der Pflege 5 (2016), no. 1, pp. 48–55.

Hähner-Rombach, Sylvelyn: Männer in der Geschichte der Krankenpflege. Zum Stand einer Forschungslücke. In: Medizinhistorisches Journal 50 (2015), no. 1/2, pp. 123–148.

Hähner-Rombach, Sylvelyn: Quantitative Entwicklung des Krankenpflegepersonals. In: Hähner-Rombach, Sylvelyn; Pfütsch, Pierre (eds.): Entwicklungen in der Krankenpflege und in anderen Gesundheitsberufen nach 1945. Ein Lehr- und Studienbuch. Frankfurt/Main 2018, pp. 195–219.

Harding, Thomas: The construction of men who are nurses as gay. In: Journal of Advanced Nursing 60 (2007), no. 6, pp. 636–644.

Heintz, Bettina (ed.): Ungleich unter Gleichen. Studien zur geschlechtsspezifischen Segregation des Arbeitsmarktes. Frankfurt/Main 1997.

Heyn, Maria: Zur Ausbildung von Krankenpflegern. In: Die Agnes-Karll-Schwester 19 (1965), p. 348.

Krankenpfleger bevölkern die Notunterkünfte. In: Deutsche Krankenpflegezeitschrift 24 (1971), p. 504.

Krampe, Eva-Maria: Krankenpflege im Professionalisierungsprozess. Entfeminisierung durch Akademisierung? In: Die Hochschule (2013), pp. 43–56.

Krett, Peter: Als Krankenpfleger auf der chirurgischen Wachstation. In: Die Agnes-Karll-Schwester 19 (1965), p. 351.

Kreutzer, Susanne: Vom "Liebesdienst" zum modernen Frauenberuf: die Reform der Krankenpflege nach 1945. Frankfurt/Main 2005.

Mackintosh, Carolyn: A historical study of men in nursing. In: Journal of Advanced Nursing 26 (1997), no. 2, pp. 232–236.

Moll, Friedrich; Schultheiss, Dirk: Medizin und Öffentlichkeit: Sexologie und medikale Sub-
    kulturen in divergenten Gesellschaftssystemen 1945–1968. In: Fangerau, Heiner; Halling,
    Thorsten (eds.): Urologie 1945–1990. Berlin 2015, pp. 61–79.
Notz, Gisela: Arbeit: Hausarbeit, Ehrenamt, Erwerbsarbeit. In: Becker, Ruth; Kortendiek,
    Beate (eds.): Handbuch Frauen- und Geschlechterforschung. Theorie, Methoden, Empi-
    rie. 2nd ed. Wiesbaden 2008, pp. 472–480.
O'Lynn, Chad E.; Tranbarger, Russell E. (eds.): Men in Nursing: History, Challenges, and
    Opportunities. New York 2007, available at: https://books.google.de/books?id=-Ag7TqTy
    IC0C (last accessed: 09/11/2018).
Pousset, Raimund: Krankenpfleger. Die schweigende Minderheit. In: Deutsche Krankenpfle-
    gezeitschrift 26 (1973), pp. 468–475.
Reimann, Hans Leo: Der Krankenpfleger. Zum Wandel eines Berufsbildes. In: Deutsche
    Schwesternzeitung 21 (1968), pp. 2–5.
Schimmelpfennig, Heinz: Der Krankenpfleger zwischen gestern und morgen. In: Die Agnes-
    Karll-Schwester 19 (1965), p. 344.
Schimmelpfennig, Heinz: Als Christ in der Krankenpflege. In: Deutsche Krankenpflege-
    zeitschrift 26 (1973), p. 47.
Scholz, Albrecht: Geschichte der Dermatologie in Deutschland. Berlin 2013.
Schwamm, Christoph: Männlichkeit und die (Selbst)positionierung von Krankenpflegern in
    der Bundesrepublik ca. 1945 bis 2000. In: Hähner-Rombach, Sylvelyn; Pfütsch, Pierre
    (eds.): Entwicklungen in der Krankenpflege und in anderen Gesundheitsberufen nach
    1945. Ein Lehr- und Studienbuch. Frankfurt/Main 2018, pp. 29–64.
Statistisches Bundesamt: Zahl der Woche vom 6. März 2012. Pressemitteilung. Wiesbaden
    2012, available at: https://www.destatis.de/DE/PresseService/Presse/Pressemitteilungen/
    zdw/2012/PD12_010_p002pdf.pdf?__blob=publicationFile (last accessed: 09/11/2018).
Tschierschke, Rudolf: Als Krankenpfleger in Finnland. In: Die Agnes-Karll-Schwester 21
    (1967), p. 46.
Ummel, Hans: Krankenpflege. Männliche Professionalität zwischen 'Händchenhalten' und
    Patientenhandling. In: Heintz, Bettina (ed.): Ungleich unter Gleichen. Studien zur ge-
    schlechtsspezifischen Segregation des Arbeitsmarktes. Frankfurt/Main 1997, pp. 67–121.
Wandel, Lothar: Als Krankenpflegeschüler in der Kinderklinik. In: Deutsche Schwesternzei-
    tung 21 (1968), pp. 10–12.
Wetterer, Angelika: Arbeitsteilung und Geschlechterkonstruktion. "Gender at work" in theo-
    retischer und historischer Perspektive. Konstanz 2002.
Williams, Christine B.: Doing "Women's Work". Men in Nontraditional Occupations. New-
    bury Park, CA 1993.
Winter, Manfred: Klinikassistent? Ein Beruf ändert sein Gesicht – vielleicht auch seine Be-
    zeichnung. In: Deutsche Schwesternzeitung 21 (1968), pp. 5–10.
Wollscheid, Albert: Die Situation des Krankenpflegers in der heutigen Zeit. In: Deutsche
    Schwesternzeitung 21 (1968), pp. 14–16.

# Negotiating Electroconvulsive Therapy (ECT) in Dutch Psychiatry: Cultural and Intraprofessional Tension over Biological Psychiatry, 1950–2010[1]

*Geertje Boschma*

## Introduction

"Yes, Electroconvulsive Therapy, ECT, I did myself, indeed, push the button. First it was applied without anesthetics", Jaap Prick stated, "but then we sometimes had problems with backbone fractures. Eventually [in the 1950s], I involved an anesthetist, he gave a light anesthetic. That was an improvement, indeed."[2] Jaap Prick, former Chef de Clinique of the Psychiatric Department at the St. Canisius hospital in Nijmegen, was one of eight psychiatrists interviewed as part of a research project on the history of ECT in the Netherlands in 2011. Prick had started his career in Nijmegen in 1947 as a so-called neuro-psychiatrist, and regularly performed ECT among other somatic treatments such as insulin therapy.[3] This paper explores the history of ECT primarily from the viewpoint of psychiatrists who continued using ECT or took it up as a treatment modality during a time period when it provoked deep controversy and public debate in the 1970s and 1980s. Using the interviews with eight psychiatrists as the primary source material as well as archival and additional primary and secondary sources, the main goal of the analysis is to explore under which circumstances the therapy was maintained despite the medical and cultural ambivalence that emerged about it.

Since its first application in Italy in 1938, ECT has provoked varied professional and public responses. Existing historiography on ECT shows how its use and side-effects have been the subject of ongoing debate.[4] Current debates

---

1   I gratefully acknowledge the junior visiting fellowship from the Descartes Centre for the History and Philosophy of Science and Humanities at the University of Utrecht, the Netherlands in 2011 supporting this research. I thank Dr. Joost Vijselaar for his guidance and the professionals for the interviews. Ethical approval for the project was obtained from the University of British Columbia Behavioral Research Ethics Board. Parts of this paper are drawn from Boschma (2015) and are used with permission from Manchester University Press.
2   Interview with Jaap Prick by author, 21 April 2011. Prick did not mention whether muscle relaxants also were used; once use of anesthetics grew common, typically a muscle relaxant was given along with an anesthetic to prevent muscle contractions during ECT. See Groenland/Kusuma (1999), p. 43. Quotes from interviewees, in this paragraph and the remainder of the paper are all from the oral history interviews. They were conducted by author in 2011, except for the interview with Bas Verwey, which was conducted by Joost Vijselaar and Josef Vos, 22 November 2006, and shared with me.
3   Neuro-psychiatrist is the translation of "zenuwarts" in Dutch, or "Nervenarzt" in German.
4   Cf. Gawlich (2018); Kneeland/Warren (2002); Nolen (1999); Sadowsky (2017); Shorter/Healy (2007); Vijselaar (2013).

centre on the effects on memory, whereas in the past, unmodified treatment sometimes resulted in fractured bones or vertebrae, as Jaap Prick pointed out as well, and which was a serious concern, also in his view.[5] In current mental health practice, ECT entails the induction of a convulsion instigated by a short electric impulse through the brain for less than a second. It is given with an anesthetic and muscle relaxant under close monitoring and, if necessary, delivery of oxygen in a well-equipped treatment room in a hospital or out-patient clinic.[6] According to current guidelines of the Dutch Association of Psychiatry depression is the primary indication for ECT with varying rates of effectiveness reported.[7] Patient or family permission and informed consent for ECT has to be obtained, according to the same guidelines.[8]

The critique that emerged most vehemently in the 1970s did not only cen-tre on the medical nature of the therapy and the way it was performed, how-ever, it also encompassed a larger cultural critique.[9] Nevertheless, the rapid and effective relief ECT brought about in some cases of severe depression or catatonia was a powerful memory, not only recalled in interviews but also featured as an important argument to hold on to the therapy at a time when the call for its abandonment grew.[10] Few psychiatric treatments have provoked such varying public responses, from fervent protest and activism in the 1970s and 1980s, vividly kept in memory, for example by films such as the world-famous "One Flew over the Cuckoo's Nest", to public acceptance and more optimistic reports over its efficacy within the last few decades.[11] Recent histori-ography highlights how its social appraisal has varied from it being embraced as a hopeful remedy bringing relief in difficult circumstances to it being re-

5   Cf. Interview with Prick; Interview with Walter van den Broek by author, 23 March 2011. See also: Gawlich (2018); Sadowsky (2017); Vijselaar (2010), pp. 193–195; Meeter et al. (2011); Nolen (1999). For a contemporary patient view on ECT: Dukakis/Tye (2006).
6   Cf. Groenland/Kusuma (1999).
7   ECT is indicated in particular for medication-resistant depression, for which antidepres-sant medications have not been effective; for depression with characteristics of psychosis it might be the primary indication: Van den Broek et al. (2010), pp. 31, 36–39. Research reports on healing effects, or effectiveness reported in terms of remission percentages, vary from 28 per cent to 68 per cent for patients with medication-resistant depression, and from 41 per cent to 91 per cent for patients with non-medication-resistant depres-sion: Van den Broek et al. (2010), p. 40. For a historical discussion of ECT efficacy: Sadowsky (2017), pp. 5–10.
8   Cf. Van den Broek et al. (2010), pp. 31–35 and 139–145. Recommendations to inform families of the risks of ECT and ask their permission were included in nursing textbooks from the 1950s (written by psychiatrists): Hamer/Haverkate (1950), p. 509; Hamer/Tolsma (1956), p. 558.
9   Cf. Braslow (1997); Vijselaar (2013).
10  Cf. Interviews with Goos Zwanikken and Joke Zwanikken-Leenders by author, 10 and 24 February 2011; Interview with Fons Tholen by author, 15 March 2011; Stegge (2012), p. 602; Nolen (1999); Koerselman/Smeets (1992).
11  Cf. Hirshbein/Sarvananda (2008). The movie is based on Kesey (1962). A few months prior to the première of "One Flew", a Dutch movie on psychiatry, "Kind van de Zon" ("Child of the Sun"), was featured in the Netherlands, which also included a scene on ECT that drew public attention to psychiatry; Van Hintum (2009).

jected head-on, characterized as a symbol, if not tool of undue oppression.[12] Gawlich also examines the use and meaning of the ECT machine itself within a socio-technological systems perspective.[13] Ethical concerns about ECT not only centred on mixed results of the therapy or a limited theoretical explanation, but also on the way its therapeutic use could be justified in a variety of ways.[14] While it was helpful to some patients, particularly in case of depression, others did not experience any relief, and the unmodified use in the earlier period of the therapy caused considerable fear. Moreover, the way ECT also was understood and used to counter excessive agitation created the risk that, without a clear therapeutic rationale, legitimate use of the therapy could shift into misuse as a disciplinary measure.[15] In most instances patients lacked power to refuse the treatment and psychiatrists' decisions typically prevailed.[16] It was not until the late 1970s that procedures for informed consent began to be developed.[17]

In the Netherlands, ECT also almost disappeared in response to public activism, but then resurged in the 1980s and 1990s, particularly in general hospitals, reflecting wider trends.[18] In the paper ECT is perceived as part of a larger psychiatric and social system in which cultural values and believes, processes of socialization and technological change, as well as hierarchical power relationships all shape ECT and its public and professional appraisal.[19] The analysis of interviews with selected psychiatrists who, as part of their focus on biological psychiatry, continued to use ECT or reestablished the treatment following a period of fierce critical psychiatric protest contributes to an understanding of the way ECT was continued as a medical practice in face of strong anti-psychiatric sentiment and public protest. At the height of protest and public debate over ECT in the Netherlands in the 1970s and 1980s it stirred deep controversy, with opponents arguing that it should be outlawed on the grounds of it being inhumane, dangerous and unscientific, figuring as a strong symbol of protest against biological psychiatry, whereas proponents, who were in the minority by then, argued in favour of its effectiveness in certain circumstances and conditions and opposed abandonment. In response, governmental advice was sought and in the mid-1980s formal ECT guidelines were issued and implemented, confirming the acceptability of its use under strict conditions, and only as a measure of 'last resort' in cases in which other therapeutic approaches had been ineffective.[20] The guidelines also stimulated

---

12   Cf. Gawlich (2018); Kneeland/Warren (2002); Sadowsky (2017); Shorter/Healy (2007); Vijselaar (2013).
13   Cf. Gawlich (2018).
14   Cf. Braslow (1997), pp. 104–117; Nolte (2017).
15   Cf. Braslow (1997), pp. 104–117; Vijselaar (2010), pp. 193–195; Shorter/Healy (2007), pp. 214–224; Rooijmans (1978).
16   Cf. Nolte (2017); Vijselaar (2010), pp. 193–195.
17   Cf. Koster: Informed Consent (1992); Witmer/De Roode (2004).
18   Cf. Van Hintum (2009); Kneeland/Warren (2002).
19   Cf. Blok (2004); Vijselaar (2013); Gawlich (2018).
20   Cf. Legemaate (1985).

the development of a stronger research base for the therapy as I will show in
the paper. The public view gradually shifted as did the medical practice and
justification surrounding ECT. The analysis concludes with an examination of
the wider acceptance of ECT during the 1990s. During that time public dispute over ECT faded and an emerging culture of evidence-based practice en-
veloped its use.[21] It is argued that the divergent perspectives on ECT emerged
within the context of wider social changes and transformations in psychiatry,
using a generational approach: how and under which social and medical influences has the continued application of ECT been negotiated in the face
of fierce political debate, conflict and protest? And how was the application
and continued use of ECT interconnected with broader developments in psychiatry? The commentaries of the interviewees provide a lens through which
larger social trends in the development of ECT can be understood, without
claiming their views are necessarily representative or comprehensive.[22]

## Background

ECT was first applied in Dutch psychiatry in 1939 and has continued to be
applied to the present day.[23] Outpatient or psychiatric clinics in general hospitals gradually have become the dominant environment for ECT in recent
decades underpinned by an expanding field of biological psychiatry and ar-
ticulation of its evidence-base.[24] The 2010 ECT guideline of the Dutch Association of Psychiatry, for example, encapsulating the contemporary evidence
supporting ECT, listed 36 ECT Centres, the majority of which were located in
psychiatric departments of general and university hospitals.[25]

　　Even so, in public memory the controversial perspectives on the treatment
lingered. When, in 2011, ECT was introduced anew in the psychiatric clinic
of the new Jeroen Bosch General Hospital in Den Bosch, for example, its
launch drew the attention from a local newspaper. The reporter pointed out
that much had changed about ECT, suggesting the controversial history of
ECT was not yet forgotten although it no longer provoked the public response
it once did.[26] For Goos Zwanikken, however, professor emeritus of psychiatry
from the Radboud University of Nijmegen, the news prompted an emotional
response. Upon reading the news he felt compelled to write a letter to Leon
Vos, the psychiatrist who was going to provide the therapy, stating: "Hon-
ourable colleague, in the Brabants Dagblad [Brabant Daily] of March 10 I
read [...] news that makes me happy: Congratulations with your decision [to

21  Cf. Bolt (2015).
22  For a review of oral history see Boschma et al. (2008).
23  Cf. Barnhoorn (1940); Barnhoorn (1941).
24  Cf. Rooijmans (2007); Bolt (2015).
25  Cf. Van den Broek et al. (2010), pp. 136, 177.
26  Cf. Van Uffelen (2011).

start again with ECT]."[27] For Zwanikken it seemed a historical moment, worth a tribute: "Accolades to you for your initiative [Vos]. Even among our medical colleagues people with guts, not afraid to take initiative are too few, unfortunately. How about, once you have given your first ECT treatment, I step by and we raise a glass? I will bring [the champagne]!"[28] For Zwanikken the news seemed an affirmation that past struggles he and other colleagues had endured to defend ECT as a viable therapeutic option had paid off. It likely also reminded him of the resistance he and others had faced in doing so, making a note of support seem fitting.

The psychiatrists who I interviewed differed by age group, educational background and time of practice, but all had taken up and conducted ECT as part of their practice at some point. At the time of the interview, they had leading roles in the field of psychiatry or had retired from such a role, either as university professors, chefs de clinique, institutional or clinic heads, or directors. For the purpose of the analysis I divided them in three generational groups although there is no strict divide. A generational lens seemed a useful frame of reference to consider significant changes in the context of practice and use of ECT over time.[29] The first group comprised the two above-mentioned psychiatrists who trained and started their careers as neuro-psychiatrists in the 1940s and 1950s and recalled the time ECT was widely used. The second group consisted of four psychiatrists who started their specialty training in the 1970s and officially registered as psychiatrists. Their training substantially differed from the former group as it pertained to ECT. During their specialty education ECT was no longer taught as a common part of practice and most of them had never heard about it during their training or learned to see it as something that was outdated. Use of ECT had dwindled and only existed within the margins of professional practice. As public debate over its use heightened during the 1970s, it became increasingly seen as abhorrent, typically no longer done. Therefore, an examination of the way and circumstances in which these psychiatrists did take up ECT illustrates the controversial context in which ECT was maintained. By means of their individual accounts the larger social process of ECT's reappraisal which ran counter to the dominant public view in the late 1970s and 1980s is highlighted. The third group consisted of two psychiatrists who provided leadership nationally in the development of ECT as an accepted part of psychiatric practice during the 1990s. During the 1990s ECT became more explicitly embedded in a culture of evidence-based medicine. While one of these two third group psychiatrists took up ECT in the 1980s at the height of public controversy, and from that viewpoint could be considered part of the second group, I included him into the third because of his engagement with continued professional development

27  Letter from Goos Zwanikken to Leon Vos, March 2011. Upon the interview with Zwanikken about his past experience with ECT as part of this research in February 2011 I received a copy of his letter to Vos on 22 April 2011.
28  Letter from Goos Zwanikken to Leon Vos, March 2011.
29  Cf. McPherson (1996).

of ECT in the 1990s.[30] I interviewed the psychiatrists among other professionals with the goal to understand the history of the continued use of ECT, and
to explore whether and how the context of general hospital psychiatry had
affected that use.[31] In this paper I focus on the way these psychiatrists understood and justified ECT within their practice.

Table 1: Interviewees' medical education, specialty training and career by generation
(in 2011)

| Name | Medical education | Psychiatrist (specialist education) | At interview 2011 |
|---|---|---|---|
| First generation: neuro-psychiatrist | | | |
| Jaap Prick | 1947, Amsterdam | 1947–1951 | 1951–1984 Conservator/Chef de Clinique, Nijmegen, Emeritus |
| Goos Zwanikken | 1952, Amsterdam | 1953–1957 | 1985–1991 Professor of Psychiatry, Nijmegen, Emeritus |
| Second generation: psychiatrist (as of 1972) | | | |
| Willem Nolen | 1973, Leiden | 1974–1978 | 2003 Professor of psychiatry, mood disorders, Groningen |
| Frans Zitman | 1972, Groningen | 1973–1977 | 2000 Professor of biological psychiatry, Leiden |
| Frank Koerselman | Approx. 1974, Amsterdam | 1976–1980 | 1997 Professor of Psychiatry, Utrecht |
| Fons Tholen | Approx. 1975, Groningen | 1976–1982 | 1993 Head of Patient Service, Psychiatric University Clinic, Groningen |
| Third generation/group: psychiatrist as of 1983* [after 'ECT guidelines'] | | | |
| Bas Verwey | 1978, Amsterdam | 1979–1983 | 1984 Head of Psychiatry, General Hospital Rijnstate, Arnhem |
| Walter van den Broek | 1985, Leiden | 1987–1992 | Head of medical education, as of 2015 Professor of evidence-based medical education, Rotterdam |

*Bas Verwey registered as a psychiatrist in 1983, and could be considered in between 2nd
and 3rd 'generation'. He did take up ECT upon his appointment in Arnhem in 1984, but
gained national influence during the 1990s, working closely with Van den Broek in the
Working group ECT Netherlands (WEN) to establish the ECT guideline for the Dutch Association of Psychiatry after 1995. Hence he is included into the third group.

30   See Table 1 for a complete overview.
31   Other professionals included nurses. For a history of ECT from the viewpoint of nurses
     see Boschma (2015); Boschma (in press).

## ECT in the 1950s and 1960s

Jaap Prick and Goos Zwanikken represented the first group, starting their careers in the late 1940s and 1950s when ECT was new and widely applied by the 1950s: "Everywhere they did ECT", Zwanikken confirmed.[32] ECT and other somatic treatments, such as insulin therapy, had generated therapeutic optimism at a time few effective treatments were available. Medical confidence in somatic, that is bodily, treatments had gained momentum in the 1920s, starting with the application of malaria fever treatment and deep sleep therapy. Subsequently, shock treatments with insulin and metrazol were introduced in the 1930s.[33] These treatments generated a comatose state in a patient using insulin, or artificially evoked a convulsion using metrazol, both of which were claimed to have a healing effect. Psychiatrists who introduced these therapies noted them as promising in terms of their treatment potential. Still, they were aware of the risk these therapies also posed.[34] The application of metrazol therapy, for example, was known for the way it could trigger a deep sense of hopelessness and disintegration in patients, sometimes described as near death experience, just before the onset of the convulsion, which caused deep fear. Some suggested that accompanying psychotherapy might mitigate such effects.[35] For similar reasons of risk reduction the use of electricity was seen as an improvement as compared to metrazol therapy, because ECT did not generate a time lag at the start of the convulsion. It seemed to generate less fear in patients and its administration was deemed better manageable.[36] During the 1950s modified use of ECT with application of anesthesia and use of muscle relaxants grew more common, although at that time use of anesthesia still came with considerable risk Zwanikken recalled.[37]

Both Prick and Zwanikken were neuro-psychiatrists. In the 1950s the specialty was viewed as an integrated field of neurology and psychiatry. Although neurology was a central component, psycho-analysis and phenomenological psychiatry became influential as well.[38] Jaap Prick favoured organic views and biomedical explanations of mental illness. He viewed psychiatric disease first and foremost as a "cerebral dysfunction" of an organic nature he explained.[39] Although trained as a psycho-analyst as well, he did not believe in the approach. Treatments were initiated from a somatic point of departure, he noted. Zwanikken was more intrigued by the philosophical angle of psychotherapy. The somatic approaches they learned about during their clinical training were quite a contrast to what they learned about psychiatry in more theoretical ori-

32  Cf. Interview with Zwanikken.
33  Cf. Van der Scheer (1941); Gijswijt-Hofstra et al. (2006); Vijselaar (2013).
34  Cf. Hutter (1941); Van der Horst (1947).
35  Cf. Van der Horst (1947); Cohen Stuart/Zeijlstra (1950). A similar argument was made for other somatic therapies.
36  Cf. Vijselaar (2010), pp. 187–195; Hutter (1941).
37  Cf. Interview with Zwanikken; Binneveld/Wolf (1985), pp. 163–167.
38  Cf. Weijers (2001).
39  Cf. Interview with Prick.

ented lectures Zwanikken recalled: "Those [theory classes] were all about phenomenological philosophy."[40] He also trained as a psycho-analyst in addition
to his specialist training as neuro-psychiatrist. Zwanikken had found these to
be two very distinct areas of practice: "Separate worlds", he recalled.[41] But he
seemed comfortable juggling both. Career-wise Zwanikken made a switch in
1959 when he, somewhat unexpectedly, gave up his position as head-assistant
in a leading university clinic to become Chef de Clinique in the largest mental
hospital in the South of the Netherlands, Voorburg, an institution with close
to 1,400 patients.[42] The career move seemed a step down in the eyes of his
colleagues, particularly the head of the university clinic, Zwanikken recalled;
in the 1950s few registered specialists went to work in mental hospitals he had
found.[43] But the salary was better, he said, and it did seem to give him an additional advantage as a (private practice) psycho-analyst: "In 1959, I was the
first psycho-analyst in the South."[44] By then, the context in which ECT was
commonly applied rapidly changed.

During the 1960s use of ECT dwindled because of the advent of psychotropic medication. "In the 50s new medication became available", Zwanikken noted.[45] He remembered how in 1953 a Belgian specialist in training
introduced chlorpromazine (Largactil) in Utrecht to the Department Head,
Professor Rümke. Prick confirmed: "Yes, because of the medication all that
[use of somatic treatments] changed."[46] Although use of medications had not
been uncommon, the particular quality of the new psychotropic medication
made a substantial difference.[47] It was found to reduce psychotic symptoms
while users remained responsive and alert, making their behaviours more
manageable, and – as it was argued – more open to psychotherapeutic interventions.[48] Others saw psychotropic medications as confirmation of organic
causes. Prick recalled: "I used to consider [the new] medications 'the singing
seed'" of psychiatry. "For me it was a confirmation of the organic nature of
psychiatry. With the medications you finally got to treat organic causes with
chemical measures."[49] Proponents of psychotherapy, however, saw medication

40  Interview with Zwanikken.
41  Zwanikken's commentary seemed to refer in particular to the way inpatient psychiatry
    and psycho-analysis formed two different contexts of practice. See also Abma/Weijers
    (2005), pp. 63–77.
42  The annual report of Voorburg for 1959 listed a total number of 1,368 patients. During
    the years 1951–1966 the institution held its largest patient population of over 1,300 pa-
    tients. Thereafter the number of patients gradually dropped: 1,225 in 1967 and reaching
    1,138 in 1970: Binneveld/Wolf (1985), p. 233. Compared to their Anglo-American coun-
    terparts Dutch 20th century mental hospitals were relatively small institutions.
43  See also Abma/Weijers (2005), p. 96, who note that in the mid-20th century the majority
    of registered specialists did not practice as institutional psychiatrists ("gestichtsartsen").
44  Interview with Zwanikken.
45  Interview with Zwanikken.
46  Interview with Prick.
47  Cf. Pieters/Snelders (2007).
48  Cf. Binneveld/Wolf (1985), pp. 165–166.
49  Interview with Prick.

as a measure to apply psychotherapeutic treatment more effectively.[50] Once use of psychotropic medications spread, the application of ECT decreased. "It became outdated", Zwanikken recalled, "in Voorburg it stopped in the late 1960s. Only sporadically it was applied."[51] Historians Binneveld and Wolf observed how the last ECT treatment in Voorburg took place in 1972.[52] In another psychiatric hospital, Vogelenzang, in the town of Bennebroek, ECT treatment was gradually discontinued in most departments during the 1960s with the last treatments applied in 1973.[53] New and different forms of psychotherapy, such as group therapy, began to dominate the field as did psychological and social explanations of mental illness.[54]

## Polarization in the 1970s and 1980s: ECT and the rise of critical psychiatry

The group framed as the "second generation" psychiatrists began their specialty training in the 1970s at a time psychiatry underwent profound change. Although the use of ECT did not entirely disappear and continued to be practiced, albeit rarely, new trainees in psychiatry were no longer exposed to it as a common part of practice.[55] Divergent explanatory frames of the nature of mental illness took on new meaning. Organic or medical-biological and psychogenetic or psychoanalytic explanations of mental illness were often held in juxtaposition, with the latter gradually growing more prominent. Proponents of the one view could be squarely opposed to those of the other.[56] Tension over "the medical model" – which opponents perceived as too narrowly focused on physiological explanations and organic disease causation or, evenly so, as a refusal to engage relationally with patients – grew during the 1960s and affected the perspective on ECT.[57]

Within this growing critical view on psychiatry, controversy over ECT took a political and activist turn in the 1970s. A critical psychiatric counter-movement emerged, invigorated by a wider counter-cultural critique resist-

---

50  The movie "The Snake Pit" (1948, directed by Anatole Litvak, producers Robert Bassler, Anatole Litvak, and Darryl F. Zanuck; distributed by 20th Century Fox) exemplifies this viewpoint. See also Vijselaar (2013).
51  Interview with Zwanikken.
52  Cf. Binneveld/Wolf (1985), pp. 164–165.
53  Cf. Van Ree: Problemen (1977), p. 594. Psychiatrist Van Ree reported one exception to the discontinuation of ECT in Vogelenzang in 1973. In 1975 one more patient received ECT upon her own explicit request. She had had ECT for depression in the past with good results. Since then ECT was no longer used. Van Ree had collected the information on ECT in response to a survey held by the National Anti-Shock Action 120 Volt (see next section).
54  Cf. Blok (2004).
55  Cf. Interviews with Frank Koerselman by author, 6 July 2011; with Willem Nolen by author, 15 March 2011; with Tholen; with Frans Zitman by author, 17 March 2011.
56  Cf. Abma/Weijers (2005).
57  Cf. Blok (2004), pp. 131–165; Interview with Louise Dols by author, 22 March 2011.

ing traditional hierarchical and paternalistic structures in society, and which increasingly drew public attention to psychiatry.[58] Around 1970 a conflict at Dennendal, an institution for mentally retarded people – then still an integral part of the psychiatric hospitals system – had already placed psychiatry in the public eye. Activist psychologists and staff occupied the institution for some time on the grounds that they resisted authoritarian structures, calling for more authenticity and cultural renewal. The conflict became headline news, causing much political turmoil and police involvement. Counter-cultural views suddenly went public as images and reports were on TV and spread in the news.[59] Soon a social and cultural critique on psychiatry and mental hospitals intensified, shared by counter-culturally minded professionals, students, institutional staff, family members and patients alike.[60] Although by no means a unified group, they resisted the alleged authoritative medical model that seemed antithetical to new psychotherapeutic insights among other points of critique.

An influential spokesperson of the critique was psychiatrist Jan Foudraine, whose widely read book, "Not Made of Wood", was published in 1971.[61] In it he questioned the notion of mental illness, inspired by four and a half years' working as a psychiatrist at the psychoanalytic centre Chestnut Lodge, in Maryland, USA, and subsequently as Chef de Clinique of a new psychotherapeutic centre, Veluweland, in the Netherlands in the mid-1960s. Challenging the idea that people suffering from schizophrenia should be called sick, as the clinical psychiatric model would have it, he argued instead that schizophrenia was better to be understood as an inherent social critique exposing the "insanity" of contemporary society. In isolating people suffering from psychosis in institutions psychiatry had taken the wrong turn, he argued, neglecting the potential psychotherapy offered to engage with them. He was inspired by international ideas on the value of therapeutic communities and an anti-psychiatric critique that already was spreading in the United Kingdom and North America.[62] His view galvanized the anti-psychiatric movement in the Netherlands, bringing it to public attention but also stirring considerable disagreement among his psychiatric colleagues, leaving some vehemently opposed to Foudraine's views, others inspired. Critique on psychiatry also grew from the side of family members and patients who were alarmed about the inadequate care in psychiatric hospitals and a critical patient movement emerged.[63]

---

58   Cf. Blok (2004). In the Anglo-American literature this movement is typically referred to as anti-psychiatry. In the recent Dutch historiography it is more typically referred to as critical psychiatry.
59   Blok (2004), pp. 28–29.
60   Cf. Heerma van Voss (1978); Fox et al. (1983); Blok (2004).
61   Cf. Foudraine (1971).
62   Cf. Foudraine (1971); Blok (2004). A similar critique in the US was voiced by Szasz (1961) among others.
63   Corrie van Eijk-Osterholt became an advocate for her hospitalized sister in the late 1950s. She published a book on her experiences and her leading role in the emerging

Around 1970 the demarcation of the professional field of psychiatry also changed. The fields of neurology and psychiatry, traditionally merged into one field of neuro-psychiatry, increasingly grew apart, with each area focusing on different types of diseases and diagnoses. Despite intra-professional tension over the relationship between the two areas, a formal split of the field into two separate specialties between the fields took place in the early 1970s.[64] The qualification of "neuro-psychiatrist" discontinued and psychiatry became a specialty on its own. Because psychotherapeutic approaches and psychosocial explanations of mental illness began to dominate psychiatry, the traditional link to neurology as an integrated field of neuro-psychiatry changed. When in 1972 a new registration law for medical specialists was enacted, registrants had to indicate whether they registered for one field or the other, which particularly among older practitioners was cause for considerable resistance.[65] The second generation interviewees, however, all trained after this change was enacted and they registered as psychiatrists.

A final influence of note on the changing field of psychiatry was the increasing use of psychotropic medication. It expanded the scope of the field with a new emphasis on biological psychiatry, envisioned, however, as a sub-field of psychiatry. In the academic hospital in Groningen, for example, Professor van Dijk, a prototypical psycho-analyst, who became head of psychiatry in 1963, supported the development of biological psychiatry.[66] He might have anticipated the relevance of this new sub-specialty to underpin use of new medications. In 1966 he appointed Herman van Praag as one of the first professors in this new area. In his new role Van Praag started biomedical research on depression, but he also maintained ECT treatment at the academic hospital's psychiatric clinic in Groningen, which he occasionally applied.[67] When Van Praag left in 1977 his successor also occasionally performed ECT and hence Groningen was one of the places where ECT never disappeared, even though few people were aware the treatment still existed and it was only rarely applied.[68] Due to the dominance of psychodynamic psychiatry the expansion of biological psychiatry was met with ambivalence, which was a noticeable influence on the careers of the second group of interviewees.

family and patient movement: Van Eijk-Osterholt (1972); Hunsche (2008), pp. 19–20; Heerma van Voss (1978).

64   Cf. Abma/Weijers (2005), pp. 94–99, 104–106, 178–179. Formal regulation of medical specialties, established in 1961 with the registry coming into force in 1972, triggered tension because criteria for registration as either neuro-psychiatrist, neurologist or psychiatrist had to be determined. By 1972 neurology and psychiatry were formalized into separate specialties, whereas registration as neuro-psychiatrist discontinued.

65   Cf. Abma/Weijers (2005), p. 156; Blok (2004).

66   Cf. Interviews with Tholen, Nolen, and Zitman.

67   Cf. Van Praag (1980); Interview with Nolen; Interview with Dols. For an analysis of nurses' involvement in ECT see Boschma (2015).

68   Van Praag's successor, Rudi van den Hoofdakker, occasionally applied ECT. Cf. Interviews with Dols and Tholen.

Adherents of the critical psychiatric movement began to organize, rally-
ing not only for better service, but also for more democratic structures and
assertion of patient rights. Many new patient organizations, self-help groups,
and alternative facilities sprung up, forming a vocal patients' movement whose
interests often intertwined with those of students in hospitals and university
psychiatric clinics dissatisfied with their training conditions. The groups interconnected in protests and action, which took multiple forms, including rallies,
petitions, and media involvement.[69] A Dutch movie on psychiatry was featured in the Netherlands in February 1975, just months prior to the première
of "One Flew" in the summer of 1975. The Dutch movie, entitled "Kind van
de Zon" ("Child of the Sun"), included a scene in which the main character
was subjected to ECT in its unmodified form.[70] In combination the films drew
considerable public attention to ECT with commentary in the newspapers
and on TV.

A few years prior, in 1973/74 the journal *Gekkenkrant* (The Mad News) had
been founded with the goal to serve as a platform for psychiatric critique and
a forum for (ex-)patients to freely voice their opinion and mobilize them into
action. When the latter went slower than anticipated out of this group a more
radical initiative emerged. In 1976, members of this group deliberately chose
ECT as a focus of their political action. Set up in parallel with the *Gekkenkrant*
but also as a distinct organization, the National Anti-Shock Action 120 Volt
(NASA) was launched that year and spread throughout 1977.[71] Activism by
this group centred on biological psychiatry which was seen as representing
the alleged repugnant "medical model", and ECT was being targeted as an essential symbol of the critique. The group took example from similar activism
in California among other states in the USA, and purposefully focused their
protest on ECT as a means to make their point.[72] Their publications about the
alleged widespread use of ECT in mental hospitals, particularly as a method
of discipline and punishment, stirred public debate and provoked further action. Also among psychiatrists many were of the opinion that adequate use
of psychotherapy had made ECT redundant.[73] A talk show on the damaging
effects of ECT broadcasted on TV in 1977 further sparked public awareness,
which already had been heightened by the 1975 movies. Professionals, activists, and patients joined into protesting the use of ECT.[74] As a proponent of
biological psychiatry, Van Praag became target of protest as well; at a sympo-

---

69  Cf. Heerma van Voss (1978).
70  Cf. Blok (2004), p. 34.
71  Cf. Blok (2004), pp. 173–182; Speciaal Voor U (1977).
72  Cf. Commentary from Flip Schrameijer, sociologist and former editorial member of the
    *Gekkenkrant*, 28 March 2011, Utrecht (seminar, notes by author); *Gekkenkrant* (The Mad
    News), nos. 20 and 22 (1977).
73  Cf. Van Ree: Problemen (1977); Van Ree: Als Voorstander (1977); Van der Post (1977);
    Blok (2004).
74  Activists included academics, ex-patients and professionals: Heerma van Voss (1978);
    Fox et al. (1983). Interview with Fried van de Ven and Joke Zwanikken-Leenders by
    author, 19 April 2011.

sium organized at the occasion of his appointment as a professor of biological psychiatry at the University of Utrecht in 1977, a smoke-bomb was thrown into the lecture hall and the police was called in. In his case activism centred on his alleged authoritarian response to students who wanted more input in their education and disagreed with his biomedical focus.[75]

ECT became an explicit object of NASA activism. During a week of organized national actions and demonstrations, for example, activists rallied at the gates of hospitals where ECT was still conducted. The NASA also surveyed hospitals to find out at which ones ECT was still conducted and it then published a "blacklist" of psychiatrists who continued to perform ECT.[76] Opinions and responses among psychiatrists were divided. Some, such as psychiatrist Van Ree, publicly agreed with the NASA action, affirming ECT was an outdated form. Once the blacklist was published only very few came out in support of ECT, although some did, beginning to publicly offer a counter-response – pointing out that the treatment could have good results.[77] A rally at the gates of the municipal hospital in Arnhem, in June 1977 formed a case in point. A local committee of the NASA action, consisting of members of the Patient League, former and current psychiatric patients of mental hospitals, and practitioners, such as a group of psychiatric nurses from the nearby Wolfheze mental hospital, assembled at the gate of the Arnhem municipal hospital demanding to stop ECT. Posted under a banner stating "Danger: Shock – Watch Out", they handed out flyers informing the public that ECT was still happening in this hospital and provided information on its damaging effects. The action was headline news in the local papers.[78]

Thomas Kraft, head of psychiatry at the Arnhem municipal hospital, was one of the few psychiatrists who took a stance against the hostility and began to openly advocate in support of ECT. Although one of the ones targeted in the NASA blacklist, a week after the rally at the gates of the hospital in Arnhem he offered a counter-point in one of the newspapers: "A Patient Can Really Recover with ECT" its headline read. In the article, Kraft pointed out how ECT was a preferred treatment above use of anti-depressants in some cases, especially for those patients who did not respond well to medications. He spoke out in favour of ECT, and explained how he regularly had used the treatment effectively over the last years. In taking this public stand, Kraft was trying to use openness about the therapy as a way to counter the critique. He stressed that in its contemporary, modified form ECT was applied with use of anesthetic and muscle relaxants, very different from the way it was portrayed in the NASA actions and in the media. He argued against abandonment of ECT because of its clinical effectiveness in some cases, in which it had really

---

75   Cf. Blok (2004), pp. 182–185.
76   Cf. Blok (2004); Speciaal Voor U (1977).
77   Cf. Van Ree: Problemen (1977); Kraft (1978); Kroft (1977).
78   Cf. GZ zet Shockbehandeling (1977); Shock-Gevaar (1977); Heerma van Voss (1978).

helped people.[79] His colleague Kroft, director of a nearby mental hospital, was among the few who publicly articulated a similar opinion in favour of ECT.[80]

Invigorated by the forceful debates in the media and professional journals, members of municipal parliaments raised critical questions, but also in the national parliament questions were raised, seeking political support to abandon the treatment.[81] In offering a counter-argument, however, Kraft had helped to set off a counterpoint in the public debate. Gradually other psychiatrists, such as Harry Rooijmans, professor of psychiatry in Leiden, who did not share the idea that ECT should be abandoned, also began to defend the use of ECT as a treatment that might be beneficial in some cases.[82] In a publication in the *Dutch Journal of Medicine* he stayed on the side of caution, but basically supported the point of view that ECT should not be withheld from severely depressed patients who might benefit from it and to be held on as a treatment option. Still, unlike Kraft, it did not seem he conducted ECT himself. Rather, in his commentary he referenced the international professional literature confirming the efficacy of ECT. Potential benefits should be carefully weighed against the risks, he offered, as every patient and case was unique. The then known facts about the therapy did not justify "the current negative publicity surrounding ECT", Rooijmans argued, although ECT still "would be a therapy one would not turn to easily. It certainly has been misused in the past", he noted.[83] He found it difficult to judge whether or not misuse might still occur, but it certainly should not be a reason to withhold the therapy from patients who would really need it, he pointed out.[84] Therefore, he hoped reason would win from "emotionally coloured publicity".[85] Very much along the lines Kraft and Kroft had outlined, the Dutch Association of Psychiatry articulated a statement in 1978 that ECT should remain available albeit under

---

79   Cf. Psychiater dr. Th. B. Kraft (1977). Kroft had made a similar point as Kraft in a public statement and suggested the establishment of an advisory committee on ECT to provide a national guideline: Kroft (1977).

80   Cf. Kroft (1977); Rooijmans (1978).

81   Cf. Kraft (1978); Kroft (1977); Rooijmans (1978); Van Ree: Problemen (1977).

82   Cf. Rooijmans (1978).

83   Rooijmans (1978), quote from p. 1671. In this article Rooijmans did not provide a source for his statement about past misuse. Whereas Rooijmans referred to "misuse in the past", his contemporary colleague, Lit noted in 1973, in a review of the (then) published scientific evidence on ECT, how, in the 1950s, ECT might have been used "too often, without critical thought and even as a measure to correct behaviour" ["te veel, kritiekloos en zelfs gedrags-corrigerend toegediend", translation GB]: Lit (1973), p. 56. As such inappropriate past use of ECT was mentioned in contemporary psychiatric literature and acknowledged by contemporaries, however, similar to Kraft (1978) and Kroft (1977), both Lit and Rooijmans did argue that such past misuse should not be a reason to completely abolish ECT because in some situations of severe depression ECT had proven to be beneficial and more effective than medication. See Lit (1973) and Rooijmans (1978).

84   Cf. Rooijmans (1978).

85   Rooijmans (1978), quote from p. 1671.

strict conditions.[86] In response to the questioning in parliament, in 1979, the state secretary of health ordered a formal advice on ECT from the National Health Council, a governmental advisory board, which included members of the medical profession, and an advisory committee was formed.[87]

In 1983, the National Health Council presented its conclusions: They advised in support of ECT suggesting the therapy should remain available, albeit under stringent restrictions – only as a last measure after other treatments, such as medications, had been proven futile. It also should be provided within proper, well equipped settings, and be based on informed consent and proper protocol. By 1985 the state government confirmed support of these guidelines and assigned the State Medical Inspectorate of Mental Health the task to set up a national registration system to track ECT.[88] The number of treatments had dropped considerably by then. Reportedly, nationally the number of ECT treatments was about 50 a year by the end of the 1970s.[89] While the new guidelines put in place restrictions, in a sense they also acknowledged ECT as an acceptable treatment even if under strict conditions.[90] Although actions and protests continued for some time, medical interest in ECT also began to expand again in the late 1980s.

### Renewed interest in ECT in the midst of controversy

As such, the second group of psychiatrists trained in the 1970s took their medical education and specialty training under very different circumstances and viewpoints around ECT.[91] Indeed, this group had learned to see it as an outdated practice and some had never heard about ECT during their medical education. The circumstances prompting their initial involvement with ECT or their shift in opinion about it provide insight in the way ECT was reconsidered in the 1980s, in part in response to the critique, but also due to a new appraisal and justification of its use.

Willem Nolen's interest in ECT developed in 1978. In that year, he was appointed as a psychiatrist at Parnassia Hospital.[92] The medical director at Parnassia "wanted to put the institution on the map", Nolen recalled, and

---

86   Rooijmans (1978), p. 1669.
87   Cf. Legemaate (1985); Rooijmans (1978). Then state secretary of health was Mrs. Veder-Smit. The committee included representation from all stake-holder groups, including opponents as well as proponents of ECT.
88   Cf. Legemaate (1985).
89   Cf. Nolen (1999), p. 6; Blok (2004), p. 174.
90   Cf. Legemaate (1985), p. 397; Gezondheidsraad (1983); Geneeskundige Inspectie voor de Geestelijke Volksgezondheid (GIGV) (1985); Interview with Annemiek Koster by author, 16 June 2011.
91   See Table 1 for an overview of the four psychiatrists comprising the second generation group.
92   Cf. Nolen (1999); the hospital's original name was Bloemendaal Hospital near The Hague, and was later subsumed under Parnassia.

proposed to establish a unit for biological psychiatry of which Nolen became head.[93] To expand his knowledge in this area, Nolen was supported to take a leave for a study trip to Denmark. Only then he became intrigued by the potential of the therapy. Prior to his Denmark trip Nolen had never heard from the "modern" way of doing ECT, with anesthesia and muscle relaxants. During his medical studies in Leiden (1966–1973) he had not learned about ECT, whereas in Parnassia, where he took his specialty training (1974–1978), all he had noticed was some older colleagues still occasionally conducting ECT, unmodified. His supervisor, however, had advised him that the treatment was outmoded and so he had never considered doing it.[94] In Denmark "I saw ECT applied in its modern form", Nolen said, and he was exposed to new research on the approach.[95] The modern application inspired him, and the way its use was supported by research had a lasting impact on his view: "I became convinced of the usefulness of ECT and found it surprising that the treatment had almost disappeared in the Netherlands, or, if it was applied – in the hospital where I worked – it was done in such an outmoded way."[96] Rather than appraising ECT based on its clinical effect alone, Nolen became motivated to also conduct empirical research on ECT for treatment of depression in the new unit at Parnassia, applied in its modern, modified form. He carefully took notice of the debate on ECT guidelines that was evolving in the Netherlands, suggesting a treatment protocol in which ECT would be used after anti-depressants had been tried.[97]

The public and political climate, however, was not conducive to Nolen's plans. Only through cautious networking and seeking review for his study protocol from peers and the State Medical Inspectorate of Mental Health was he able to proceed with research. Nolen's plans soon became target of political activism, and his research was questioned. Upon the opening of the new unit for biological psychiatry at Parnassia in 1980, the Mobile Police Unit had to provide assistance to protect the grounds and facilitate the opening ceremony by the state secretary of health. Nolen continued to follow the national debate on ECT. He also engaged in discussion with some members of the Council's advisory committee on ECT, among others with psychiatrist Van Ree, who had joined the committee while taking a stance against ECT. In a public statement in 1977 Van Ree supported NASA's call for prohibiting ECT, but upon further study of the literature, a review of clinical records in his home institution, and likely being exposed to other views within the committee, he changed his mind taking a dramatic turn in position.[98] Nolen and Van Ree decided to jointly publish two review articles on the efficacy and

---

93  Interview with Nolen.
94  Cf. Nolen (1999), p. 4.
95  Cf. Interview with Nolen; Nolen (1999), p. 4.
96  Nolen (1999), p. 5.
97  Cf. Interview with Nolen; Nolen (1999).
98  His initial stance against ECT is published in Van Ree: Problemen (1977); Van Ree: Als Voorstander (1977).

ethics of ECT respectively, arguing in support of maintaining ECT as a treatment option.[99] Nolen made sure he was among the audience when the advice from the National Health Council (1983) was discussed in state parliament in 1984.[100] To indicate how controversial the climate around ECT had become, in the interview Nolen explained out how colleagues from the Psychiatric Clinic in Groningen had been hesitant to publish several articles they had prepared on ECT's effectiveness and side-effects out of fear for negative publicity.[101] At a symposium on ECT hosted in Groningen in 1984, shortly before the report of the National Health Council was discussed in parliament, police was called in for assistance.[102] When, a year later, at the occasion of the publication of the governmental guidelines, Nolen hosted a conference on ECT in Parnassia with all stakeholders involved, including the hospital's patient council, a smoke-bomb was thrown into the conference centre and police was involved as well.[103]

Fons Tholen first learned to conduct ECT when he was appointed as psychiatrist at the Psychiatric Clinic in Groningen in 1982. ECT had never been discontinued in that clinic, he confirmed, but it was rarely applied.[104] While he was working at the same clinic during his training as psychiatrist some years prior, he had not been involved with the therapy at all, he recalled. Conducting ECT he learned from Van Praag's successor, Rudi van den Hoofdakker. In the early 1980s he became part of a group who started a retrospective dossier review to begin to look at ECT outcomes, also with the view to begin to establish a research base on ECT. Eventually the Groningen group engaged with a larger national study on ECT, once systematic registration of the treatment was set up and treatment protocols began to be formalized in the mid-1980s after the government had issued guidelines in 1985, Tholen recalled.[105] Political as much as scientific reasons triggered new interest in ECT research.

A clinical influence prompting renewed interest in ECT were disappointing experiences with the new anti-depressants, in that sometimes suicide risk increased during the time it took for such medications to take effect, which typically was several weeks. Increase in suicide rates, particularly in cases of acute depression was an important reason to reconsider the application of ECT. In cases of acute depression ECT worked much faster according to psychiatrists who remembered its effect.[106] It also could be effective in other situations of rapid deterioration of a patient's status. Tholen, for example,

99   Cf. Nolen/Van Ree (1982); Van Ree/Nolen (1982).
100  Cf. Interview with Nolen.
101  Cf. Nolen (1999), p. 5.
102  Cf. Interviews with Nolen and Dols.
103  Cf. Interview with Nolen.
104  Interview with Tholen.
105  Interview with Tholen.
106  Interview with Zwanikken. Koerselman described how witnessing the rapid, positive effect of ECT on one of his patients made a strong impression and contributed to his shift in opinion about ECT: Koerselman/Smeets (1992).

vividly recalled one patient's rapid improvement: "I remember one patient",
he noted, "who just laid in bed, looking at the ceiling [...], in catatonic stupor.
After the ECT he walked again, across the hall, looking at the paintings."[107]
Zwanikken confirmed, "you had to see it."[108] Zwanikken in fact revised his
earlier, 1970s view on ECT as an outdated mode of treatment because of
disappointing experiences with anti-depressants. After he had experienced
some devastating outcomes of cases in which patients on anti-depressants had
committed suicide, he was ready to reintroduce ECT in Voorburg. But even
raising the idea provoked a storm of protest.[109] It was not until 1985, upon
his appointment as professor of psychiatry in Nijmegen, that he was able to
reinstate ECT at the Radboud University Hospital, likely also encouraged
by the new governmental guidelines which had been accepted by that time.
Still, his initiative caused heated debate and public action, also in Nijmegen.
One activist placed an obituary of the new professor in the local newspaper.
Zwanikken recalled how he had police involved to investigate the source of
this threat to make sure it did not come from within the clinic, which it did
not.[110] A critical group in Nijmegen, The Nuts Foundation, organized a public
debate on "The return of ECT", which drew over 200 attendants. Protests
held on throughout the 1980s.[111]

Starting or continuing to apply ECT in the 1980s was therefore a complex
process, which Bas Verwey also discovered when he took up practice as head
of psychiatry in Arnhem in 1984, succeeding Thomas Kraft who had never
given up on using ECT in his practice. ECT had not been a topic of interest
during Verwey's training as psychiatrist in Leiden. His education had included
one session on ECT, Verwey recalled, but it was introduced mostly as a practice of the past, perhaps still done in certain places, but without any suggestion that it would have much relevance for their current practice.[112] Harry
Rooijmans, his professor in Leiden who taught the session, may have felt
compelled to familiarize his students at least with the concept. As mentioned,
Rooijmans had been one of the few psychiatrists who had made a nuanced
statement in support of ECT at the height of public controversy and published
on the matter in 1978, right after the NASA actions.[113] Five years later, in
1983, the year Verwey registered as a psychiatrist, and the year in which the
National Health Council had formulated their official advice on ECT, Rooijmans commented, likely with some relief that his view was supported: "ECT
cleared from blame (?)."[114] Within this context, the session he offered the
students may indeed have been one in which he shared his views on the rele-
vancy of the therapy, but perhaps also assuming that it rarely would be used.

107 Interview with Tholen.
108 Interview with Zwanikken.
109 Cf. Binneveld/Wolf (1985), pp. 216–218.
110 Cf. Interview with Zwanikken.
111 Cf. Legemaate (1985), p. 397; 'Terugkeer van de Elektroshock' (1986).
112 Interview with Bas Verwey by Joost Vijselaar and Josef Vos, 22 November 2006.
113 Cf. Rooijmans (1978).
114 Rooijmans (1983).

Kraft on the other hand, who Verwey was to succeed, was one of the psychiatrists who had hands-on experience with performing ECT. As noted above, Kraft had spoken publicly in support of ECT, pointing to its usefulness in severe cases of depression. In the newspaper interview conducted in response to the public action against him, he carefully laid out ECT's potential benefits drawing on his own experience with the therapy. In another publication in a professional journal he confirmed his standpoint with reference to the international scientific literature in support of ECT, and was known among colleagues for still practicing it.[115] Kraft received referrals from around the country, Verwey recalled.[116]

Kraft was very much interested to transfer his skill to Verwey, who had never thought of the possibility of learning to do ECT before he arrived. On the day Verwey was going to be introduced to his practice, Kraft had scheduled patients for ECT on the morning of Verwey's arrival. "First thing Kraft said when I walked in on my first day", Verwey recalled, was: "'let's just first do the ECT. Have you ever seen that?' 'No', I answered, 'I have never seen it.'"[117] Verwey remembered: "He said, just put on your white coat. We went to a treatment room where typically one or two patients would be shocked. The head nurse was already standing by and the anesthetist entered the room as well, to give the anesthetic right there in the treatment room. Then we did ECT."[118] Likely aware that there might be the possibility Verwey would object to this training, Kraft did ask him whether he had any objection. "I did not", Verwey remembered, "but I also never had imagined this would happen." Verwey's surprise likely reflected the way ECT still was anathema in the early 1980s, most often not a therapy a new practitioner might consider doing. More likely, they would consider it one that was "no longer done". Verwey knew about ECT though, and was prepared to take a stand: "I did not object to it, because my father was neuro-psychiatrist, and he had done ECT. He often had told me how he thought it was a useful treatment, and had been able to effectively help quite a few patients that way."[119] Still, Verwey also realized he did not have the knowledge, and therefore did express some hesitance when Kraft asked him if he wanted to learn ECT: "I said, well, I can't just push the button, can't I?" But Kraft had scheduled ample time, "and so we did it together. He instructed me on which button to push, and how to handle it thereafter."[120] On his first day, Verwey had performed ECT.

Despite Kraft's support and initial training, however, once Verwey went about applying ECT on his own following Kraft's retirement, he did run into difficulties – there simply was not much information available on how to best apply the therapy. Verwey was clearly socialized differently about ECT than

115  Kraft (1978).
116  Interview with Verwey.
117  Interview with Verwey.
118  Interview with Verwey.
119  Interview with Verwey.
120  Interview with Verwey.

his predecessor and likely because of the existing controversy over ECT he felt unsure he was doing the right thing, or rather, whether he was doing things right. He soon encountered a problem. He discovered the hard way that the equipment Kraft had handed down to him seemed outdated and no longer safe to use. He first noticed he was dealing with an outdated machine while conducting ECT on a patient, and the machine failed – equally threatening was the response from the technician he had called in for assistance. The technician not only condemned the equipment right away, but also took the machine to the desk of the hospital director, pointing out to Verwey that he was not supposed to use this equipment anymore and should not even conduct ECT. It seemed the technician was aware ECT had become controversial and did not think using the machine was appropriate. Verwey likely was well aware the incident could threaten his reputation and so he felt somewhat in a panic when he contacted Kraft for advice. Kraft's response subsided his immediate fear: "Kraft said, yes, there still is a brand new machine in the closet – I bought it once when we had some extra money available and it hasn't been used. Unbelievable – fantastic." The relief Verwey must have felt still came through in his words. At least for the immediate moment, Verwey was able to retain his reputation (and control) as a psychiatrist practising ECT. He continued to treat patients and resisted the technician's response suggesting he should no longer do this. He even found the local dealer of Siemens, the company where the machine had been bought – a Siemens Konvulsator – although getting the most recent user instructions was not easy either. The company's initial response also was that these machines were no longer used, but then they did provide Verwey with a user guide.

Siemens Konvulsators were indeed used in several institutions in the Netherlands, but more commonly used was the Elther machine, produced since the early 1940s by a Dutch engineering company Cohen Stuart N. V. Electro Medische Apparaten (Electro Medical Equipment). This company had designed the first Elther machine in close collaboration with the psychiatrists who first conducted ECT in the 1940s, and thereafter the company regularly had produced new versions of the Elther machine, adapting to new technological and professional insights on how the therapy could best be performed. Into the 1970s this was the most commonly used machine in the Netherlands although demand for it had dropped severely once use of medication had gained momentum.[121] Verwey did get the Siemens machine to work though, and worked with it for a number of years. He likely also obtained the support from the hospital director.

Still, having resolved the immediate problem and delving into the literature about ECT did not relieve Verwey from a deeper worry that he needed more knowledge and more assurance the equipment and procedure was adequate: "I thought, oh dear, what am I doing here?"[122] In hindsight he com-

---

121 Cf. De Valk (2009), pp. 5–6. For a history of ECT machines until the 1950s see also Gawlich (2018).
122 Interview with Verwey.

mented: "The machine and the way it was done still lacked a certain level of sophistication, [the idea] that you would simply adjust the machine and then it was supposed to work well – I found that a bit over the top, actually ... and, of course, I began to read about it."[123] Although Kraft had given him all the literature he had gathered on the topic, and which had been a good start, in subsequent years Verwey began to expand his knowledge, orient himself on newer equipment and started to network with other colleagues more openly, nationally and internationally. He became aware that in several other countries ECT was more widely applied. In the Netherlands however, the context was still tense, and Verwey did not know much about who else conducted ECT. There was a risk involved in being open about it, he conveyed in the interview.[124] When asked who else might have applied ECT at that time, he somewhat hesitantly noted, "... [in] Vlissingen maybe, [...] and in Groningen perhaps – but they were not very public about it. Nobody advertised such things at that time", he stated. He then mentioned how Nolen had started to do ECT in Parnassia, but he reiterated: "[but] I did not know that at that time."[125] Few psychiatrists had up-to-date skills, and therefore, psychiatrists like Nolen and Verwey who were motivated to continue ECT, had to carefully build their proficiency and knowledge on the newer insights by networking, reading and building connections.

Verwey recalled how he attended several international conferences and was able to network with colleagues also interested to orient themselves on international developments, which boosted his confidence. In the late 1980s he attended an international conference in Athens where he met Max Finck, one of the leading American scholars on ECT, who then invited him to visit, which he indeed did in the early 1990s.[126] He found Finck's work most helpful. In 1992 he attended the first European symposium on ECT and also began to publish on the performance of ECT in his own hospital.[127] From the 1990s onwards Verwey became a national leader himself on the development of general hospital psychiatry and ECT. In 1991 he was appointed member and later chair of the section on general hospital psychiatry within the Dutch Association of Psychiatry. Soon he also networked with a colleague in Amsterdam to further consolidate his expertise in ECT. This colleague, Willem Wennegar, was interested to start using ECT in his practice in the Valerius Clinic in Amsterdam. Verwey recalled how he went on a study trip to the US in the early 1990s with Wennegar where they visited several ECT Centres and took an accredited ECT course.[128] Verwey then made a point of also visiting a supplier of ECT machines available in the US. He learned about the North-American models Thymatron and MECTA. From the late 1980s

---

123 Interview with Verwey.
124 Interview with Verwey.
125 Interview with Verwey.
126 Interview with Verwey.
127 Cf. Verwey (1991); Verwey (1992).
128 Interview with Verwey.

onwards, when application of ECT increased again in the Netherlands the latter models were the most commonly used.[129] Likely their visit was made at the time when three hospitals in Amsterdam considered to re-introduce ECT.[130] Similar to Nolen, Verwey and Wennegar sought consultation through international contacts.

Frans Zitman and Frank Koerselman did in fact not engage with ECT until the late 1980s, quite some time after the start of their careers as psychiatrists and after the formal governmental guidelines on ECT had been issued. Zitman became head of the psychiatric outpatient clinic at the Leiden University Hospital upon his registration as psychiatrist in 1977. In 1984 he was appointed associated professor in biological psychiatry at the same university.[131] ECT was not practiced in Leiden. Verwey who had trained and practiced in Leiden as well, had the same experience. Zitman first encountered actual performance of ECT when he was appointed as a new professor of biological psychiatry in Nijmegen in 1988. He learned ECT from Zwanikken's team in Nijmegen. Local circumstances were a crucial influence on the process of reappraising ECT in the 1980s. As Verwey's comments also indicated, awareness of who else in the country might perform ECT was minimal and not necessarily publicly shared because of the controversial status of ECT. During his training as psychiatrist he had never been exposed to it, but working in Nijmegen where Zwanikken had re-introduced ECT shifted Zitman's views. "I was evidence-based avant la lettre", he mentioned, "you have to do what works. I had looked at the literature", he said, "and thought it was a useful treatment."[132] By then Nijmegen's clinical environment in psychiatry indeed fostered the use of ECT again.[133] This change in context also affected Koerselman.

Koerselman became involved with ECT in 1988 as well. In that year the regional inspector of mental health in the province of North-Holland contacted several groups of psychiatrists in Amsterdam to consider reintroducing ECT as a treatment option, as it was no longer offered anywhere in the province. Koerselman joined an ECT steering group that was formed and membership in that group helped him to reframe his perspective on ECT. Another decisive influence on his shift in perspective was a clinical experience with one of his patients he experienced during this time. The patient who suffered from a severe psychotic depression with delusions of being dead refused any

---

129 Cf. De Valk (2009), p. 20. An in-depth examination of ECT machine manufacturing and promotion is beyond the scope of this paper; comparison of industrial manufacturing of ECT machines vis-à-vis pharmaceutically produced anti-depressants also needs further research beyond the scope of this paper. The expansion of pharmaceutical interest in psychiatry has been examined by Healy (2012). Both therapies intersect with medical prescription practices.

130 Cf. Koerselman/Smeets (1992).

131 Cf. Interview with Zitman.

132 Interview with Zitman; Zitman (1991).

133 About a decade later Zitman reinstated ECT at Leiden University, upon appointment as professor in 2000.

form of treatment while his health rapidly deteriorated. The patient was transferred to a hospital in Rotterdam where he received ECT, which Koerselman had a chance to witness. Once he observed the rapid improvement of the patient, he realized his negative view on ECT had been unfounded.[134]

An autobiographical account of his engagement with ECT in Amsterdam he co-published with a colleague in 1992 illuminated how his engagement with ECT in the late 1980s was indeed a process of reappraisal of ECT, a shift from his previous perspective imbued with anti-psychiatric critique. After joining the steering group and having witnessed the way ECT had improved the condition of his desperately ill patient, his view changed from considering ECT as a symbol of undue medical power, as he had learned during the 1970s, to one in which not considering ECT was in fact seen as an undue acceptance of medical powerlessness preventing psychiatrists from seeing ECT as a potential healing tool and making them complicit in withholding severely depressed patients from available treatment. Once he had shifted his view in this way, such powerlessness could be condemned as a false stance, doing more harm than good in case of encountering patients with severe depression, because it effectively held psychiatrists back from applying ECT.[135] Partaking in the ECT reintroduction process thus instilled him with motivation to learn and incorporate ECT in his practice.

From the accounts of the second group of interviewees it seemed the 1980s was a pertinent period of transformation of ECT practice. On the one hand ECT was a target of protest, whereas on the other it became an object of re-evaluation as a potentially useful procedure with efficacy in some cases. In combination the interviewees' comments suggest that reliance on published evidence, quiet persistence informed by clinical experience, that is, continued exposure to patients desperately suffering from severe depression not easily resolved by any other means, and professional and international networking were essential influences in laying the foundation for a new acceptance of ECT. Furthermore, even though throughout the 1980s ECT continued to provoke protest, affirmation resulting from a cautious, yet positive governmental advice on ECT confirmed in 1984 and issued as official governmental guideline a year later, held considerable authority, and spurred renewed interest in ECT.[136]

Involvement of the State Medical Inspectorate of Mental Health further added to a context of acceptance of ECT. Still, analysis of the interviews suggests that one other influence was of crucial importance in shifting the practice around ECT in the late 1980s. The emerging policy pressure to provide scientific evidence in resolving questions or problems of professional practice gained momentum during the second half of the 20th century and seemed another crucial factor in the way psychiatrists began to support continued

---

134 Cf. Koerselman/Smeets (1992), p. 133.
135 Cf. Koerselman/Smeets (1992), pp. 132–133.
136 Cf. Legemaate (1985); Nolen (1985); Koerselman/Smeets (1992); Interviews with Nolen, Tholen, Zitman, and Verwey.

use of ECT with new research evidence. Empirical research on ECT as of the mid-1980s also contributed to the stabilization of ECT.

## Evolving research on ECT as of the mid-1980s and into the 1990s

By the late 1980s a habit of conducting empirical research to support the efficacy of ECT by scientific means and evidence began to be taken up to justify the incorporation of ECT as an acceptable part of psychiatric practice. It could be argued that this shift was part of a wider social change in which strategic processes of objectification and quantification or standardization according to a protocol began to structure and underpin professional practice and governmental and political decision-making, also in matters of health and medicine.[137] Dutch psychiatrists began to add empirical studies on ECT to the international professional literature, using statistical methods to demonstrate efficacy based on outcomes, scores on depression scales for example, borrowed from approaches in clinical psychology and other fields in the social sciences.[138]

Embracing empirical studies grounded in statistical analysis was a new phenomenon in psychiatry in the late 20th century, according to Harry Rooijmans, who in 2007 reflected on the evolution of scientific research in psychiatry by looking back on his own career.[139] When he entered the field of psychiatry at the University of Groningen in the mid-1960s "psychiatry was predominantly a literary, philosophical (phenomenological) subject", he noted, "systematic, empirical research to test hypotheses was only emerging in the periphery of the field."[140] The beginning research climate in Groningen in the 1960s seemed to have been inspiring to him. In his reflection he mentioned Van Praag's dissertation on Monoamine Oxidase Inhibitors (anti-depressants) in 1962, later appointed in Groningen as professor in biological psychiatry, and the epidemiologically oriented dissertation research of Rob Giel in 1965, who later became a lead professor in social psychiatry in Groningen, as examples of new steps towards a more empirically based psychiatry. Within biological psychiatry empirical approaches began to be used to study the therapeutic efficacy of pharmacological interventions as Van Praag's example illustrated.[141]

---

137 Cf. Bolt (2015), pp. 67–85; Abma/Weijers (2005), p. 173; Sadowsky (2017).
138 Up until the 1980s literature reviews and reports on ECT by Dutch psychiatrists typically referenced international literature, but few Dutch studies existed prior to the 1980s: Kraft (1978); Rooijmans (1978); Nolen (1999). On the rise of empirical studies in psychiatry see also: Abma/Weijers (2005), pp. 173–175; Rooijmans (2007).
139 Cf. Rooijmans (2007).
140 Rooijmans (2007), quote from pp. 10–11.
141 Rooijmans (2007). Exploring the emergence of advice, exchange of information and collaboration between pharmaceutical companies and psychiatrists in developing strategies and approaches to medication use and prescription was beyond the scope of this paper. Binneveld/Wolf (1985), p. 166, report however how Voorburg's director Woltring

As such, the new studies on the efficacy of ECT in the 1980s could be interpreted as exemplars of this newer trend. I will discuss two examples of this development in the 1980s with regard to ECT. The first is the clinical study on ECT conducted by Nolen, which resulted in his PhD dissertation published in 1986.[142] A second example is a study on experiences of practitioners, patients and family members with ECT set up under the auspices of the State Medical Inspectorate of Mental Health in 1987 and coordinated by Annemiek Koster.[143] Koster oversaw the Inspectorate's voluntary ECT registration system established following the 1985 governmental guidelines on ECT and she was invited to also coordinate the study.[144] Especially the latter study had meaning beyond the statistical outcomes. It also was a case example of a community-building endeavor within a larger social network in which practitioners were brought on board to standardize ECT practice supported by protocolization and systematic collection of empirical evidence. All twelve sites where ECT was conducted at that time joined the study. These sites also set to work to develop a unified protocol to follow the new guidelines, issued in 1985, which not only stipulated that ECT was only to be used in case of "'therapy-resistant' depression, i.e. not responding to medications, or of (lethal) catatonia", after other measures had been tried, but also that its use "should be indicated by two psychiatrists, should be given after informed consent from the patient is obtained, and should only be given in properly equipped centres".[145] In addition, systematic reporting of each procedure to the Inspectorate was expected, using a registration system. Due to such system, which entailed systematic reporting by psychiatrists of the results of each procedure based on a standardized ECT registration form and a given proto-

and his colleagues in the 1950s consulted with the medical staff of the pharmaceutical branch of the company Organon in nearby Oss about the appropriateness and side-effects of new psychotropic medications, especially anti-depressants, and guidance was provided by means of a literature review conducted by the company's medical staff upon Woltring's request because the psychiatrists found the stream of information coming to them about the new medications overwhelming. Whether such connections resulted in further research collaboration or support needs further examination, as well as how such relationships might have developed elsewhere.

142  Cf. Nolen (1986).
143  Cf. Geneeskundige Inspectie voor de Geestelijke Volksgezondheid (GIGV) (1991).
144  The State Medical Inspectorate of Mental Health is the translation of "de Geneeskundige Inspectie voor de Geestelijke Volksgezondheid", most commonly referred to as the GIGV. In this paper I also refer to it as the "Inspectorate". Koster: Visies (1992); Interview with Koster; Geneeskundige Inspectie voor de Geestelijke Volksgezondheid (GIGV) (1987).
145  Nolen (1999), p. 5; Geneeskundige Inspectie voor de Geestelijke Volksgezondheid (GIGV) (1985); Interview with Koster: She noted that the registration system was voluntary. Because ECT was deemed an acceptable medical therapy there was no legal foundation for obligatory registration. The Inspectorate transferred oversight of ECT to the psychiatric profession starting in 1995.

col at each site, a culture adaptable to research-based practice was, inadvertently perhaps, put in place.[146]

Nolen started his study inspired by the research context he encountered in Denmark in 1978. Comparable research centres in biological psychiatry were only gradually emerging in the Netherlands and none of them focused on ECT research.[147] Van Praag, the new research chair in biological psychiatry, for example, conducted research on anti-depressants, not on ECT. In Copenhagen Nolen met a fellow who had just translated in English the results of an Italian study on ECT, showing positive effects of ECT in patients who had not responded to the anti-depressant imipramine.[148] Nolen began to rethink the idea that psychotropic medications had made ECT obsolete.[149] He first re-introduced ECT in Bloemendaal in its modern, modified form after completing a training on ECT in Denmark.[150] In the 1980s he started to set up his own study, designed to examine the effect of ECT if use of anti-depressants did not seem to work. This design was already in anticipation of the guidelines under discussion in the advisory committee of the National Health Council.

In anticipation of potential protest Nolen had his research proposal reviewed by experts, the Inspectorate, and Parnassia's already existing patient advisory council.[151] It was an effective strategy he found, because indeed an activist group "Stop the Biopsychiatry" questioned his study, which in turn resulted in questions by members of parliament, some of whom he actually knew. Because his proposed study was reviewed by the Inspectorate, however, Nolen was able to conduct his research. Rafaelsen, the head of the Danish research centre was one of the reviewers of his proposed protocol. In contrast to the approach suggested by the Dutch governmental guidelines, Rafaelsen considered the approach to first treat a patient with all existing pharmaceutical therapies prior to applying ECT not the most appropriate from an ethical standpoint, in that a potentially effective treatment was withheld from a patient for too long. In Denmark the attitude was that a patient who would not respond to anti-depressants but might benefit from ECT should be treated with it right away. On the other hand, Rafaelsen concurred that the Dutch situation was an advantage from a research point of view in that a series of treatments could be tested with ECT applied as the measure of last resort.[152] That was indeed the way Nolen set up his study: he treated 90 patients with

146 Geneeskundige Inspectie voor de Geestelijke Volksgezondheid (GIGV) (1987); Geneeskundige Inspectie voor de Geestelijke Volksgezondheid (GIGV) (1991); Interview with Tholen; Interview with Koster.
147 Van Praag's research in Groningen was one example. His successor Rudi van den Hoofdakker was one of the academic supervisors of Nolen's dissertation; Interview with Nolen.
148 Cf. Interview with Nolen; Nolen (1999), p. 4.
149 Cf. Nolen (1999), p. 4.
150 Cf. Nolen (1999), p. 5.
151 Cf. Interview with Nolen.
152 Cf. Interview with Nolen. Several Dutch psychiatrists held a similar view. For a detailed overview see Slooff/Van Berkestijn/Van den Hoofdakker (1982).

anti-depressants according to the established medication protocol, whereafter nine patients were treated with ECT and of those six experienced recovery, using statistical analysis of scores on identified outcome measures. At the time Nolen completed his study the context surrounding ECT was still precarious and resulted in an empirical, protocolized, but still guarded approach.[153]

Although Nolen's study constituted one of the first empirical studies on ECT in the Netherlands, published in 1986, interestingly he himself did not identify it as such.[154] In a historical overview of ECT he wrote in 1999, he referenced his study only in passing when stating that upon acceptance of the 1985 governmental guidelines: "ECT took its place in the Dutch protocol of treatment of depression – [applied] if all regular treatments [with anti-depressants] would not be effective." Although this statement succinctly summarized the approach of his study, its title did not include ECT, suggesting the study was about treatment of depression with different types of anti-depressants and "other biological treatment methods".[155] The only 'other' method included in the study was ECT.[156] It might be that the still tense climate in the country around ECT at the time made it more feasible to identify the study as one on treatment of depression, without mentioning ECT explicitly in the title. It also is possible that the title foreshadowed the focus of Nolen's career. Evaluation of anti-depressants was the direction in which Nolen would develop his research and he became a specialist in pharmacotherapy of mood disorders.[157]

The second example of a study establishing the efficacy of ECT was the one initiated by the State Medical Inspectorate of Mental Health (GIGV) and coordinated by Annemiek Koster. In addition to overseeing the voluntary registration of ECT treatments upon the acceptance of ECT guidelines in 1985, the Inspectorate also initiated research using statistical analysis of the ECT registration data according to epidemiological principles. By instigating a study on experiences with ECT of patients, family members and practitioners the Inspectorate contributed to the justification of ECT. Annemiek Ko-

---

153  Cf. Interview with Nolen. See also Blok (2004), pp. 174–189 on anti-psychiatric critique on ECT and biopsychiatry.

154  Nolen (1986).

155  Nolen (1999), p. 5. Nolen's 1986 study was titled: "Behandeling van depressie, strategieën bij de keuze van antidepressiva en andere biologische behandelmethoden" ("Treatment of depression, strategies informing the choice of anti-depressants and other biological therapies").

156  Nolen (1999), p. 5: at that point, in 1986, regular pharmaceutical treatments that had to be tried prior to using ECT included tricyclic anti-depressants, lithium, and monoamine oxidase inhibitors (MAOIs).

157  Nolen (2008). In 1993 Nolen obtained an academic position at the University of Utrecht and was appointed Professor of Psychiatry (Mood Disorders) in Groningen in 2003. In his publications he regularly acknowledged the funding received from pharmaceutical companies for his research on psychopharmaca for mood disorders. He kept a critical outlook on this treatment modality though. In looking back on the use of pharmacotherapy in mood disorders in a review in 2008, Nolen noted how fifty years of development of this therapy had not necessarily brought the solutions in treatment of mood disorders hoped for in the early development of this therapeutic modality.

ster, psychologist and social epidemiology researcher in mental health, who had just been appointed at the Inspectorate in 1986, was assigned the task of setting up the ECT registration and the research.[158] Starting research as part of registration was stimulated by the Head of the Inspectorate, Jan van Borssum Waalkes who was a psychiatrist by background.[159] Because debate and controversy over ECT tended to continue Van Borssum took the initiative to start research with the aim to develop a fuller picture of ECT particularly from the perspective of patients and family members, Koster explained to me. She knew Van Borssum from a previous study she had coordinated – a national, multi-centre evaluation of (ex-)patient experiences from seven Dutch psychotherapeutic communities.[160] She used the framework of this previous study to set up a similar project on experiences with ECT, this time simultaneously evaluating the experiences of three groups of stakeholders. Koster had been hesitant to agree to this task, she recalled.[161] If it had not been for the encouragement of Van Borssum she perhaps never would have embarked on it: "Initially I did not want to do this study, I hardly knew anything about ECT, and thought just as many did, 'who still does this?'" she recalled.[162] Still, Van Borssum convinced her that ECT should remain available as a therapy and the idea to ask patients and family members for their perspectives and experiences with ECT was also his.[163] Convinced by his enthusiasm for a study, Koster set up a longitudinal cohort study to monitor results and carefully surveyed the experiences with ECT among the three groups. The process not only facilitated data gathering on ECT, but the state-funded research also underscored the importance of the development of evidence in supporting policy and practice and, in this case, in diverting public protest by gathering the opinions of people who underwent the procedure themselves. In addition, it facilitated community-building and new skill development around the therapy.[164]

The ECT registration procedure included submission of a standard registration form, filled out and submitted by the practitioner for each case in which the therapy was applied, recording a set of standard items on the patients, the procedure, and the number of treatments. The viewpoints and experiences of the patients and family members were gathered, using personal interviews as well as scores on several instruments to measure levels of depression. Systematically examining the interview data in comparison with scores on depression scales filled important gaps in the information available on

---

158 Cf. Geneeskundige Inspectie voor de Geestelijke Volksgezondheid (GIGV) (1987).
159 Cf. Bakker (2010), pp. 61–78; Interview with Koster.
160 For Koster's CV: Koster: Visies (1992), p. 171; Interview with Koster.
161 Interview with Koster.
162 Interview with Koster.
163 Interview with Koster.
164 Interview with Koster; Geneeskundige Inspectie voor de Geestelijke Volksgezondheid (GIGV) (1987); Geneeskundige Inspectie voor de Geestelijke Volksgezondheid (GIGV) (1991); Zitman (1991).

ECT, Koster recalled.[165] The cohort was formed based on all reported cases from the twelve sites where at that point ECT was conducted, from April 1986 to the end of 1987, constituting about 100 cases.[166] In each case, the patient was invited to participate, as were one of their family members and the practitioner. Koster conducted the interviews, which took place across the country. Data were collected during a period of five years with each patient and family member being interviewed three times, once before ECT and twice, at one week and at three months, following the treatment, the report of which was published in 1991. The report underscored the usefulness of the procedure as perceived by all three groups and confirmed ECT's efficacy. It also confirmed ECT was used as a measure of last resort.[167] Once Koster had completed the report, the Inspectorate supported a secondary analysis of the data, which formed Koster's dissertation. In the latter she examined in more depth the question to what degree patients were able to judge the effect of their own treatment, as well as differences in judgments between the groups and in relation to the scores on the depression scales. The analysis also informed questions around informed consent, on which Koster reported as well.[168] The main findings confirmed agreement in opinions and scores within and between the three groups of participants about the initial expectations as well as the effect of ECT in terms of functioning. About two thirds of the patients and families were positive about the patient's functioning afterwards which correlated with more positive expectations prior to ECT, about 27 per cent were indifferent and about 7 per cent negative.[169] In a detailed discussion of the findings Koster noted that indifferent might indicate non-positive, considering the tendency, especially among elderly patients, to be grateful and the unequal position of patients and physicians.[170] Still, the study confirmed the value of including patient and family viewpoints. The results also suggested that the implicit agreement about the dire condition of the patient prior to ECT seemed an important frame of reference in judging the evaluation of ECT among all three groups.

Drawing from the Inspectorate report, a year later the Dutch Association of Psychiatry issued more specific directions for practitioners with regard to indication, informed consent and ECT procedures.[171] Locally, each site where ECT was offered had to set up a systematic approach for monitoring ECT and reviewing the indications and application of the procedure. It was

---

165 Interview with Koster.
166 Cf. Geneeskundige Inspectie voor de Geestelijke Volksgezondheid (GIGV) (1987); Geneeskundige Inspectie voor de Geestelijke Volksgezondheid (GIGV) (1991); Koster: Visies (1992).
167 Cf. Geneeskundige Inspectie voor de Geestelijke Volksgezondheid (GIGV) (1991).
168 Cf. Koster: Visies (1992).
169 Cf. Koster: Visies (1992). For a detailed summary of the findings see pp. 131–153. The study population included 98 patients with a mean age of 61 years (77 women and 21 men), p. 145.
170 Cf. Koster: Visies (1992), p. 152.
171 Cf. Van Bemmel et al. (1992); Nolen (1999), p. 6.

a new way of showing accountability about medical procedures which was
a relatively new phenomenon in the culture and practice of medicine at the
time. Zitman, for instance, recalled how he had been involved with forming
a clinical committee to evaluate and monitor the indications for ECT in Nijmegen.[172] He published a detailed review of the 1991 Inspectorate's study
report in a professional journal.[173] At that point, the group in Nijmegen did
not conduct research on ECT. It was introduced as a clinical program, he
remembered. Data were provided to the national group, but no independent
research was conducted on site. A similar system was set up in Groningen.[174]
ECT research grew more common as of the 1990s, likely facilitated by the
system of data collection that had been put in place. Verwey for example,
initiated an analysis of all ECT treatments at the Arnhem hospital, which
he published in 1991, with support from his former supervisor Rooijmans
from Leiden.[175] The national study seemed to have stimulated a network of
ECT practitioners who also valued the exchange and publication of evidence
as a core part of their practice.[176] It could be argued that the governmental
initiative to monitor and study ECT empirically, triggered by the tumultuous
protests over ECT, facilitated (and financed) systematic ECT registration. In
turn registration stimulated research expansion and lay a foundation for an
evidence base in line with the culture of providing scientific evidence which
had gained momentum, also in medicine, by the end of the 20th century.[177]

## ECT in the 1990s – new prominence of biological psychiatry and a culture of evidence

In the 1990s biological psychiatry became a more prominent part of psychiatry and the use of ECT expanded. A last upheaval of protest against ECT
occurred in 1990, when three Amsterdam hospitals were being invited by the
Inspectorate to start ECT in the province of North-Holland. The therapy had
not been offered in the province for a while. The initiative triggered intense
protest, not only in the media, but also in a court case in which activists
argued that ECT violated the human right of bodily integrity as well as international law against physical abuse. Their claim was not upheld in court,
however, although it drew wide support also from practitioners.[178] In the hospital where Koerselman directed the psychiatric clinic, for example, half of
the clinic's nurses resigned overnight in protest.[179] Despite the commotion,
Koerselman used the walk-out as an opportunity to appoint a new group of

---

172  Cf. Interview with Zitman.
173  Cf. Zitman (1991).
174  Cf. Interview with Tholen.
175  Cf. Verwey (1991); Interview with Verwey.
176  Cf. Slooff/Van Berkestijn/Van den Hoofdakker (1982).
177  Cf. Bolt (2015).
178  Cf. Koerselman/Smeets (1992).
179  Cf. Interview with Koerselman.

nurses who were in support of ECT, he recalled.[180] Upon the outcome of the court case, the steering group and the agencies planning on introducing ECT continued to provide public information and steering group members attended an open forum discussion as well.[181] After a while the protest died down, while the Inspectorate once more emphasized the accepted guidelines.

Heading into the 1990s, ECT had become an integral part of biological psychiatry in all provinces. This shift in practice and perspective was particularly noteworthy in the careers of Verwey and Van den Broek. I describe them as the third generation interviewees, although Verwey could be considered to be part of both the second and third group.[182] They jointly led the transfer of the existing governmental registration system on ECT to the psychiatric profession as of 1992 and became national leaders in promoting the professional status and the public image of ECT during the 1990s. Initiatives were channeled through the Dutch Association of Psychiatry. As a leader within the section on general hospital psychiatry within this Association (since 1990 and chair since 1995) Verwey collaborated with Walter van den Broek to work with the Inspectorate towards professional self-regulation of ECT.

Walter van den Broek took his specialty training as a psychiatrist from 1987 until 1992 at the Medical Centre of the Erasmus University in Rotterdam, whereafter he was appointed as a psychiatrist at the Medical Centre and soon became head of medical education. He learned about ECT in the midst of his education as psychiatrist, when one of his mentors, Jan Bruijn, introduced the therapy at Erasmus in 1989. Van den Broek was one of the specialists who learned to conduct ECT and made it a focus of his research. Following its introduction, research on ECT was taken up in the department at Erasmus to enhance its empirical, evidence base.[183] Similar to Verwey, Van den Broek also went to the US to take a course in ECT.[184] In 2004 he undertook dissertation research jointly with his colleague Tom Birkenhäger, conducting a detailed examination of ECT outcomes of a group of patients who first had been treated with anti-depressants, an approach quite similar to the one Nolen had first used in the mid-1980s, and which had remained the basis of Dutch ECT treatment guidelines.[185] Van den Broek also regularly published on ECT outcomes.

Because the state registration process was a voluntary system, and the 1991 report had supported ECT as a useful medical procedure, the Inspector-

180 Interview with Koerselman.
181 Cf. Koerselman/Smeets (1992).
182 Nolen withdrew from publicity and debate over ECT in the early 1990s and turned to research on anti-depressants. He mentioned how for years he was involved in all public debates around ECT but felt it was time to leave further advocacy on ECT to others: Interview with Nolen.
183 Cf. Interview with Van den Broek.
184 Interview with Van den Broek. Van den Broek did not state where he went to take a course.
185 Cf. Van den Broek/Birkenhäger (2004); Van den Broek et al. (2010); Interview with Van den Broek.

ate decided it would discontinue its involvement with ECT registration after completion of the study.[186] Legally there was no longer a need to maintain registration by the Inspectorate, a point also clarified in the 1991 report.[187] The accountability to maintain ECT standards should become a professional responsibility using self-regulation similar to other medical procedures and mandates. Enacting this policy, the Inspectorate started negotiations with the Dutch Association of Psychiatry and the parties agreed that a transfer process would be initiated starting in 1995.[188]

As a professional body, Van den Broek recalled "we did not want to give up the ECT registration because it generated valuable data and information."[189] When the Inspectorate decided to discontinue the monitoring, "we decided to maintain the registration and inspection and set it up within our own Association with support of the Association's Office. Registration of cases [became] simpler, we developed an online reporting system to facilitate it", Van den Broek noted.[190] From these statements it can be gathered that within the profession the registration data was recognized as a valuable source of legitimization of ECT and as a way to underscore its efficacy, both of which were fitting with the emerging culture of evidence-based medicine.[191] To facilitate the transfer, in 1994 a committee was set up in collaboration with the Dutch Association of Psychiatry, called the "Landelijke Evaluatie-commissie ECT (LEE)" (National Evaluation committee ECT), which would oversee the transfer, and of which Koster would remain coordinator and secretary.[192] The role of the LEE was to oversee and support the Association in setting up a system of self-regulation and quality control.[193] Another outcome of the negotiation was that the delegated transition process coordinated by the LEE would be financially supported by the Inspectorate, including the detachment of Koster. The existing registration was maintained, including the registration form, although the number of questions on the form were expanded to collect additional data, Koster remembered.[194] During this time the reported number of performed ECTs steadily increased, from 102 cases reported in the GIGV study from April 1986 to the end of 1987, to 273 cases reported to the LEE in 1998.[195]

---

186  Cf. Interview with Koster.
187  Interview with Koster; Geneeskundige Inspectie voor de Geestelijke Volksgezondheid (GIGV) (1991).
188  Interview with Koster.
189  Interview with Van den Broek.
190  Interview with Van den Broek. See also Van den Broek et al. (2010).
191  Cf. Bolt (2015).
192  Cf. Interview with Van den Broek and with Koster.
193  Cf. Landelijke Evaluatie-commissie ECT (LEE) (1996); Landelijke Evaluatie-commissie ECT (LEE) (1997).
194  Interview with Koster.
195  Cf. Landelijke Evaluatie-commissie ECT (LEE) (2000), p. 15; Koster: Informed Consent (1992), p. 71; Interview with Koster.

Simultaneously, from its part the Dutch Association of Psychiatry started a Working group ECT Netherlands (WEN) in 1994, as counterpart to the LEE and organizationally structured as a sub-group of the Association's general hospital psychiatry section chaired by Bas Verwey. The WEN, initiated and co-chaired by Van den Broek and Verwey would set up and coordinate the system of self-regulation, promote it among the practitioners, and develop an evidence-based practice guideline. In this capacity they had an instrumental role in further standardizing ECT practice and the development of an evidence-based ECT guideline which governed the professional self-regulation of ECT from 2000 onwards. The reporting system was reworked into an online submission process, and the evidence-based guideline was published as the formal Association's ECT guideline in 2000, and updated again in 2010.[196]

Van den Broek and Verwey were keen to maintain the existing ECT registration system, but for new reasons: "We thought stopping [registration] would be a shame because of the evidence it provided", Van den Broek pointed out.[197] Maintaining the registration facilitated the establishment of an evidence base to support data collection and quality assurance of ECT. Performance results could also be used to address public concerns that were still lingering, they found. To address the latter, the Association also published a brochure on ECT meant to inform the public as well as patients and families who were prescribed ECT.[198] Both Verwey and Van den Broek were convinced of the efficacy and safety of ECT in indicated cases, but public ambivalence over the procedure had not disappeared. "The image of ECT still needs work, there still is concern among the public, but these [concerns] are not based in facts", Van den Broek noted.[199] The registration remained similar to what it was, "but it is now online, easier, and we keep track of all treatments this way and are able to develop an annual performance report. I am in favour of making the report publicly available, that way everybody will be able to compare their local or individual situation to the national average, that's the ideal", he stated.[200]

By 2000, the WEN took over control of the registration, provided courses on ECT for psychiatrists, wrote a handbook, and issued and updated the ECT guideline: "this newest ECT guideline really has been coming from the profession itself – these are evidence-based, scientific", Van den Broek emphasized.[201] At the time of the interview, the group was working to establish a system of agency visitation to further assure quality: "That is the latest devel-

196 Cf. Geneeskundige Inspectie voor de Geestelijke Volksgezondheid (GIGV) (1991); Landelijke Evaluatie-commissie ECT (LEE) (1996); Landelijke Evaluatie-commissie ECT (LEE) (1997).
197 Interview with Van den Broek.
198 Cf. Interview with Van den Broek.
199 Interview with Van den Broek.
200 Interview with Van den Broek.
201 Van den Broek/Leentjens/Verwey (1999); Nederlandse Vereniging voor Psychiatrie (2000); Van den Broek et al. (2010).

opment", Van den Broek noted.[202] Steady increase of use as well as bureaucracy marked the application of ECT since the transfer. "Despite the increase
in number of locations where ECT was performed [by the end of the 1980s],
we did not get any less but actually more patient referrals for ECT in Arnhem", Verwey observed.[203] At the time of the interview with Verwey in 2006,
he mentioned that nationally over 300 patients were treated annually, which
was a further increase compared to the number reported by the LEE in the
late 1990s. In addition to his contributions to the handbook and guideline
development, Verwey's team in Arnhem regularly reported on their research
and exploration of ECT indications.[204] To Verwey and Van den Broek, the
steps taken by the profession as well as the continued research on ECT con-
solidated the therapy as a self-regulated, evidence-based medical practice.

By the end of the 20th century ECT had been folded into a culture of
evidence-based practice. The increased use seemed to reflect a renewed professional and public trust in the procedure. New media reports on the practice
had shifted in tone and its public portrayal depicted a more positive image.[205]
The increased use of ECT had not necessarily lowered use of anti-depressants
or other pharmacotherapeutics.[206] Rather, within the biological psychiatric
context ECT seemed incorporated as an integral part of a depression protocol, basically consolidating the process set in motion in the late 1980s. The
social climate and public response, however, had turned into one of increased
acceptance, underscoring how ECT and the public and medical response to it
reflected the larger social structure and culture of which it was part.

## Conclusion

The generational analysis of psychiatrists' experiences with ECT showed how
the scientific justification for ECT shifted from one primarily resting on clinical justification and medical authority alone, to one justified by empirical
research and a wider set of strategies to communicate its efficacy. This shift
in scientific justification is not merely a story of medical success, but rather a
reflection of the way medical care has been pushed into a new way of scientific justification, and onto a new platform of public negotiation that involved

---

202 Interview with Van den Broek.
203 Interview with Verwey.
204 Cf. Interview with Verwey; Stek/Beekman/Verwey (1997); Verwey/Van den Broek/
    Mueller (1998); Verwey/Van Waarde/Mueller (2003).
205 Cf. Van Hintum (2009).
206 Cf. Van den Broek et al. (2010), pp. 147–152: The 2010 ECT guidelines recommend
    use of anti-depressants as follow-up therapy ("nabehandeling") upon completion of ECT
    treatment, p. 149. For critical analyses of the increase in use of anti-depressants and phar-
    macological research on anti-depressants see Dehue (2008); Healy (2012). Also Nolen
    has reported concern over the limited outcomes of anti-depressants over time: Nolen
    (2008).

multiple stakeholders.[207] The eventual acceptance of ECT was not an isolated event, but intimately reflected larger social and medical developments in psychiatry and in society at large. During the latter half of the 20th century, particularly after 1970, psychiatrists were pressured to negotiate the justification of their work based on new terms, and ECT formed an early case example. While during the 1970s ECT became a symbol of psychiatric critique and counter-cultural protest against authoritarian structures and biological reductionism in psychiatry, during the late 1980s the public perception and scientific culture surrounding ECT changed. Personal accounts of psychiatrists who either continued or took up ECT practice during this time of controversy and transition reflected this larger social change. Although clinical arguments about the efficacy of ECT in case of devastating and pharmacotherapy-resistant depression figured as an important influence in the controversy over ECT, public accountability and transparency of the way the treatment was performed grew in importance. Building upon a state-supported registration system put in place in 1985, practitioners responded in new ways, and to more stakeholders involved, including patients, families, and allied personnel. Patients joined protests, but eventually also became stakeholders in a therapy that seemed effective for some. It seemed the strategic move of the State Medical Inspectorate of Mental Health to not only include practitioner perspectives but also patients' and family members' experiences in a public account of ECT practice underscored a shifting perspective on ECT. It also made research a more powerful policy factor in the debate. The shift to research-based practice formed new dependencies from the part of psychiatrists, such as a larger influence and pressure of the pharmaceutical industry in the development of the protocol of depression treatment and more pressure to be publicly held accountable regarding the prescription and application of ECT. A conservative approach to the number of indications for ECT also characterized the Dutch context of ECT performance. The public upheaval and protest of a critical counter-cultural and patient movement shook up psychiatrists' expert-based medical authority, and nearly stopped ECT use in the late 1970s. Establishing strict conditions was a way to retain ECT in the face of deep public controversy and protest. Rather than intra-professional tension alone, however, a broader cultural transformation of which psychiatry was part shifted the perspective on ECT from the late 1980s onwards. The continued use of ECT was grounded in a new dominance of biological psychiatry which gained momentum towards the end of the 20th century. Ambivalence over the efficacy of anti-depressant medication also contributed to a reassessment of ECT. Increased use of ECT was supported with new empirical research strategies and scientific justification. As a result of these dynamics ECT was folded into a new medical culture of protocol and evidence-based practice

---

207 Cf. Achterhuis (1980); Tonkens (2003). For an analysis of the shifting demand for medical accountability as well as patient autonomy during the course of the 20th century in the US: Tomes (2016). See also Bolt (2015); Sadowsky (2017), especially the latter's discussion of efficacy of ECT.

that dominated medicine at the turn of the 21st century. It appears on the one hand, the public and clinical confidence in ECT increased in the 1990s, while on the other, the control, or power so you will, over its application became dependent on a broader range of interested groups.

## Bibliography

*Oral history interviews (Author's private collection)*

Interview with Bas Verwey by Joost Vijselaar and Josef Vos, 22 November 2006.
Interviews with Goos Zwanikken and Joke Zwanikken-Leenders by author, 10 and 24 February 2011.
Interview with Willem Nolen by author, 15 March 2011.
Interview with Fons Tholen by author, 15 March 2011.
Interview with Frans Zitman by author, 17 March 2011.
Interview with Louise Dols by author, 22 March 2011.
Interview with Walter van den Broek by author, 23 March 2011.
Interview with Fried van de Ven and Joke Zwanikken-Leenders by author, 19 April 2011.
Interview with Jaap Prick by author, 21 April 2011.
Interview with Annemiek Koster by author, 16 June 2011.
Interview with Frank Koerselman by author, 6 July 2011.

*Literature*

Abma, Ruud; Weijers, Ido: Met Gezag en Deskundigheid. De Historie van het Beroep Psychiater in Nederland. Amsterdam 2005.
Achterhuis, Hans: De Markt van Welzijn en Geluk. Baarn 1980.
Bakker, Catharina T. (ed.): Terug naar de Basis. Geschiedenis van het Staatstoezicht voor de Inspectie van Vandaag. Utrecht 2010.
Barnhoorn, Johannes Anthonius Joseph: Mededelingen Over de Toepassing van de Convulsietherapie Door Middel Van Electroshock. In: Nederlands Tijdschrift voor Geneeskunde 84 (1940), pp. 290–300.
Barnhoorn, Johannes Anthonius Joseph: Convulsietherapie Door Middel Van Electroshock. In: Psychiatrische en Neurologische Bladen 45 (1941), pp. 279–287.
Binneveld, Hans; Wolf, Rob: Een Huis met Vele Woningen. 100 Jaar Katholieke Psychiatrie, Voorburg 1885–1985. 's-Hertogenbosch 1985.
Blok, Gemma: Baas in Eigen Brein: Antipsychiatrie in Nederland 1965–1985. Amsterdam 2004.
Bolt, Timo: A Doctor's Order. The Dutch Case of Evidence-based Medicine (1970–2015). PhD Diss. Univ. of Utrecht. Apeldoorn 2015.
Boschma, Geertje: Beyond the Cuckoo's Nest. Nurses, Electro-Convulsive Therapy and Dutch general hospital psychiatry. In: Fealy, Gerard; Hallett, Christine; Dietz, Susanne Malchau (eds.): Histories of Nursing Practice. Manchester 2015, pp. 100–122.
Boschma, Geertje: Electroconvulsive Therapy (ECT) and Nursing Practice in the Netherlands, 1940–2010. In: European Journal for Nursing History and Ethics [in press].
Boschma, Geertje et al.: Oral History Research. In: Lewenson, Sandra; Krohn-Herrmann, Eleanor (eds.): Capturing Nursing History. A Guide to Historical Methods in Research. New York 2008, pp. 79–98.

Braslow, Joel: Mental Ills and Bodily Cures. Psychiatric Treatment in the First Half of the Twentieth Century. Berkeley 1997.

Cohen Stuart, M. H.; Zeijlstra, H.: Over beleven bij Shockbehandeling. In: Folia psychiatrica, neurologica et neurochirurgica Neerlandica 53 (1950), pp. 470–480.

De Valk, Melissa: Het Erfgoed van de Electroshocktherapie in Nederland, 1939–1975 [Unpublished Master's Thesis]. Univ. of Utrecht 2009.

Dehue, Trudy: De depressie-epidemie. Amsterdam 2008.

Dukakis, Kitty; Tye, Larry: Shock. The Healing Power of Electroconvulsive Therapy. New York 2006.

Foudraine, Jan: Wie is van Hout … Een Gang door de Psychiatrie. Bilthoven 1971 [English edition: Not made of Wood … A Psychiatrist Discovers His Own Profession. New York 1974].

Fox, Becky et al.: Psychiatrische Tegenbeweging in Nederland. Amsterdam 1983.

Gawlich, Max: Eine Maschine, die wirkt. Die Electrokrampftherapie und ihr Apparat. Paderborn 2018.

Geneeskundige Inspectie voor de Geestelijke Volksgezondheid (GIGV): Richtlijnen Over Electroconvulsie-Therapie 1985. Staatstoezicht op de Volksgezondheid. Leidschendam 1985.

Geneeskundige Inspectie voor de Geestelijke Volksgezondheid (GIGV): Ervaringen met elektroconvulsietherapie (ECT). Deel 1: Onderzoeksopzet. Rijswijk 1987.

Geneeskundige Inspectie voor de Geestelijke Volksgezondheid (GIGV): Ervaringen met ECT, een inventarisatie van oordelen en ervaringe met elektroconvulsietherapie (ECT). Deel 2: Resultaten. (=Onderzoeksreeks 6) Rijswijk 1991.

Gezondheidsraad: Advies inzake electroconvulsietherapie. 's-Gravenhage 1983.

Gijswijt-Hofstra, Marijke et al. (eds.): Psychiatric Cultures Compared. Psychiatry and Mental Health Care in the Twentieth Century. Amsterdam 2006.

Groenland, T. H. U.; Kusuma, A.: Anesthesie bij elektroconvulsietherapie. In: Van den Broek, Walter W.; Leentjens, Albert Franciscus Gerardus; Verwey, Bas (eds.): Elektroconvulsietherapie. Houten 1999, pp. 37–47.

GZ zet Shockbehandeling Niet Stop. NASA-project in Arnhem. In: Arnhemse Courant (7 June 1977).

Hamer, Bernard Christiaan; Haverkate, J. H. (eds.): (Schermers') Leerboek bij het Verplegen van Geestes- en Zenuwzieken. 8th, revised ed. Amsterdam 1950.

Hamer, Bernard Christiaan; Tolsma, Frederik Jacob (eds.): Algemeen Leerboek voor het Verplegen van Geestes- en Zenuwzieken. 9th, revised ed. Leiden 1956.

Healy, David: Pharmageddon. Berkeley 2012.

Heerma van Voss, Arend J.: De Geschiedenis van de Gekkenbeweging: Belangenbehartiging en Beeldvorming Voor en Door Psychiatrische Patienten, 1965–78. In: Maandblad Geestelijke Volksgezondheid 33 (1978), pp. 398–428.

Hirshbein, Laura; Sarvananda, Sharmalie: History, Power and Electricity: American Popular Magazine Accounts of Electroconvulsive Therapy, 1940–2005. In: Journal of the History of the Behavioral Sciences 44 (2008), no. 1, pp. 1–18, DOI: 10.1002/jhbs.20283.

Hunsche, Petra: De Strijdbare Patiënt: Van Gekkenbeweging tot Cliëntenbewustzijn – Portretten 1970–2000. Amsterdam 2008.

Hutter, A.: De Electrische Krampbehandeling van de Endogene Melancholie. In: Nederlands Tijdschrift voor Geneeskunde 85 (1941), pp. 3317–3321.

Kesey, Ken: One Flew Over the Cuckoo's Nest. New York 1962.

Kneeland, Timothy W.; Warren, Carol A. B.: Pushbutton Psychiatry: A History of Electroshock in America. Westport, CT 2002.

Koerselman, Frank; Smeets, Rob: ECT in Amsterdam: Een Persoonlijk Verslag. In: Maandblad Geestelijke Volksgezondheid 47 (1992), pp. 131–140.

Koster, Annemiek M.: Informed Consent bij Elektroconvulsietherapie. In: Tijdschrift voor Psychiatrie 34 (1992), pp. 70–77.

Koster, Annemiek [M.]: Visies op ECT. Een vergelijking tussen oordelen van patiënten, familieleden en behandelaren over elektroconvulsietherapie. PhD Diss. Erasmus Univ. Rotterdam 1992.

Kraft, Thom: Mythen en misverstanden rondom de electroshocktherapie. In: Maandblad Geestelijke Volksgezondheid 33 (1978), pp. 106–112.

Kroft, L.: Elektro-shock in de actualiteit. In: Tijdschrift voor Ziekenverpleging 30 (1977), no. 15, pp. 695–702.

Landelijke Evaluatie-commissie ECT (LEE): Verslag over 1995–1996. Rijswijk 1996.

Landelijke Evaluatie-commissie ECT (LEE): Verslag over 1997. Den Haag 1997.

Landelijke Evaluatie-commissie ECT (LEE): Verslag over 1998–1999 [preliminary draft; obtained from Annemiek Koster, LEE Coordinator, 1995–1999]. Den Haag 2000.

Legemaate, Johan: De Electroshocks, 1979–1985. In: Maandblad Geestelijke Volksgezondheid 40 (1985), pp. 397–402.

Lit, A. C.: Electroshock en Slaaponthouding. In: Tijdschrift voor Psychiatrie 15 (1973), pp. 56–64.

McPherson, Kathryn: Bedside Matters. The Transformation of Canadian Nursing, 1900–1990. Toronto 1996.

Meeter, Martijn et al.: Retrograde amnesia after electroconvulsive therapy. A temporary effect? In: Journal of Affective Disorders 132 (2011), pp. 216–222, DOI: 10.1016/j.jad.2011.02.026.

Nederlandse Vereniging voor Psychiatrie: Richtlijn electroconvulsietherapie. Amsterdam 2000.

Nolen, Willem A.: Electroconvulsietherapie: Aanvaardbaar op Voorwaarden. In: Maandblad Geestelijke Volksgezondheid 40 (1985), pp. 295–300.

Nolen, Willem A.: Behandeling van depressie, strategieën bij de keuze van antidepressiva en andere biologische behandelmethoden. PhD diss. Univ. of Leiden. Assen 1986.

Nolen, Willem A.: De Geschiedenis van de Electroconvulsietherapie (ECT) in Nederland. In: Van den Broek, Walter W.; Leentjens, Albert Franciscus Gerardus; Verwey, Bas (eds.): Elektroconvulsietherapie. Houten 1999, pp. 1–7.

Nolen, Willem A.: Vijftig Jaar Farmacotherapie Van Stemmingsstoornissen. Zijn De Verwachtingen Uitgekomen? In: Tijdschrift voor Psychiatrie 50 (2008), pp. 111–116.

Nolen, Willem [A.]; Van Ree, Frank: Electro-convulsieve therapie: 'Ja … Maar …'. In: Tijdschrift voor Psychiatrie 24 (1982), pp. 23–35.

Nolte, Karen: Shock Therapies and Nursing in the Psychiatric Clinic of the University of Würzburg in the 1930s and 1940s. In: Hähner-Rombach, Sylvelyn; Nolte, Karen (eds.): Patients and Social Practice of Psychiatric Nursing in the 19th and 20th Century. Stuttgart 2017, pp. 135–152.

Pieters, Toine; Snelders, Stephan: From King Kong Pills to Mothers's Little Helpers – Career Cycles of Two Families of Psychotropic Drugs. The Barbiturates and the Benzodiazepines. In: Canadian Bulletin of Medical History 24 (2007), no. 1, pp. 93–112.

Psychiater dr. Th. B. Kraft. Patient Kan Echt Beter Worden met ECT. In: Arnhemse Courant (2 July 1977).

Rooijmans, Harry G. M.: Electroshockbehandeling. In: Nederlands Tijdschrift voor Geneeskunde 122 (1978), pp. 1669–1671.

Rooijmans, Harry G. M.: Electroconvulsie Therapie: Van Blaam Gezuiverd (?). In: Nederlands Tijdschrift voor Geneeskunde 127 (1983), pp. 1973–1974.

Rooijmans, Harry [G. M.]: De Verwetenschappelijking van de Psychiatrie. In: Van Balkom, Ton et al. (eds.): Scientification of Psychiatry. Utrecht 2007, pp. 9–16.

Sadowsky, Jonathan: Electroconvulsive therapy in America. The Anatomy of a Medical Controversy. Abingdon; New York 2017.

Shock-Gevaar. Pas Op. In: De Nieuwe Krant. Dagblad voor Arnhem en Omgeving (27 June 1977).

Shorter, Edward; Healy, David (eds.): Shock Therapy: A History of Electroconvulsive Treatment in Mental Illness. Toronto 2007.

Slooff, Cees J.; Van Berkestijn, Johannes W. B. M.; Van den Hoofdakker, Rudi H.: Electroshock. Therapeutische effecten. In: Tijdschrift voor Psychiatrie 24 (1982), pp. 531–555.

Speciaal Voor U: De Zwarte Lijst (Van Artsen Die Shocken). In: Speciaal NASA Klapnummer van de Gekkenkrant 22 (June 1977), pp. 10–12.

Stegge, Cecile aan de: Gekkenwerk: De Ontwikkeling van het Beroep Psychiatrisch Verpleegkundige in Nederland, 1830–1980. Maastricht 2012.

Stek, M. L.; Beekman, A. T. F.; Verwey, Bas: Electroconvulsie Therapie in de Behandeling van Depression in ouderen. In: Tijdschrift voor Gerontologie en Geriatrie 28 (1997), pp. 106–112.

Szasz, Thomas: The Myth of Mental Illness. Foundation of a Theory of Personal Conduct. New York 1961.

'Terugkeer van de Elektroshock': Een Verslag van het Openbaar Debat op 26 Juni 1986 in het Kolpinghuis te Nijmegen, Stichting De Nuts. Nijmegen 1986.

Tomes, Nancy: Remaking the American Patient. How Madison Avenue and Modern Medicine Turned Patients into Consumers. Chapel Hill, NC 2016.

Tonkens, Evelien: Mondige Burgers, Getemde Professionals. Utrecht 2003.

Van Bemmel, A. L. et al.: Electroconvulsietherapie. Aanbevelingen voor Indicatiestelling, Informed Consent en Uitvoering. Nederlandse Vereniging voor Psychiatrie. Utrecht 1992.

Van den Broek, Walter W. et al.: Richtlijn Electroconvulsietherapie. 2nd ed. Utrecht 2010.

Van den Broek, Walter [W.]; Birkenhäger, Tom: Treatment of depressed inpatients: Efficacy and Tolerability of a four-step treatment algorithm. PhD diss. Erasmus Univ. Rotterdam 2004.

Van den Broek, Walter W.; Leentjens, Albert Franciscus Gerardus; Verwey, Bas (eds.): Elektroconvulsietherapie. Houten 1999.

Van der Horst, Lambertus: De Behandeling met Electroshock. In: Nederlands Tijdschrift voor Geneeskunde 91 (1947), pp. 3069–3073.

Van der Post, Louk: Electroshocktherapie, waarom nog? In: Maandblad Geestelijke Volksgezondheid 32 (1977), pp. 688–694.

Van der Scheer, Willem M.: De Resultaten van de Shockbehandeling Met Insuline en Cardiazol Bij Dementia Praecox. In: Psychiatrische en Neurologische Bladen 45 (1941), pp. 252–278.

Van Eijk-Osterholt, Corrie: Laat ze het maar voelen. Amsterdam 1972.

Van Hintum, Malou: Met een stroomstoot uit de put. Elektroshock. In: De Volkskrant (11 July 2009), Sectie Intermezzo, pp. 22–23.

Van Praag, Herman (ed.): Handbook of Biological Psychiatry. New York 1980.

Van Ree, Frank: Problemen rond ECT. In: Tijdschrift voor Psychiatrie 19 (1977), pp. 591–599.

Van Ree, Frank: Als Voorstander van een Verbod. In: Tijdschrift voor Ziekenverpleging 30 (1977), no. 16, pp. 762–763.

Van Ree, Frank; Nolen, Willem [A.]: Voorwaarden voor het toepassen van ECT. In: Maandblad Geestelijke Volksgezondheid 37 (1982), pp. 1162–1173.

Van Uffelen, Tilly: Reinier start met stroomtherapie. In: Brabants Dagblad (10 March 2011), Brabantsdagblad.nl, Sectie Den Bosch, p. 26.

Verwey, Bas: Electroconvulsietherapie in een perifeer ziekenhuis. In: Nederlands Tijdschrift voor Geneeskunde 135 (1991), pp. 1694–1697.

Verwey, Bas: Europese electroshock. Verslag van 'First European Symposium on ECT. Critical history – future trends,' Oostenrijkse ECT-research Society, 26–28 March 1992, Graz, Austria. In: Maandblad Geestelijke Volksgezondheid 47 (1992), pp. 1126–1129.

Verwey, Bas; Van den Broek, Walter [W.]; Mueller, M. E. T. M.: ECT. Vaak te laat geïndiceerd? In: COBO-bulletin 31 (1998), no. 2, pp. 22–30.

Verwey, Bas; Van Waarde; J. A.; Mueller, M. E. T. M.: Depressie. Stoppen of doorgaan met ECT? In: COBO-bulletin 36 (2003), no. 2, pp. 37–40.

Vijselaar, Joost: Het Gesticht. Enkele Reis of Retour. Meppel 2010.

Vijselaar, Joost: 'A Hole in the Armour of Dementia Praecox.' Somatic Cures within the context of Psychiatry in Multiplicity. In: Schmuhl, Hans-Walter; Roelcke, Volker (eds.): Heroische Therapien. Die Deutsche Psychiatrie im internationalen Vergleich 1918–1945. Göttingen 2013, pp. 168–184.

Weijers, Ido: De Binnenhuisarchitecten van de Nederlands Verzorgingstaat. Menswetenschappers en Doorbraak. In: Gewina 24 (2001), pp. 196–206.

Witmer, Johannes M.; De Roode, Robinette: Implementatie van de Wet Geneeskundige Behandelingsovereenkomst (WGBO). Van Wet naar Praktijk, Deel 2: Informatie en Toestemming. Koninklijke Nederlandse Maatschappij tot bevordering der Geneeskunde (KNMG). Utrecht 2004.

Zitman, Frans: Ervaringen met ECT. In: Nederlands Tijdschrift voor Geneeskunde 135 (1991), pp. 1669–1670.

# Mothers on Children's Wards: Conflicts in German Paediatric Care from the mid-1950s to the late 1970s

*Sylvelyn Hähner-Rombach* †

## Introduction

Paediatric nursing developed in its own special way within the history of nursing in Germany. With the rise of paediatrics in the 19th century[1], the establishment of paediatric wards (1829/30 at the Charité Hospital in Berlin) and children's hospitals (Paris 1802, the first university children's hospital at the Charité in Berlin in 1894), alongside a high number of infant deaths (i.e., 20 per cent in a birth year died within the first year of life[2]), the paediatricians saw the need for nurses with special qualifications to care for this vulnerable group of patients. Thus, the paediatrician Arthur Schlossmann (1867–1932) began to train the first baby nurses in 1898 in Dresden in the baby clinic that he founded.[3] Paediatric nursing, which was initially limited to babies and infants, began its independent development.

Already in 1917, the Prussian government provided a state examination for baby nurses[4], a year later the first baby and infant nurses passed their exams after a one year long training course. In 1923, in most German states the training was expanded to two years.[5] In 1930/31 the training for baby and infant nurses was uniformly organised by the state for the whole country.[6] However, paediatric nursing, as this partial discipline was now explicitly called, was only included in the statutory regulations on nursing in 1957.[7] For that reason many paediatric nurses regard 1957 as the beginning of their profession.

During the time period I am analysing here, only West Germany, Austria and Switzerland offered independent training in paediatric nursing care.[8]

### Sources

For this article I mainly drew on the journal *Deutsche Schwesternzeitung* (German Journal for Nurses), which has been published regularly since 1948. During the period in question, it was the most important journal across various organisations and was also used for publications in paediatric care. In 1971, it

---

1    Cf. Peiper (1958), pp. 217–229; Seidler/Leven (2003), pp. 203–205.
2    Cf. Neumann (2005), p. 746.
3    Blessing (2013).
4    Cf. Neumann (2005), p. 748.
5    Cf. Neumann (2005), p. 748.
6    Elendt (1992), pp. 33–34.
7    Cf. Gesetz über die Ausübung des Berufs der Krankenschwester, des Krankenpflegers und der Kinderkrankenschwester (Krankenpflegegesetz) [Act on Nursing Care] (1957).
8    Cf. Stemann (1969), p. 259.

changed its name to *Deutsche Krankenpflegezeitschrift* (German Journal of Nursing) to also address and include male nurses. Since 1993, it has been published to the present day under the title *Pflegezeitschrift* (Nursing Journal). In addition to the *Deutsche Schwesternzeitung*, there were other journals that were published by individual organisations such as the "Agnes-Karll-Verband", or associations such as the German Red Cross, or by the unions such as the Union for Public Services, Transport and Traffic ("Gewerkschaft Öffentliche Dienste, Transport und Verkehr", ÖTV). Yet, since nearly all organisations, associations and unions also used the *Deutsche Schwesternzeitung* to share their opinions or report about their work, this journal reflects a broad spectrum of the field.

Of course, journals also have their limitations, as we all know. Not every contribution the editors received was published and the selection criteria for the publications were not communicated to the public. It is not known whether and to what extent the content was edited. Furthermore, the journals often do not provide insights into the everyday experiences, practices, or personal problems on the job. Exceptions are the letters by the readers, yet these were usually very short. Other so-called ego-documents such as journals, correspondences, memoirs are rare in nursing care and need to be researched. This is an area for oral history. The emotional connection between nurses and children with all inherent conflicts – in particular the relationship to the mothers of the babies in their care – can only be addressed in personal interviews, if at all, because the files and printed sources only provide limited answers. For that reason, we have begun to conduct interviews with former paediatric nurses and parents, if applicable, and if possible also with male paediatric nurses. First results of these interviews are also included in this article.

*Epistemological interest*

The history of paediatric nursing is one of the under-explored areas within German history of nursing. There is no substantial work for the time after 1945.[9] Yet, paediatric nursing is suitable for a historical analysis for several reasons. On the one hand, it is easier to track down the relationship between the nurses and the patients in their care than is possible in other areas in nursing history. On the other hand, paediatric nursing presents some specific features that I will subsequently briefly summarise: they both sharpen the eye for the history of nursing and also reveal its distinctions.

Even more so than nurses in adult care, paediatric nurses seemed to embody the ideal of caring attention, motherliness etc., especially because as carers of babies, infants, and children they were in very close contact with them. Thus, they often carried their small, crying patients along while they com-

9    For the time before 1945 the number of works is also manageable. See Elendt (1992); Blessing (2013). To contribute the filling this research gap, in November 2017 I started a research project on the history of paediatric nursing in West Germany with the regional focus of Baden-Württemberg. This paper is part of this research.

pleted other tasks. For that reason, paediatric nurses are particularly prone
for a gender specific analysis. With a few exceptions[10], they were unmarried
until the 1970s when the delayed "introduction" of married paediatric nurses
happened. Paediatric nurses regarded themselves as caring substitutes for the
absent mothers who were usually only allowed access to the wards, and thus
to their child, twice a week for one, or at most two hours. In many houses they
were, however, not allowed to pick up their children during the visit but could
only look at them through a window. The children in the care of paediatric
nurses became in a sense "their" children. This is the result of all the interviews I have conducted so far with paediatric nurses. These close relationships
were enhanced by the fact that in the time period under investigation the
nurses spent a lot of time with the children in the patients' rooms, so they engaged with them much more – or had to engage with them because children
cannot take care of themselves to the extent that adults can. The paediatric
nurses felt a particularly high responsibility for their patients as the children
could not necessarily speak or communicate the way adults can; they were
dependent on the nurses who monitored them closely and encompassingly
and served as a mediator between them and the doctor.

These specifics seem to be particularly fruitful for a gender specific analysis because here, several groups of women met each other in conflictual situations: On the one end, there were the unmarried and thus childless nurses
with a distinct professional image, and on the other end of the spectrum were
the married mothers of possibly more than one child who potentially also
worked. Mothers who worked were regarded with suspicion not only by conservative politicians and doctors at the time, but also by many nurses. Their
"professional celibacy" excluded the possibility of becoming mothers themselves until they left the job to get married. Mothers and nurses furthermore
competed for the ill child, a fact that is hardly ever confessed, because due
to his or her admission to hospital, the child had become more the nurse's
responsibility than the mother's. Mothers' attempts to gain more access to
their ill children, and the disposition of some (both male and female) doctors
who favoured this for medical and/or psychological reasons, resulted in many
attempts to prevent this from the side of the nurses. Yet, these did not form a
homogeneous block either. There was the group that tried to keep the mothers away as much as possible, there were those nurses who fought for opening
up the wards to the mothers, and finally there was the rather silent group of
undecided and doubtful nurses.[11]

---

10   In the *Deutsche Krankenpflegezeitschrift*, the follow-up journal of the *Deutsche Schwesternzeitung*,
     there was a brief article in 1973 with a photograph of the first male paediatric nurse in
     Bavaria. Cf. Bayerns (1973), p. 506. After he had learned a trade he had taken care of
     old people in a home for a year, then pursued a three-year long training programme as a
     nurse, and finally added the specialised training in paediatric nursing for 18 months. Dur-
     ing the same time, the first male paediatric nurse was trained at the Olgahospital in Stutt-
     gart. In other houses, men were only trained as nurses on the ward for infectious diseases.
11   Since men entered this profession only later we can merely ask them about wards that
     had been closed to parents for a longer time period or that allowed only limited access

While the debate on opening paediatric wards for mothers or parents is quite specific even within the history of nursing, the inherent conflicts that I will address in more detail later on led to more open and more frequent discussions of the self-perception of the nurses with regard to their importance to the patients and their view of the children's relatives than was the case with other nurses. That means that in these discussions we can find information about the relationship between the nurses and their patients, i. e., the children, and the relationship between nurses and relatives.

Some doctors perceived mothers or parents on the children's ward also as a problem, but they argued that it was an inconvenience for the nursing staff. In other words, with this diversion they were able to hardly ever address their own insecurities caused by the presence of parents when they performed clinical tasks. I will neglect the doctors who favoured opening the wards for mothers or even admitting them together with the children and who became vocal early on in the context of hospitalisation damage[12], in subsequent years even more so. My focus is on the nurses rather than the doctors.

The voices of the mothers cannot be adequately considered here because they were hardly ever included in the sources that are available and have been analysed. To remedy this gap, I will draw on the interviews again. From England we have excerpts of 50 letters by parents that report from the 1950s onwards about the expanding of the visiting hours or the simultaneous admission of mothers.[13] For the German time period under investigation we have only one letter by a mother who reports from memory about the traumatic experience of being separated from her son due to longer hospital admissions.[14]

## Mothers in hospital

When contemporary journals, literature, and the press discussed the topic of mothers in the hospital, most often two models were considered that were not, however, completely mutually exclusive: a) admitting children with their mothers and b) expanding the visiting times for mothers or parents.

In many cases, mothers were also offered to stay because some of them could not visit on a daily basis because of the distance between home and

---

such as the intensive paediatric unit of the city hospital Stuttgart that grants parents access only at certain hours.

12  For instance, in the interdisciplinary medical journal *Medizinische Klinik* (Medical Clinic), the paediatrician Köttgen from Mainz published in 1958 an article on the "Verkümmerung als Folge von Pflegeschäden beim Kind" (in English: Atrophies due to the nursing care damage in children). Cf. Köttgen (1958). He addresses here the early examples of hospitalisation damage that were observed at the beginning of the 20th century and the pioneering role the Anglo-Saxon areas played here. In the 1970s publications on the damages caused through hospitalism increased in the German speaking world. Cf. Troschke (1974); Robertson (1974); Biermann (1978).

13  Cf. Krankenhäuser und Kinder aus Sicht der Eltern. In: Robertson (1974), pp. 101–153.

14  Private archive Annegret Braun, Letter by H. F. to Annegret Braun from 20/08/2017.

hospital, lack of public transport etc. When we think of co-stay we must, however, not think of the rooming-in facilities[15] that were provided later. Rather,
these were simple accommodations in neighbouring rooms, empty rooms in
the nurses' accommodations etc. Until the mid-1980s individual rooms for
mothers and children were the exception; most hospitals did not have the
capacity for that. In 1974, the foundation hospital for children in Stuttgart, the
Olgahospital, enabled the first ward for parents to stay with their children in
Southern Germany.

The model for opening the wards and letting the mothers stay came
mainly from England; in later years, references to the US were also made.
In 1957, the Ministry of Health in the UK commissioned a specially formed,
interdisciplinary committee that included members from paediatrics, surgery,
psychiatry, general practice, administration, nursing and a neutral lady from
the outside to issue a report on the "Welfare of Sick Children in Hospital".
In 1959, this report was published under the title "Platt Report"[16] and included several recommendations for hospitals of which three "caused the biggest stir"[17]: It proposed that visiting children should be possible without any
time restrictions, mothers of children who were less than five years old should
receive the option to stay with their child, i.e., stay with them at the hospital
the entire time, and it demanded that the training of doctors and nursing staff
should take into account and implement the needs of children. Independent
of the Platt Report, individual English paediatricians had begun to set up
mother-child units. At the same time, there were also attempts to install paediatric nursing at home.[18] In the US, Switzerland, and in Bosnia there were
pioneering projects at the same time to allow mothers into the hospital.[19]

*How the discussion evolved among German nurses*

With the first mention of the topic, it was immediately presented as an argument. This happened in the *Deutsche Schwesternzeitung* in 1955. The headline
of the article was phrased as a question: "The child at hospital being cared
for by the mother?" ("Das Kind im Krankenhaus von der Mutter betreut?")[20]
The report began with a critical statement that the Senior Nurse Annemarie
von Klitzing from Munich, an influential figure at the time, had written as a
response to an article from the *Nursing Mirror* from November 1954.[21] The

---

15   The so-called "rooming-in" is mainly known from maternity wards and was transferred
     to the children's wards as well.
16   The leader of the investigation was the surgeon Sir Harry Platt; hence the name "Platt
     Report". Cf. Robertson (1974), p. 93.
17   Robertson (1974), p. 93.
18   Cf. Robertson (1974), p. 95. In Troschke we find a detailed international overview over
     the literature. Cf. Troschke (1974), chapters 3.1. and 3.2.
19   Cf. Biermann (1978), p. 7.
20   Cf. Klitzing (1955); Gillett (1955).
21   On Annemarie von Klitzing see Klitzing (1997).

original article was printed in translation next to her opinion piece. Numerous contrary letters from readers followed. The article in the English journal had reported on a successful "new experiment with daily visiting times" at the Bristol Royal Hospital for Children.[22] The article was illustrated with four photographs from the ward that showed parents or mothers with their children in the patient rooms. Klitzing also included these illustrations in her critique that already raised the most important issues that were repeatedly addressed in the ensuing debate and that I will analyse later on. Klitzing's critique of the English "experiment" began with the note: "In several European countries and in the US, paediatric hospitals have begun to allow multiple hours for a mother or father to visit their sick child and engage or care for him or her in other ways – thus making a virtue out of necessity."[23]

While this quote also speaks of America, all articles in the *Deutsche Schwesternzeitung* address English examples. The reason might be that the nurses had closer and more effective ties to their colleagues in England rather than the US. By contrast, doctors who favoured the opening of children's hospitals drew instead on the North American model.[24]

The second piece of evidence in the *Deutsche Schwesternzeitung* is a brief message from 1959 without any commentary. It describes a report that Dr. James Robertson completed for the British Ministry of Health. In response to this "report" that is probably identical to the "Platt Report" mentioned above, the Ministry decided that "mothers of infants are allowed to take part in caring for their children at the hospital if the doctors desire this."[25]

The English paediatric psychologist Robertson had published in 1958 a book titled "Young Children in Hospital" that was published in German in 1974 as part of the series "Beiträge zur Psychologie und Soziologie des kranken Menschen" (Articles on the psychology and sociology of sick people). This series was published by Gerd Biermann and Jürgen von Troschke who had themselves published a piece on children in the hospital in 1978 and 1974, respectively.[26] The English consultant and his work were thus known among clinicians but also by paediatric nurses.

In 1964 an article in the *Deutsche Schwesternzeitung* drew again on English examples. The *Nursing Times* had published an article in 1963 that reported on an experiment at the Royal Alexandra Hospital in Brighton in 1959. Here, the experiment was not to expand visiting times but an attempt to "set up, as a trial, a small area with eight beds for mothers and children in which both

22  Gillett (1955), p. 146.
23  Klitzing (1955), p. 145.
24  This was the case at the Olgahospital Stuttgart. Cf. private archive Sylvelyn Hähner-Rombach, interview with Annegret Braun. The report of a nurse who worked for about four years at the neonatal intensive care unit in Offenbach also mentions the "first positive experiences in the US" as the reason for the expansion of visiting hours in 1972. Cf. Arnold-Ullinger (1978), p. 52.
25  Die Mutter (1959), p. 309.
26  Cf. Troschke (1974); Biermann (1978).

have a little space for themselves that was separated through a glass wall".[27]
The article described the whole procedure but also how mothers were being
prepared for the stay so that they knew both what to expect and also what was
expected of them.

In another article from the *Deutsche Schwesternzeitung* from 1966 we learn
that in Newcastle-upon-Tyne there had been such a ward for much longer,
namely since 1925.[28] Just as in Brighton, the mothers here were informed
about the rules and expectations. At the same time, there was the option of
extended visiting times for those mothers and fathers who could not take up
the offer of staying with their children.

The topic was introduced in the *Deutsche Schwesternzeitung* in 1955 and
did not stop in the following years until the end of the 1970s – until the open-
ing-up in West German hospitals was no longer a major exception, i. e., when
the situation had changed to a degree that the measures could not be undone
anymore, and the discussion lost its heat or had become obsolete.

*Agents*

The participants in the debates were foremost mothers and fathers who wanted
to accompany their children to the hospital. Some of them were organised in
the Action Committee: Child in Hospital ("Aktionskomitee Kind im Krankenhaus"). In 1968, a women's group in Frankfurt had started this committee
"to change the situation of sick children and their parents in the hospital".[29]
Ten years later, in 1978, there were action groups already in 54 cities in West
Germany.[30] The action committee did not only consist of parents but also
paediatric nurses, doctors and representatives of other health professions.
Furthermore, the action committee conducted eager lobbying and ensured
its presence in the press. For instance in November 1979 the journal *Eltern*
(Parents) that had been founded in 1966 published a list of hospitals in West
Germany that were open for full day visits (111 hospitals) and a list of hospitals that allowed mothers to stay with their children (150 hospitals). These lists
had been created by the action committee.[31]

Secondly, the paediatric nurses were agents who did not have their own
professional representatives[32] during the time under investigation and were a
very heterogeneous group. While they did not make the decisions in the hos-

27  Kind und Mutter (1964), p. 247.
28  Schwester Ingrid Schmalzl (1966).
29  Aktionskomitee Kind im Krankenhaus: http://root.akik.de/phocadownload/akik-chronik
    09.pdf (last accessed: 17/10/2018).
30  Cf. Aktionskomitee (1978).
31  Cf. Kind im Krankenhaus (1979), p. 56.
32  In 1980, the Working Group of Paediatric Nurses ("Arbeitskreis der Kinderkranken-
    schwestern", AKK) was founded that registered itself two years later in the register of
    associations. In 1991, the AKK evolved into the Professional Organisation of Paediat-
    ric Nurses ("Berufsverband der Kinderkrankenschwestern und Kinderkrankenpfleger",

pital, they had to be convinced if the co-stay of mothers was to be successful. The chief physician made the decision, but the supporting consultants and doctors were similarly important. The latter had gained their open perspective often during stays abroad – and mainly, as mentioned above, in the US. Due to the specific epistemological interest of this current article, they will not be further analysed. Other agents were the providers and funders of hospitals who will likewise not be considered here.

*The positions: pro and contra*

Looking at the views, there were certainly overlaps between doctors and nurses. Doctors who did not want to have parents constantly looking over their shoulder or engaging them in discussions joined the nurses who spoke out against the increasing presence of mothers.

Pro
These were the nurses for whom opening the paediatric wards to parents was an important matter and who cooperated with the doctors who voted in favour of an increased presence of parents. These nurses often had already suffered from the consequence of the limited visiting times during their training: screaming and unhappy children on the one side of the window and desperate mothers and helpless fathers on the other side, in the middle the nurse who was supposed to calm down both sides.

   We have to remind ourselves of the specific situation of German paediatric nurses, the main aspects of which I already mentioned above: Professional celibacy, the large significance of (medical) monitoring of the children, the role of the nurse as a mediator between child and doctor, nurses as substitutes or even replacements of the mother, and the competition between the nurses for the children's "affection" (keyword: "most popular nurse") and their poorly developed professional self-confidence. We repeatedly find reference to "little" and "big" nursing care with the "little" nursing care, i.e., paediatric nursing, counting for "less". For instance in an article from 1954 we read: "During the last decades we paediatric nurses had to fight a lot for the equality between us and nurses in adult care. We were regarded for a long time as 'second class nurses'."[33]

   The nurses' disposition towards opening the wards depended also on different factors, as Senior Nurse Stemann described in 1967: first, there was the disposition or view of the chief physician, i.e., whether he regarded psychological aspects higher than clinical work or vice versa. The chief physician tipped the balance. Second, the opinions depended both on the available space and a well-working routine. Many wards had simply not enough room

---

   BKK). Cf. Berufsverband Kinderkrankenpflege e. V.: https://www.bekd.de/der-bekd-ev/ geschichte-des-berufes-und-des-berufsverbandes/ (last accessed: 17/10/2018).
33   Oberschwester Maria Plieninger (1954), p. 124.

in the tightly occupied patient rooms because frequent visits had not been part of the planning when the hospitals were built. If there was to be a chair next to each bed one could hardly move anymore. Reducing the number of beds in the rooms would have resulted in a lower capacity for admissions, which was not desirable. According to Senior Nurse Stemann, a routine that was set in stone could have made it harder for a nurse to "imagine a different regime than the usual processes on the ward". Finally, the lack of staff had a huge effect for the forming of the opinion. Through the expansion of theoretical training through the Act on Nursing Care in 1957, this became even worse among the students.[34] The Senior Nurse also noted that while the Act on Nursing Care included psychology and pedagogy in the training, this new knowledge had to be more strongly integrated into the work at the wards to successfully face the challenges that the new openings would entail.

Contra
The nurses who rejected the idea used arguments on various levels. Often, they justified their opinion with medical-hygienic, psychological, and professional-political arguments. Furthermore, they mentioned the additional work these extended visits caused.

Medical-hygienic arguments

The arguments that drew on the sciences were presented already from the very beginning. They included the danger of introducing infectious diseases through parents and other relatives because of the missing protective clothing. The pathogens could come from a domestic environment that the hospital could not control, or from the public transport in particular if the visitors were still in their coats when they stood next to the bed in which they "had just used the tram".[35] Furthermore, according to this justification, with extended visiting times the visitors would not just bring in the dirt from the streets on only two days of the week but every day. This would have meant far more efforts in keeping the ward clean which was also one of the nurses' tasks.

Psychological arguments

Arguments that drew on the, at the time, young discipline of psychology were used for both the children and the nurses. The increase of the children's pain of separation from twice to seven times a week was one of the main arguments. We already read in 1955: "Do not many children daily experience new sadness and excitement when the mother or father have to go home again?"[36]

34  Stemann (1967), p. 581.
35  Klitzing (1955), p. 145.
36  Klitzing (1955), p. 145.

The nurses were the ones who would have had to calm the children again. The argument continued that this situation would also be difficult for children who received fewer visits than others. Their suffering would be increased from two to seven days.

In addition, the nurses mentioned some parents' problematic reactions to "fulfilling orders and measures that they would not understand and would possibly regard as superfluous or painful for their child".[37] This also included that the nurses – and the doctors – felt that they were constantly monitored by the parents or mothers. The visitors' increasing questioning of the daily life at the hospital and the alleged criticism about the conditions at the hospital or the ward was also seen as a burden.

The parents' presence also resulted in an increase of the danger for nurses to be involved in problematic family affairs which they at times found burdening. Knowing the children's social or family environment was not regarded as important for nurses at the time.

A psychological argument from later days (when visiting times had mainly been expanded everywhere) was the pressure for parents who were not able to come for daily visits or stay at the hospital because of time or other reasons. For instance, a survey with parents at the university hospital Hanover in 1980 had the result that "some parents are basically not able to visit their child every day. Because of their environment they feel a moral pressure to stay with their child for the whole day. The parents thus experience a certain psychological and physical burden that can be transferred to the child in hospital."[38]

The different frequency of visits of the children at a ward could result in sadness and disappointment in those children who received fewer visitors. If there was a sudden interruption of previously daily visits, the "pain of separation" could have even stronger effects since "the child had established no relationship to the nurses".[39] The observation implied, however, that the relationship between the nurse and these children was generally less strong. It would be noteworthy to investigate this further.

Some statements also included arguments regarding the effects on the sibling who had to spare their mother when she spent more time with the sick child: "If a mother moves completely or for the most part into the hospital she creates a sensitive gap in her family." The passage continues that this could result in "abnormal attitudes among the siblings as we know it from an only child when a brother or sister is born".[40]

37  Klitzing (1955), p. 145.
38  Koppe/Gebensleben (1980), p. 713.
39  Koppe/Gebensleben (1980), p. 713.
40  Stemann (1967), p. 581.

Professional-political arguments

In 1967, Senior Nurse Dietlinde Stemann from Hamburg conducted a survey with ten senior nurses from various hospitals. The goal was to learn more about the attitude of their houses concerning the extension of visiting times. The following concerns with regard to the nurses' roles emerged:

> The nurse is worried about the separation of powers. She rightfully argues that it will be only her job to perform those measures that the child does not voluntarily agree to do. This is not an expression of jealousy but gets to the heart of care: blending the unpleasant with the friendly aspects so skilfully that the child accepts the one to receive the other.[41]

After handing over basic care to the mother, the nurse lost (physical) contact with the child. Monitoring the patient was also disturbed because of the mother's presence – both aspects had been main motivations to become a paediatric nurse in the first place. The nurses were thus left with the unpleasant and fear-inducing tasks because "everything that is fun such as playing, feeding, and bathing the mother will do".[42]

In 1979 this point was picked up again. Reviewing her experiences after one and a half years of letting mothers stay in a paediatric hospital in Hamburg, one nurse noted:

> our former task to care for the child and serve as a mediator between child and doctor has been pushed into the background. While administering therapies for the patient we are no longer the person the child relates to at the sickbed. This insight is hard for many nurses because the child experiences the nurse now only when she performs unpleasant tasks.[43]

That means that for some nurses their concerns became reality, at least partially.

Additional workload for the nurses

While enabling more contact between mother and her sick child was regarded as desirable, in 1955 the following statement was published: "Do not try to make this idea that is compelling for many reasons more attractive for the nurses by making them believe their workload would be made 'easier' through the help of the mother. The opposite is true."[44]

In her description of a failed experiment with unlimited visiting hours, the author evokes an image of demanding mothers who spoiled their children, undermined the doctor's orders, at times brought along other children to visit and left a mess behind that the nurses had to clean up. Similarly, the situation is portrayed twelve years later in 1967 in another commentary:

41   Stemann (1967), p. 581.
42   Private archive Annegret Braun, Braun (1979).
43   Rundtischgespräch: Mütter im Kinderkrankenhaus (1979), p. 676.
44   S. W. (1955), p. 304.

> From experience we know that mothers usually have uncountable extra desires and that they expect an open ear for both important and also unimportant questions [...] All of this means a bigger burden for the nurse and can result in the child being caught in a field of tensions.[45]

Dealing with mothers whose behaviour in the nurses' eyes could be overly anxious and helpless but also uninterested or ignorant and demanding, or who acted on their own authority could be quite demanding for the nurses. The additional time for conversations, answering questions, and providing information was substantial in comparison to visits that occurred for three or four hours a week. This argument has also to be read in the context of increasing staff shortages. Thus, a nurse who in principle favoured opening the wards to the mothers, acknowledged in 1979 that she and her colleagues had hoped early on after mothers were allowed to stay with their children that they would now have more time for those children whose parents could not stay with them all day. However, this was not the case. Letting the mothers stay had not brought relief but the need for more time to talk to them. How to talk to parents and learning to understand the parent's perspective were skills that had to be acquired first.[46]


*Reasons for opening the wards*


In 1955 the nurse Gertrud Maas responded to Annemarie von Klitzing's negative commentary, arguing already then that the separation of mother and child in hospital could cause suffering and subsequent developmental and educational problems in the child. One of the main arguments for opening the wards was to minimise or prevent these effects. Maas began her response with the statement: "Yes! I want to say a joyful Yes to a daily visiting hour for children [...]"[47], before addressing the individual arguments Annemarie von Klitzing had presented. She did not ignore the difficulties but presented suggestions on how to deal with them. "I know from many years of experience that it is much easier to care for children without the constant influence of parents who are often scared, at times unreasonable and occasionally even consciously repugnant." According to her, this aspect was part of the "area of education and leadership for which each nurse should have a calling anyway and in which she should be trained".[48] One remedy could also have been to schedule such treatments at times when no visit from parents was to be expected who – and here Maas referred to the article about Bristol – were only visiting in the late afternoon or evening. The most important counter-argument, namely the daily repeated agitation when the parents had to go home, she also regarded "as the most dangerous moment", but: "Nurses

---

45   Stemann (1967), p. 581.
46   Cf. Rundtischgespräch: Mütter im Kinderkrankenhaus (1979), p. 676.
47   Maas (1955), p. 241.
48   Maas (1955), p. 241.

with pedagogical skills will be able to happily divert these and will calm the children [...] both physically and mentally."[49] Maas finished her argument as follows:

> I think it is right for a mother to have one or two hours to play with her child and give him or her all the familiar help that retains the close relationship between them. Then she should say good-bye with the promise to 'come back tomorrow'. If a child, even a very small child, experiences that this promise is true and that it only has to sleep one time between the get-togethers it will be calm and content.[50]

In 1967, i.e., twelve years later Gertrud Maas wrote again to the *Deutsche Schwesternzeitung* on the topic and pointed out how helpful it could be for the therapy to integrate the mother and how useful the conversation with her could be:

> Small children are very conservative. Each change of habit means a loss for them. It is simply impossible to learn of such things during a doctoral admission exam or during a very busy visiting hour. For that you need regular contact with the mother. How many children's tears, how much agitation (and sedatives) could be saved, how much effective help for the development of the child could be provided.[51]

Using sedatives in children before the visiting times was mentioned only by this nurse in the *Deutsche Schwesternzeitung* though. The interviews with paediatric nurses reveal however that unsettled or screaming children often received sedatives prophylactically before the visiting hours – possibly to avoid upsetting the mother or to ensure "peace" in general. The nurses did not seem to have had a problem with administrating sedatives to children (for instance, the neuroleptic medication atosil). While only the doctors were allowed to prescribe medication, the interview partners revealed that the ward nurse decided on the administration when no doctor was present. That was not regarded as a problem either.

Another nurse pointed out, also in 1967, additional consequences of limited visiting times that were unbearable for many nurses.

> I share the opinion that the visiting times as they currently happen in most paediatric hospitals must be revised. Until now nurses have been loathing them. Twice a week crowds of people are standing in front of the windows or in the door-frames to the patient rooms. Inside there is a turmoil because of crying children, outside the parents are in turmoil. Often, no true communication is possible and many parents go home unsatisfied.[52]

She supported the idea to remedy the situation by introducing daily visiting times. In her letter she also discussed arguments against the expansion of visiting times. "We have to vigorously encounter the often heard complaint 'I cannot work when I am constantly being observed.' A paediatric nurse should have enough self-confidence that she does not experience the parents as annoying observers."[53]

49  Maas (1955), p. 241.
50  Maas (1955), p. 241.
51  Maas (1967), p. 87.
52  Schwester R. M. (1967), p. 138.
53  Schwester R. M. (1967), p. 138.

In addition she called for a positive attitude towards the parents in whose situation one should put oneself. Finally she voted for allowing parents of severely ill children to stay with them day and night which, according to her, was already possible in some hospitals. Apparently she had gained such experience.

> At night-shift I was always happy when parents took up this offer and I knew that the child was also being observed by a relative. I could take care of the other children more calmly because I knew that I would be immediately informed if the condition of the child should change.[54]

Finally she suggested to take parents into account when building new hospitals so that space for their visits could be included during the planning of the rooms.

Developments in nursing care at the time in general also showed effect, including changes to the working hours. The increasing introduction of working in shifts, which was highly controversial, resulted in different nurses taking on the care, which had a significant impact on the relationship between nurses and the child patients. While in the old working model only one nurse was responsible for her patients during the day, the new shift system meant that it was two. One Senior Nurse shared in 1967 her conviction that the time was over that a child was exclusively taken care of by "his or her" nurse. The child was by now surrounded by many people "amongst whom only the mother is the only constant and calming factor".[55] This alone was reason enough in her opinion to allow mothers onto the wards.

The decision of the city council in Munich to allow mothers to stay with their children resulted in 1966 "again in fierce discussions" according to the *Deutsche Schwesternzeitung*.[56] The longer commentary by nurse W.K. on the topic began with the observation that the admission and the stay at the hospital was difficult for a small child due to the separation from the mother and the different environment. Then she asked whether the usual visiting time of twice a week for an hour would be enough with regard to the important mother-child-relationship. Typical arguments against the more frequent presence of the mother she countered with the self-critical question of whether it was not actually the case that the structure of the hospital operation that the nurses had organised and that was allegedly disrupted by the many visits "was possibly not the right thing for the small patients?"[57] The counter arguments – the difficult adjustment to the hospital, introduction of infections – even resulted in "advising parents against visiting their child at all to ease the transition".[58]

---

54  Schwester R.M. (1967), p. 138.
55  Stemann (1967), p. 581.
56  Schwester W.K. (1966), p. 509. The decision of the city council in Munich to establish the new children's hospital in Munich-Harlaching as a mother-child-hospital with daily visiting times and the opportunity for parents to stay was discussed in all professional circles and the West German press. There were also reports about it in Stuttgart.
57  Schwester W.K. (1966), p. 510.
58  Schwester W.K. (1966), p. 510.

Subsequently she listed all the known reasons for expanding the visiting times: that the child's recovery would benefit from more frequent visits, that mother and nurse could exchange notes and that the mother could receive advice for the time after the stay at the hospital. In her mind, all of these were valid arguments for daily visiting times.

Senior Nurse Elisabeth Leist from the University Hospital Heidelberg reported in 1968 about her experiences of many years with mothers who had stayed together with their sick children and had offered to help on the ward "no matter with what" by themselves. "Years ago we already utilised this offer for our house. We accommodated the women – whose number was always limited – provided meals and appointed them, depending on their skills and knowledge, for four to six hours every day."[59]

"Domestic activities" ("hausfrauliche Arbeiten") for instance in the dining hall were suitable. In the remaining time, these women, including also grandmothers, had the opportunity to visit their children or grandchildren.

> We have had good experiences with this set-up. All women were grateful for this good will and we, on the side of the hospital, were grateful for the help offered because in all cases the help from the mothers and grandmothers could be felt. It was important for all mums whose children were without exception severely ill that they were in the immediate vicinity of the child and to be part of the group of people in the house where the child was a patient.[60]

At times the connection to the mothers and grandmothers did not stop after the stay at the hospital was over. We could add that the offer to help did not hurt the reputation of the children's hospital in the wider population as the free labour was probably not regarded as a problem at the time.

In subsequent years the number of reports and opinion pieces by paediatric nurses in the *Deutsche Schwesternzeitung* on opening up the hospitals dramatically dropped. One reason was probably that the hospitals increasingly had expanded visiting times[61] and the nurses had gotten used to the new settings or had looked for work elsewhere. From the middle of the 1970s we have the report mentioned above by a nurse from Offenbach about her four years of experience in a neonatal intensive care unit that had expanded visiting times. After she had weakened all of the counter-arguments, she talked mainly about the changed role the paediatric nurse had due to the presence of the mother.

> It has often been said that with this new structure the nurse can no longer build a relationship to the patient, that she would only be providing food and administering therapies. [...] In my opinion and experience we still have plenty of opportunity to build a relationship with the little patients. It always depends on how the nurse herself maintains the contact.[62]

59  Leist (1968), p. 366.
60  Leist (1968), p. 366.
61  The emphasis is on increasing, i. e., it was still not generally the case. Thus, in 1979 an article was published in the *Deutsche Krankenpflegezeitschrift* that referred to a refusal to expand visiting times. Cf. Keuth (1979).
62  Arnold-Ullinger (1978), p. 54.

She also considered it to be the nurse's task to check on the mothers, especially as this could have an impact in the child after being discharged. The nurse's work would also benefit from this. Her conclusion left no doubt: Despite some difficulties, none of the nurses wanted to return to the old structure.

During the interviews with former paediatric nurses in the larger area of Stuttgart one nurse reported that, after she had worked on an open ward, she could never "go back". When she wanted to work in her job again after her children were old enough, she started at a hospital in her area. Soon she stopped because the old visiting rules still applied there. She could not and did not want to tolerate the consequences of the restrictive visiting times.[63]

## Voices of the Mothers

As mentioned at the beginning of this article, statements by the mothers on the individual management of visiting times are (still) rare apart from the official statements by the Action Committee: Child in Hospital.

At least in the *Deutsche Schwesternzeitung* there were two very different positions. The first is from 1955 and referred to the opinion piece by Senior Nurse Klitzing on the English model of expanding visiting hours. The letter came from a former paediatric nurse who had by now become a mother herself and hence was no longer working. The writer introduced herself as a "hybrid", i. e., both as a mother and, though no longer working, professionally socialised as a paediatric nurse. She completely agreed with Klitzing's negative view and emphasised some points in particular. In terms of hygiene, one "could never […] let in members from all demographic backgrounds" and only very few mothers would comply with the dietary rules ("Essensvorschriften"). She continued asking why, if the mothers did not wear any protective gear ("Schutzkittel"), the nurses were still supposed to wear a uniform and she claimed that more frequent visits would delay the recovery. Finally she wrote the following:

> Our child certainly went through a lot in the last year: two operations and after the first one very bad pneumonia – and all of that at the age of two years. At least we always showed ourselves behind the window and when I saw that the child was in a good mood and I could leave knowing all was well, I was always glad, as hard as it was.[64]

What happened inside her when she saw her child in an unhappy mood she does not discuss in the journal.

The other example is from a mother who tried to raise awareness about the mothers' situation with the nurses. In 1979, the *Deutsche Krankenpflegezeitschrift* printed a letter by an anonymous mother that she had written to the nurses of the ward where her child had been. After thanking the nurses again for their

---

63  Private archive Sylvelyn Hähner-Rombach, Interview with M. N. on 16/01/2018.
64  Kollan (1955), p. 242.

work she discussed her fears and the emotions from when she had stayed at the hospital with her child.

> In addition to the stress because of my sick child, I needed to adapt to the nurses' expectations and I constantly felt that I was actually highly unwelcome. There was a bed for my child but where was I supposed to sleep? My child received meals but there was nothing for me. Suddenly I felt very insecure and everything that I would usually and normally do for my child was suddenly a problem. Was I allowed to take the temperature, change nappies, feed and calm down and cuddle my child or did I have to wait for instructions?[65]

The letter was supposed to create an understanding in the nurses for the mothers' situation and also for mothers that had been classified as "unreliable". The mother addressed the competitive situation between mother and nurse and said in hindsight that a good collaboration between mothers and nurses would have been possible "if both had been brave enough to approach one another more openly rather than just staying side by side".[66] She reflected on the relationship to the nurses on a very high level. She did not report on any problems that arose later. Unfortunately, there are also tragic examples for that. For instance, one mother wrote to the former nurse Annegret Braun that her son, who had been in hospital for months as a child and whom she had hardly been allowed to visit, was restricted in his later psychological development and finally committed suicide. She blamed the separation between herself and her son for this.[67]

## The process of opening-up. Example: Stuttgart

Some hospitals only expanded the visiting hours, others enabled parents to stay with their children, and yet other hospitals began with trial models on some wards. One such hospital was the Olgahospital in Stuttgart, a foundation hospital for children that did not yet belong to the civic hospitals at this point in time.

Already in 1966 letting mothers stay with their sick children was publicly discussed in Stuttgart when the local press reported on the civic children's hospital in Munich-Harlaching that had made this possible from July 1966 onwards.[68] The administration of the hospital informed both chief physicians at the civic children's hospitals about the coverage in Stuttgart immediately on the next day. The manager informed the mayor's office that both "shared the opinion that – apart from a few justified exceptions (e.g., a dying older

---

65   Brief einer Mutter (1979), p. 679.
66   Brief einer Mutter (1979), p. 679.
67   Private archive Annegret Braun, Letter by H. F. to Annegret Braun from 20/08/2017.
68   Cf. Mütter dürfen (1966). The *Süddeutsche Zeitung* reported that the decision by the health select committee in Munich was controversially discussed in the hospitals. These articles also circulated in the city council in Stuttgart.

child)[69] – housing mothers of sick children in the civic paediatric hospitals would not be an option"[70]. The chief physicians mentioned the "catastrophic shortage of space" and "consideration for our staff" as reasons. Indeed, the constant shortage of staff also affected the paediatric nurses who listed these shortages as one of the reasons for rejecting the idea of expanding the visiting times. The usual visiting times in the civic hospitals in Stuttgart were on Wednesdays and Saturdays or Sundays between 3.30–4.30 pm, i.e., one hour each. In the Olgahospital, they were for two hours twice a week. In special cases, exceptions were permitted but had to be authorised by the doctor. While the shortage of rooms was also undeniable, there were no efforts made to find solutions.

Three years later, in 1969, representatives of the Action Committee: Child in Hospital sent a telegram to the President of the German Association of Cities and Towns and requested that the Association should discuss the topic. The administration in Stuttgart had a letter on the issue by the German Association of Cities and Towns. In July 1969, the health select committee of the German Association of Cities and Towns declared, however, that the decision on letting mothers stay at the hospital must remain with the doctor and it justified the decision with calling it a therapeutic problem.

Let us return to the Olgahospital. There at the beginning of the 1970s, a daily visiting time for children and a weekly evening visiting time for working parents were introduced.[71] In 1971, the first ward that was opened to the mothers was the neonatal intensive care unit. That this ward in particular was the first one, even though the fear of infections may have been even bigger than at other wards, was due to the team of doctors and a group of paediatric nurses. The latter were a young generation of nurses who had largely completed their training together and who agreed to demand more visiting times because they shared negative experiences with the restrictive hours. A special quality of the group was also that they had very well prepared their follow-up project of inviting parents of sick children to stay at the ward.

> When we as a team of nurses decided to found a ward for mothers[72] to stay, we prepared for months. We went through group-dynamic processes to understand what happens inside the other and to learn to deal with adults. We had been focused on children only, not on adults. At the beginning there were problems, but I have to say that we managed to sort it all out.[73]

69  Emphasis "older" from me as there seems to have been a difference with younger children.
70  Stadtarchiv Stuttgart, Bestand 19/1 Hauptaktei Gruppe 5, lfd. No. 1827, Administration of the children's hospitals and children's homes to the mayor's office, 26/07/1966.
71  Stadtarchiv Stuttgart, Bestand 19/1 Hauptaktei Gruppe 5, lfd. No. 1827, note for the file, Administration of the children's hospitals and children's homes, Betr. Besuchszeiten in den Kinderkrankenhäusern, 27/11/1970.
72  That means they managed to welcome mothers at the ward and integrated them into the care.
73  Frau Braun. In: Kind im Krankenhaus (1979), p. 83.

They also found support in the head of the department at the time, Dr. Gert-rud Hieronimi, who had previously worked in a children's hospital in the US where it had long been normal for mothers or parents to stay with their children.

In a retrospection from 1979 by one of the paediatric nurses[74] in Stutt-gart who had pushed for introducing a ward that allowed parents to stay ("Eltern-Mitaufnahme-Station") and had worked on its implementation, she summarises the arguments for the opening very clearly:

–   On the one hand, paediatric nurses should exhaust all opportunities to help sick children. Experience had shown that children whose parents/mothers were often present stayed in hospital for less time than the others.
–   The mothers gained more quickly the routine of caring for their child, which they could do subsequently independently at home. In addition, the recovery process was accelerated.
–   Collaborating with the mothers would also be a joy, nurses would gain satisfaction when they experienced how much help they could offer to the mothers through expert advice, sensitive counselling and personal conver-sations. Furthermore dealing with adults was also intellectually stimulat-ing.
–   The nurses learnt so much more about the child and his or her family and could adapt their care more individually.

The nurse voted for an "open ward system", i. e., that mothers were no longer to be reduced to being extras or unskilled helpers but that they had a right to receive complete information and "would not be sent out in difficult situations because in these moments the child needs them most". She continued that a care schedule should have been worked out with the mothers "that they could use for orientation" and that specifically outlined "where her area of responsi-bility is, what type of care she will take on, where she supports the nurse and which tasks must only be performed by the nurse".[75] This list immediately makes clear that the opening of the ward did not mean having less work but that the focus was foremost to do more for the children.

Mothers at the neonatal intensive care unit were also offered to stay, but overnight they could only sleep in a room in the nurses' home. Four such rooms in total were available. At the "Eltern-Mitaufnahme-Station" where par-ents were allowed to stay with their children there were ten mother-child-units for the whole ward. However, it became evident that some parents could not pay the costs (100 German marks per night) or did not have the time for various reasons to stay for 24 hours. To address the issue of the costs, the mothers were offered fold-up beds that only cost a small fee.[76] Many mothers only stayed at the hospital for the first two to four nights because by then the

74   Private archive Annegret Braun, Braun (1979).
75   Private archive Annegret Braun, Braun (1979).
76   Frau Braun. In: Kind im Krankenhaus (1979), p. 59.

children had gotten accustomed to their new environment or they felt better. Hence, the offer to use fold-up beds was more attractive for lots of mothers than the expensive mother-child-units.

After the experiences at the neonatal intensive care unit had been so positive and the demand from the parents rose, other wards at the Olgahospital also expanded their visiting hours. Accepting mothers onto the wards was, however, not everywhere possible at this hospital. At the ward for paediatric surgery, this option was still not available in 1984 as a letter from March of that year reveals.[77] This particular mother wanted to and was supposed to nurse her newborn baby while it was on the surgery ward but there was no bed or day bed for the mother when she had to stay at the ward overnight.

The opening policy of the Olgahospital finally resulted in a pressure for the civic children's hospitals to give up resistance, adapt, and also extend visiting hours.

It is noteworthy here that the acceptance of parents began at a time that was marked by the cost containment laws even though many parents had to bear the costs by themselves. Despite the attempts by the legislators to reduce the costs for hospital stays, the model was implemented step by step because parents or mothers would no longer have tolerated a refusal. In 1976, Baden-Württemberg introduced a regulation that in case a medical certificate about the medically necessary accommodation of an accompanying person was provided, the extra costs were part and thus covered in the general hospital and nursing charges for the patient.[78] If there was no medical certificate, the mother (parent) had to bear the costs by herself. In the hospitals in Baden-Württemberg these ranged from 20 to 120 German marks per day.[79]

*Reactions to the opening*

For some nurses, the opening of the wards or the invitation to let parents stay marked a success. These were often the ones who had suffered from the limited visiting time, because they could barely cope with the unhappy parents on the one side and the crying children on the other side of the window. They argued mainly for the well-being of the children and talked less about different operational processes.

Other nurses were sceptical but got on with it; in some cases they even got used to the new structure and even discovered the advantages. Yet other nurses left paediatric nursing once the wards were opened up. They regarded the opening as a fundamental change of their profession that they did not want to or could not support. However, these nurses no longer shared their

---

77  Private archive Annegret Braun, Letter by R.B. to Annegret Braun from 31/03/1984. I thank Annegret Braun for the permission to look at the files.
78  Cf. Kind im Krankenhaus (1979), p. 7.
79  Kind im Krankenhaus (1979), p. 83.

opinion in the *Deutsche Schwesternzeitung* or the *Deutsche Krankenpflegezeitschrift*, respectively. We only know of them through the reports of paediatric nurses who experienced that time. Further interviews can help to close these gaps.


## Conflicts

As I have illustrated above, oppositions and controversies cannot exclusively erupt or be localised within one profession. The conflicts that ignited around the issue of expanding visiting times for mothers/parents began with changed perceptions and interpretations of symptoms in babies and children in hospital. The "psychological hospitalism" that had been first "discovered" in children living in children's homes – analogous to the "infectious hospitalism" – goes back, apart from very few exceptions, to the 1930s (B.J. Beverly, René A. Spitz 1936)[80], but was hardly reviewed at the time. During the 1950s retrospective investigations on the late effects of traumatisations through hospital stays began and soon after scientists also started to study the behaviours during the stay on the ward.[81] These investigations were started in the new neighbouring sciences of medicine (psychoanalysis, psychology, sociology, psychosomatics) rather than in medicine itself. The lines of conflict did not all run along the professional lines, i.e., in this case doctors vs. psychologists or doctors vs. nurses, even though in the last-mentioned constellation doctors had more power to make decisions than nurses.

Inquisitive vocational school teachers reviewed the investigations mentioned above and introduced their knowledge about the consequences of hospital stays into the curriculum of paediatric nursing schools. Now, it became increasingly clear that the child at hospital did not "wobble"[82] into sleep but that this "wobbling" was a serious symptom of deficits in emotional care. Simultaneously, reports from England about the practical expansion of visiting times for mothers introduced the topic also into German paediatric nursing. Another factor that certainly influenced the development was that a new generation of paediatric nurses entered the wards: these had not grown up during the NS time nor had they been taught by teachers who had been socialised during this time. The movement of 1968 slowly also affected nursing care. These nurses were no longer willing to put up with the images of misery during or after visits and they argued for the abolition of old regulations.

At the same time, the so-called second women's movement in the Federal Republic of Germany changed the mothers' behaviour: they increasingly did not want to accept their passive or helpless position. They had been long enough perceived as a "picture of crying misery" by the nurses. These changes

---

80  Cf. Troschke (1974), pp. 15–16. René Arpad Spitz (1887–1974) was a doctor and psycho-analyst who taught also psychiatry and psychology in the US.
81  Cf. Troschke (1974), chapters 3.1. and 3.2.
82  This was the interpretation of the children's rocking movements at the time.

all resulted in shifts in the care for the (paediatric) patients by doctors because of the stronger role of relatives. This development must also be regarded in the context of the medical critical movement of the 1970s which also strengthened the confidence of patients and their relatives alike.

For paediatric nurses and mothers to come together, the nurses also had to undergo a development. The medical-hygienic and psychological arguments against an expansion of children's wards for mothers revealed an image of women on the side of paediatric nurses that strongly drew on the male view of women outside of the hospital: it suggested that mothers were irresponsible, egotistical, and ignorant in their love for their child; they caused disorder, brought dirt into the hospital, had time-consuming extra desires, undermined doctors' orders and thus threatened the children at the hospital. Finally, with their visits in the hospital they simultaneously neglected their other children at home. In this context, paediatric nurses were the "better" substitute mothers since they waved the flag of (male) sciences and prepared the paediatric patients for the measures the doctors and nurses had to perform. Their care for the patients did not collide with the realisation of the necessity of unpleasant procedures. While the mothers had the tendency to disrupt the operations at the hospital, nurses largely ensured the smooth running of affairs. They received a thank-you from the doctors when the chief physicians refused the expansion of the visiting hours referring to burden for the nurses. Thus, the conflicts did run along the gender demarcations but with the paediatric nurses having adopted the male view.

The professional political counter-arguments of paediatric nurses indicate a very limited area of tasks that was completely guided by the doctors' expectations. Simultaneously, they suggest a reduced image of the patients that was solely clinical and did not allow any psychosomatic and/or psychological perspectives.

The nurses only began to act when they were able to move away from the old understanding of the profession that had been coined for them, and when they began to imagine their own areas of responsibility that went beyond being a loving carer and doctor's assistant. Now, they were no longer (merely) a "substitute mother" and doctor's assistant but also the children's advocate, and adviser and educational counsel for the mothers or parents. They were able to compensate their loss of power and partial loss of meaning through the larger area of tasks they had chosen themselves. Those nurses that did not want to or could not participate in these changes either did not see the new options or they did not regard them highly enough. They only saw the loss of power and/or emotional connection to the children. For some the profession had changed too much and they no longer wanted to work in it. These nurses left paediatric nursing.

## Conclusion

When not promoted by the nurses, open wards resulted in the mothers feeling very unwelcome there. Those doctors and nurses who wanted to implement extended visiting times knew this very well. In some circumstances this meant that these doctors and nurses had to work hard to convince their colleagues.

Opening the wards, however, also followed the laws of the market. For instance, one hospital director in Bavaria reported that the hospital had to open up because of a decline in staff and demands from the parents in public.[83] Yet, when the laws of the market were removed, the old hierarchical structures took over again. For instance, currently parents are only allowed to visit their children at specific times at the paediatric intensive care unit in the children's hospital in Stuttgart even though involving parents on the neonatal intensive care units had received positive reviews already in 1977.[84] In this case, the cause is not with the nursing staff but the management team consisting of doctors. Nursing staff does not have a uniform position and parents have not yet been pro-active. This means that changes that had been perceived as positive for mothers or parents and also for the child can be undone if the medical directors decide to do so.

## Outlook

The current article still contains several gaps. One of them is the inclusion of the perspective of male nurses, i. e., their view of mothers and fathers during their work on paediatric wards and their relationship to children. I am referring to the question as to whether they also had the feeling that these were "their" children. Furthermore, the mere fact is of interest that male nurses were present at all in a field (nursing) that had previously been exclusively female. We can gain further insight into the latter issue through interviews with (former) paediatric nurses who had still experienced the "entry" of men into paediatric nursing and also through interviews with the first male paediatric nurses who ploughed a lone furrow.

I had also already mentioned that the view of the mothers and fathers of the children in hospital must be more strongly considered in the analysis. In the postwar years in Germany, the conservative distribution of gender roles demanded that women were mothers full-time; working mothers were regarded with high suspicion.[85] For the mothers there was also the question to what extent the hypotheses from psychology and psychiatry on the significance of the early mother-child-relationship on the development of the

---

83  Cf. Karte (1985). Another example is the "rooming-in" on maternity wards that was introduced at the end of the 1970s. Cf. Heidiri (2015).

84  Cf. Gerhard (1977).

85  Cf. on England Davis (2012), chap. 7.

personality affected their desire to be with their child, if possible, for most of the time.[86]

Furthermore, the retrospective view of contemporary witnesses on their stay at hospital as a child when the mothers or parents only had very restrictive visiting hours would be insightful here. Moving forward with this project I hope to close these gaps to a large extent.

# Bibliography

*Archives*

Private archive Annegret Braun

Braun, Annegret: Kind im Krankenhaus – Mitaufnahme von Müttern. Esslingen 1979.
Letter by H. F. to Annegret Braun from 20/08/2017
Letter by R. B. to Annegret Braun from 31/03/1984
Private archive Sylvelyn Hähner-Rombach
Interview with Annegret Braun
Interview with M. N.
Stadtarchiv Stuttgart
Bestand 19/1 Hauptaktei Gruppe 5, lfd. no. 1827

*Published sources*

Aktionskomitee "Kind im Krankenhaus" e. V. In: Biermann, Gerd (ed.): Mutter und Kind im Krankenhaus. Ein Situationsbericht aus der Bundesrepublik Deutschland. München; Basel 1978, pp. 124–125.
Arnold-Ullinger, Barbara: Erfahrungen einer Kinderkrankenschwester mit dem "Offenbacher Modell". In: Biermann, Gerd (ed.): Mutter und Kind im Krankenhaus. Ein Situationsbericht aus der Bundesrepublik Deutschland. München; Basel 1978, pp. 52–55.
Bayerns erster männlicher Kinderkrankenpfleger. In: Deutsche Krankenpflegezeitschrift 26 (1973), p. 506.
Biermann, Gerd (ed.): Mutter und Kind im Krankenhaus. Ein Situationsbericht aus der Bundesrepublik Deutschland. München; Basel 1978.
Brief einer Mutter an Kinderkrankenschwestern. In: Deutsche Krankenpflegezeitschrift 32 (1979), p. 679.
Die Mutter im Krankenhaus. In: Deutsche Schwesternzeitung 12 (1959), p. 309.
Gerhard, Jan: Mütter pflegen Frühgeborene. Erfahrungsbericht aus einer Frühgeborenen-Intensivstation. In: Deutsche Krankenpflegezeitschrift 30 (1977), pp. 347–351.
Gesetz über die Ausübung des Berufs der Krankenschwester, des Krankenpflegers und der Kinderkrankenschwester (Krankenpflegegesetz). Vom 15. Juli 1957. In: Bundesgesetzblatt (1957), Teil I, Nr. 31 vom 18.07.1957, pp. 716–719, available at: https://www.bgbl.de/xaver/bgbl/start.xav?start=//*%5B@attr_id=%27bgbl157s0716.pdf%27%5D#__bgbl__%2F%2F*%5B%40attr_id%3D%27bgbl157s0716.pdf%27%5D__1519122414036 (last accessed: 17/10/2018)

---

86   During the 1980s this perception resulted on the so-called "new motherliness".

Gillett, S.M.: "Zeit zum Bemuttern". Von Sister S.M. Gillett aus dem *Nursing Mirror*, ins Deutsche übersetzt von Schwester Edith Fischer. In: Deutsche Schwesternzeitung 8 (1955), pp. 145–146.

Karte, Helmut: Mutter und Kind im Krankenhaus. Eine kritische Betrachtung aus ärztlicher Sicht. In: Deutsche Krankenpflegezeitschrift 38 (1985), pp. 601–604.

Keuth, Ulrich: Maximal liberalisierte Besuchsregelung in der Kinderklinik. In: Deutsche Krankenpflegezeitschrift 32 (1979), pp. 673–675.

Kind im Krankenhaus. Dokumentation über eine Fachtagung am 10. Oktober 1979 in Heidelberg. Stuttgart 1979.

Kind und Mutter im Kinderkrankenhaus? Nursing Times 1963, 841. In: Deutsche Schwesternzeitung 17 (1964), pp. 247–248.

K[litzing], A[nnemarie] v[on]: Das Kind im Krankenhaus von der Mutter betreut? In: Deutsche Schwesternzeitung 8 (1955), p. 145.

Klitzing, Annemarie von. In: Wolff, Horst-Peter (ed.): Biographisches Lexikon zur Pflegegeschichte. "Who was who in nursing history." Berlin; Wiesbaden 1997, pp. 104–105.

Köttgen, U.: Verkümmerung als Folge von Pflegeschäden beim Kind. In: Medizinische Klinik 53 (1958), pp. 1–7.

Kollan, Luise: Eine Mutter schreibt dazu. In: Deutsche Schwesternzeitung 8 (1955), p. 242.

Koppe, Sigrun; Gebensleben, Susanne: Hat die liberalisierte Besuchszeit im Kinderkrankenhaus nur Vorteile für unsere Kinder? In: Deutsche Krankenpflegezeitschrift 33 (1980), pp. 712–714.

Leist, Elisabeth: Mutter und Kind im Krankenhaus. In: Deutsche Schwesternzeitung 21 (1968), p. 366.

Maas, Gertrud: "Das Kind im Krankenhaus von der Mutter betreut?" In: Deutsche Schwesternzeitung 8 (1955), pp. 241–242.

Maas, Gertrud: Zum Thema: Die Besuchszeit in der Kinderklinik aus der Sicht einer Kinderkrankenschwester. In: Deutsche Schwesternzeitung 20 (1967), pp. 87–88.

Mütter dürfen bei Kindern im Krankenhaus bleiben. In: Stuttgarter Zeitung (22 July 1966).

Oberschwester Maria Plieninger: "Zur kommenden Ausbildung der Kinderschwestern". In: Deutsche Schwesternzeitung 7 (1954), pp. 123–124.

Rundtischgespräch: Mütter im Kinderkrankenhaus. Beitrag von Karin Hülse. In: Deutsche Krankenpflegezeitschrift 32 (1979), pp. 676–677.

Schwester Ingrid Schmalzl: Mutter- und Kindabteilung. In: Deutsche Schwesternzeitung 19 (1966), pp. 26–27.

Schwester R.M.: Zum Thema Die Besuchszeit in der Kinderklinik aus Sicht der Kinderkrankenschwester. In: Deutsche Schwesternzeitung 20 (1967), p. 138.

Schwester W.K.: Die Besuchszeit in der Kinderklinik aus der Sicht einer Kinderkrankenschwester. In: Deutsche Schwesternzeitung 19 (1966), pp. 509–510.

Stemann, Dietlinde: Kind und Kinderkrankenhaus. In: Deutsche Schwesternzeitung 20 (1967), pp. 580–582.

Stemann, Dietlinde: Berufsprobleme in der Kinderkrankenpflege. In: Deutsche Schwesternzeitung 22 (1969), pp. 259–260.

S.W.: Die Mutter als Betreuerin im Kinderkrankenhaus. Eine weitere Zuschrift. In: Deutsche Schwesternzeitung 8 (1955), pp. 304–305.

*Literature*

Blessing, Bettina: Kleine Patienten und ihre Pflege. Der Beginn der professionellen Säuglingspflege in Dresden. In: Geschichte der Pflege 2 (2013), pp. 25–34.

Davis, Angela: Modern Motherhood. Women and Family in England, 1945–2000. Manchester 2012.

Elendt, Erika: Das kranke Kind und seine Pflegerin. Zur Geschichte der Kinderkrankenpflege in Jena von 1917–1987. Jena 1992.
Heidiri, Adrian Maria: Die Erfindung der natürlichen Geburt. Diskurs um Geburtshilfe
(1976–1983) – neue Frauenbewegungen, Gynäkologen und Hebammen zwischen Sicher-
heit und Selbstbestimmung. Wiss. Arbeit als Bestandteil der Prüfung für das Lehramt, His-
torisches Seminar der Univ. Freiburg/Brsg. 2015, available at: https://freidok.uni-freiburg.
de/data/11619 (last accessed: 17/10/2018).
Neumann, Josef N.: Kinderheilkunde. In: Gerabek, Werner E. (ed.): Enzyklopädie Medizin-
geschichte. Berlin; New York 2005, pp. 743–749.
Peiper, Albrecht: Chronik der Kinderheilkunde. 3rd ed. Leipzig 1958.
Robertson, James: Kinder im Krankenhaus. Mit einer Dokumentation von 50 Elternbriefen.
München; Basel 1974.
Seidler, Eduard; Leven, Karl-Heinz: Geschichte der Medizin und der Krankenpflege. 7th ed.
Stuttgart 2003.
Troschke, Jürgen von: Das Kind als Patient im Krankenhaus. Eine Auswertung der Literatur
zum psychischen Hospitalismus. München; Basel 1974.


*Internet*

Aktionskomitee Kind im Krankenhaus: http://root.akik.de/phocadownload/akik-chronik09.
pdf (last accessed: 17/10/2018)
Berufsverband Kinderkrankenpflege e. V.: https://www.bekd.de/der-bekd-ev/geschichte-des-
berufes-und-des-berufsverbandes/ (last accessed: 17/10/2018)

Conflicts due to Changes in Social Conditions

# From Wars on the Wards to Harmonious Hospitals: British Nursing Sisters' Pursuit of Collaboration on Active Service in the Second World War[1]

*Jane Brooks*

## Introduction

British nursing sisters of the Queen Alexandra's Imperial Military Nursing Service (QAs) went to war between 1939 and 1945 having been trained in a system that privileged the male doctor, his position, his work and his authority.[2] According to Sister Mary Morris, doctors, especially consultants were treated as superior beings: "junior nurses must never presume to talk to a Consultant."[3] Messages were to be given to the staff nurse, who would tell the ward sister, who would then relay the message to the doctor. On active service overseas, with limited numbers of medical officers and hundreds of thousands of men requiring medical and surgical treatment, such hierarchical work patterns were virtually untenable. Nevertheless, the need to relinquish the medical hegemony and adopt more collaborative work patterns was not easy for all doctors. To begin to adopt a less deferential attitude towards their medical colleagues was not always easy for the nurses either.

The medical officers of the Royal Army Medical Corps (RAMC) were used to working with their RAMC orderlies; men who had either chosen to engage in hospital work, were unfit for combat duties or were conscientious objectors. In the First World War an ill or injured soldier's first point of contact would have been with a male orderly in a Field Dressing Station.[4] In far-flung war zones and close to the frontline, orderlies worked directly under the control of the medical officers performing many of the nursing duties that otherwise would be undertaken by trained nurses. As female nursing sisters were posted to ever-more dangerous areas of the globe during the Second World War, medical officers needed to re-negotiate the hitherto simple hierarchy between them and their male orderlies, who were ordinary soldiers or non-commissioned officers into working relationships with professionally trained women officers, creating more complex lines of command. Never-

---

1    I should like to thank Manchester University Press for giving me permission to use some of the themes and data from my recently published monograph, "Negotiating Nursing: British Army Sisters and Soldiers in the Second World War".

2    Even after nurses were awarded commissioned officer status in 1941, nurses in the Royal Navy, Army and Air Force continued to carry the title Nursing Sister, rather than titles such as Captain, Lieutenant or Squadron Leader. There is no implied reference to women of religious orders contained in the title.

3    IWM, Documents.4850: Morris, Mary: The diary of a wartime nurse, 17 September 1940, p. 38.

4    Hallett (2009), p. 15.

theless, as the war progressed many primary sources demonstrate medical and nursing officers realised that "the most important person in the equation was the patient, not the nurse and not the doctor".[5] A trope that personified the context of war in which the common good was more important than the individual.[6] The patient as a fighting man was essential to the machine of war, especially in zones where it was difficult to post fit men quickly. Medical and nursing officers needed to heal men to return them to battle. Whilst some doctors and nurses on active service did continue to maintain the traditional professional boundaries, many realised that in order for soldiers' treatments to be effective and to increase the speed of recovery, all members of the medical team needed to develop more collaborative working relationships.[7]

Susan Grayzel argues that the First World War "gave rise to the expression 'home front' dividing the necessary labor [sic] of civilians (gendered feminine) from that of 'war front' soldiers (gendered masculine)".[8] The manner in which air power brought war to the home nation established the idea that the Second World War was a "people's war" in which all members of the nation were part of a unified identity, whether male or female. Yet, Sonya O. Rose exposes the fragility of the idea of unity in a system in which women's position was always subordinated to the war effort, whereas the fighting man was the war effort.[9] In the same way, the fragility of the concept that the various members of the medical services worked with each other as members of a professional citizenry is exposed in this article. The geographic location of the hospital or casualty clearing station (CCS), specifically its distance from 'civilisation' was frequently the issue when the nurses' autonomous working and extension to their roles were enabled or disbarred. Furthermore, medical officers had significant power that nurses could rarely undercut. This meant that if the doctor did not wish to relinquish his power, the opportunity for the nurses to affect their position was limited, often by their ability to play what has since been called the "doctor-nurse game".[10] In this game the nurse may only be successful if she can negotiate around the positions of power and authority by appearing passive to them.[11] The power of masculine authority was to have far reaching consequences at the end of the war. On demobilisation medical men had access to financial support for postgraduate study and whether married or not they could return to their hospital or community practice, sure of their prestige. There were no such opportunities for the majority of the nursing sisters, many of whom married and left nursing altogether as hospitals would not employ married nurses.

5   Brooks: Negotiating (2018), p. 151.
6   Rose (2003), p. 108.
7   Bolton (1986), p. 195.
8   Grayzel (2012), p. 3.
9   Rose (2003), p. 2.
10  Stein (1968), p. 101. The analysis of the interaction between doctors and nurses described as a 'game' has been used in a number of essays on relationships between the two professions. See for example Stein/Watts/Howell (1990); Larson (1999); Weaver (2013).
11  Wytenbroek (2015), p. 107.

The purpose of this article is to examine the conflicts on active service that nurses managed between themselves and the doctors with whom they worked and the manner in which the exigencies of war encouraged a more collaborative approach to patient care. It is also an essay about gender negotiations. The expectation that women would be subordinate to their male colleagues will be explored. I shall argue that the expectations of the male military in general and the medical officers in particular were inconsistent to the point of the impossible. Faced with multiple contradictions in expectations, the nursing sisters needed to negotiate carefully their position as women officers, professional nurses and single ladies in a hyper-masculine arena – the war zone.[12] The article begins with a brief analysis of the use of personal testimony. This is followed by an account of the nature of war and conflict. The system in which nurses and doctors were trained and worked itself caused conflict. Nurses were trained in subservience, whilst medical staff were taught to expect obedience and deference.[13] These professional hierarchies were firmly situated in what were highly gendered lives, which placed the nurse as female as subservient to the doctor as male. The nursing profession itself was strictly bound on hierarchical lines with limited engagement between nurses of different status. The article therefore follows the discussion of war and conflict with an exploration of the multiple points of conflict experienced by female nurses who were posted on active service overseas. However, as is demonstrated in the primary source material used, it was clear to many nurses and doctors on active service overseas, such hierarchies were neither helpful nor necessary. The essay will therefore examine in detail the methods and episodes of collaboration between the professions, notwithstanding the contingency of such collegiality.

## Methods and methodology

The chapter uses a range of personal testimony and the influential medical and nursing press of the day, including the *British Medical Journal*, the *Nursing Times* and the *American Journal of Nursing*. It is the personal testimonies however that frame the work. Despite censorship and self-censorship, British Army nursing sisters on overseas service wrote detailed diaries, as well as letters to friends, families and their Matron-in-Chief, Dame Katharine Jones. Some of the diaries were written for personal reasons, but have since been published,[14] others were used to create memoirs in the nurses' later years.[15] A number of

12  For a full and detailed analysis of British Army nurses' negotiations, see Brooks: Negotiating (2018).
13  Limbert (1933).
14  During the research for the wider project from which this article comes, an abridged version of Mary Morris' diary was published. See Morris (2014).
15  The testimonies of two nursing sisters, Sisters Catherine Hutchinson and Catherine Butland, used for this article come from unpublished memoirs. Although it has not been possible to locate any diaries or correspondence from which these accounts may have

oral histories were also taken for the wider project from which this article is taken. Oral history as a research method has been subject to a number of criticisms, not least in relation to the problem of memory,[16] the unequal nature of the interview structure,[17] and critically for this study the 'colouring' of the memory with post-war experiences.[18] Yet as oral historians such as Lynn Abrams, Geertje Boschma and Penny Summerfield acknowledge, the value of oral history lies in the relationship between the interviewer and interviewee.[19] When the interviewer has professional or personal points of contact with the person they interview, the richness of the story can be brought to the fore.[20] Thus as a nurse, I was able to ask questions that non-nurses would not consider. Both written and oral testimonies used in this article offer the nurses' personal accounts of war and their place in it. It is acknowledged that the personal testimonies used may not always create the most accurate and 'factual' picture of the nurses' war.[21] However, given the paucity of source material about nurses and their war experiences in the public domain, they provide a window through which their lives can be witnessed.

## Conflict

*War and conflict*

The nature of war is to maim and kill. Indeed, "war depends upon large number of people being prepared to slaughter large numbers of other people."[22] But the Second World War led the warrior impulse to kill to new heights.[23] The global nature of the Second World War brought peoples into conflict that had previously been allies and brought people into a war from all corners of the planet. Friends and neighbours were set against each other as fascism took hold of continental Europe with devastating results of an unimaginable level. Such a war was unlike any other previous war, the level of conflict superseding people's imagination.

originated, they contain such detail about not only the exciting moments, but also the mundane that it is reasonable to assume they were written from some accounts created at the time.

16  Marwick (2001), pp. 135–136.
17  Olson/Shopes (1991), p. 189.
18  Rose (2003), p. 25.
19  Boschma et al. (2008), p. 84; Abrams (2010), p. 66; Summerfield (1998), p. 83.
20  Dickinson (2015), p. 10; Brooks: Negotiating (2018), p. 10. For a detailed discussion of researcher identity in nursing history, see for example Boschma/Grypma/Melchior (2008).
21  For an excellent discussion on the use of women's diaries as a source material for women's history, see for example Hanson/Donahue (1996).
22  Bourke (2001), p. 1.
23  Brooks: Negotiating (2018).

It was also the first war in which the medical services were viewed as critical to the allies' success. As Mark Harrison argues, the medical service was understood to be an essential weapon in the bid to maintain healthy, fighting men.[24] The knowledge that better patient outcomes could be achieved if men were treated close to the moment of injury or illness, meant field hospitals and CCSs were created near the fighting.[25] Senior military figures appreciated that this need for an immediacy of care demanded trained and skilled practitioners, both medical and nursing. Thus, for the first time, a critical mass of female military nurses was posted to battle zones to salvage men and heal their minds and bodies.[26] Whether the nurses' hierarchical and frequently divisive training had prepared them for the challenges these opportunities offered is less certain.

### Creating conflict: divide and rule

The nursing sister who went to war between 1939 and 1945 had trained in a system of harsh discipline, long hours and strict hierarchies.[27] In her autobiography of her nurse training in the mid-1930s, Janet Wilks recalled the friendship that developed between Nurse Bates – a second-year student – and herself when she was on her very first ward. However, such friendships were not guaranteed[28], nor were they easy with erratic split-shift patterns and little time off when other young people would be socialising[29]. A system that ensured the most junior nurses were cut off from the outside world and were taught they were "the lowest of the low",[30] guaranteed that student nurses had very limited

---

24  Harrison (2004), p. 2.
25  Anderson (2011), p. 76.
26  For a full and detailed discussion please see Brooks: Negotiating (2018), p. 2; Brooks: Not only (2018).
27  Susan McGann and colleagues argue that the harshness of the regime was exacerbated by the inability to employ sufficient nurses to ease the burden of work. They cite The Association of Nurses' claim that 50 per cent of entrants to nursing never completed their training and that 38 per cent left in their first year. Such a high turnover meant that matrons were continually re-supplying the hospital wards with ever more inexperienced staff thus adding even further to the workload and strain of care. McGann/Crowther/Dougall (2009), p. 97.
28  Wilks (1991).
29  Elsie Davies, oral history interview 2012. In Sheila Bevington's "Nursing Life and Discipline", based on her research into the lives and conditions of nurses, she maintains that although students or student nurses show 'greater vitality' when they work a three-shift system in which they had long periods away from the wards for rest, socialisation and study, the system was not universally popular with ward sisters and staff nurses. The more prevalent and far less popular split-shift pattern gave student nurses time off during the day, but only after they had already appeared for work, negating useful time away from ward work. Bevington (1943), p. 29.
30  Roma Heaton, oral history interview 2013.

access to any sort of power. Nurses were called by their surnames,[31] except the very best of friends, a method reminiscent of boys' schools, but which precluded intimacy. As Barbara Keddy and colleagues argue with reference to Canadian nurse training, if the workers were divided then they could not revolt.[32] Nurses were expected to stand when a doctor entered the room and hold the door open for all adults.[33] Elizabeth Morris who began her training at The London Hospital, Whitechapel in 1944, recalled student nurses were "taught when we were allowed to look at a consultant [doctor] or to say 'good morning'".[34] Both Mary Morris and June Hamilton who commenced their nurse training at a west London hospital in 1943 said that as student nurses they were barred from talking to medical students. Hamilton maintained if you were caught, "it was bad luck".[35]

Mid 20th-century Britain broadly retained an ideology of professional and gender hierarchy. The 1928 Equal Franchise Act in Britain may have given women the same rights to vote as men, but this did not mean their lives were equal.[36] Caitriona Beaumont maintains that women may have been assured of their rights as citizens, but their citizenship was predicated on their value in the home as wives and mothers.[37] Women of Britain were conscripted into war-work from 1941, many taking on work that was traditionally seen as 'men's work'.[38] This was however, 'only for the duration' and they were invariably paid less than men, even when they did the same job. Indeed, as men started to enter the nursing profession, they were usually employed in lower grade positions, but paid more than their female nurse colleagues – something that angered many, including the Royal College of Nursing.[39] The male medical profession was fearful of competition from female doctors and considered the possibility of working under "female authority an unbearable affront".[40]

---

31    Private archive Jane Brooks, Foster, Susan (pseudonym): Personal correspondence with Jane Brooks, 8 September 2013; UKCHN, Morris, Elizabeth: Personal correspondence with Jane Brooks, 14 August 2013.

32    Keddy et al. (1992–1993). It is acknowledged that there are some significant differences between the Canadian system and the British one at the time. Canadian hospitals employed very few trained nurses, using the 'student' labour to staff the wards. However, there were a number of distinct similarities too, particularly in the discipline expected of student nurses and the limited power they were afforded by the system.

33    Anonymous, oral history interview (no date).

34    UKCHN, Morris, Elizabeth: Personal correspondence with Jane Brooks, 14 August 2013. It is acknowledged that the position of consultants was quite different to all other professionals in the hospital. As honorary physicians and surgeons they gave their time in voluntary hospitals for free and were therefore treated with much greater deference. According to Mayhew, for example, McIndoe was known as either 'The Boss' or 'God' at East Grinstead. Mayhew (2010), loc1162.

35    Hamilton, oral history interview 2011.

36    Beaumont (2001).

37    Beaumont (2000).

38    Rose (2003), p. 109.

39    McGann/Crowther/Dougall (2009).

40    Dyhouse (1998), p. 123.

Despite attempts by the nursing leadership to assert nursing's professional status, the general requirement of nurses to maintain a supportive and subordinate role to the medical men was reinforced therefore by both gender and profession. The position of military nurses may have been an elevated one compared to their civilian counterparts,[41] but they were structured by similar gendered and professional boundaries. Nursing sisters had been given relative rank in the First World War and were awarded commissioned officer status in 1941, but their promotion prospects were poor.[42] Most remained at junior officer level in stark contrast to the male medical officers.[43] The nursing sisters of the British Army had considerable obstacles to overcome in order to develop the collaborative approaches to care that they felt were necessary to salvage men for battle.

### Professional conflicts

Sister Barbara Collins had been on active service in Sierra Leone for just over three months when she wrote to her parents of the frustrations of war service:

> Florence Nightingale had no more difficulties in Crimea than we are having out here – lack of organisation, lack of equipment and lack of co-operation is enough to make you weep [...] However, I am only in it 'for the duration' and I shall resign then. If there is another war, nothing would induce me to nurse with the RAMC.[44]

The difficulties with the lack of equipment and organisation notwithstanding, Collins' annoyance with the RAMC is significant. Most of the personal testimonies used for this article attempt to make much of the cordial relations between the nursing sisters and medical officers. However, occasionally diaries and letters home allow the realities of conflict to appear. Sister Betty Parkin was highly critical of one doctor with whom she worked who felt that the patients' diets were his responsibility: "No small items, such as eggs, two ounces of brandy or a tin of milk, escaped his notice. Pleas that they were needed for the small emergency supply that all sisters kept went unheard."[45] Parkin's annoyance at the interference of a medical officer in patient feeding was understandable. Nurses had been in charge of patients' diets since the early days of reformed nursing in the 19th century. Nurses were trained in 'invalid cookery'

---

41   This analysis of the differing status between civilian and military nurses was raised in the radio programme 'Frontline Females', BBC Radio 4 on 11 April 1998 & 18 April 1998: These two programmes formed the primary source material for Starns (2000).

42   Jones (2005), p. 262.

43   Whilst there were differences between the Canadians and the British, where issues of gender and profession intersected, they were remarkably similar. Cynthia Toman cites a medical officer in the Royal Canadian Army Medical Corps moving from lieutenant to lieutenant colonel in nineteen days, whereas a nursing sister went on active service as a lieutenant and came home at the end of the war a lieutenant. Toman (2007), p. 94.

44   UKCHN, Collins, Barbara: Letters home from Sierra Leone, 1940–1941, 30 November 1940.

45   Parkin (1990), p. 115.

and expected to be able to make nutritious drinks and supplements.[46] An article to the *Nursing Times* in 1935 addressed all nurses when its author asked, "How to give nourishment in a digestible and agreeable form to restore the health [...]?"[47] If during the Depression of the 1930s the price to be paid for the family's food was a political motivator for women,[48] by the Second World War, women held genuine power as arbiters of the family diet who restricted food waste and managed war time rations.[49] That a male medical officer should stymie this important female nursing responsibility would understandably be a point of conflict. Although even with the increased autonomy that active service offered nurses, there was little that Parkin could do to assert what she felt was her professional responsibility.

There were more difficult wars to manage on the wards, ones that affected patient care and potentially led to harm. Some of the most vivid of these come from the diary of Sister Esther (Helen) Luker. Luker was a St. Thomas' Hospital nurse, having trained at the nursing school founded by Florence Nightingale. Given the international importance of this nurse training school, unlike many hospital training schools across Britain, it could afford to choose only the very best candidates.[50] In her war diary, she wrote of the pleasure she found working with a St. Thomas' Hospital medical officer, which "needless to say helped towards the smooth running of the ward!".[51] However, other medical officers are criticised for their officious ways or putting patients at risk. On Tuesday 5 November 1940, her diary reports that both she and her colleague Sister H. "are getting so fed up with Col W. – it's frightful".[52] Two days later she wrote, "Col W. demands tea at 4.30 pm to my intense annoyance – & then I have mine".[53] One month later on 16 December, "We do heaps of dressings with Col W. to superintend!.".[54] Prior to the war complex wound dressings

---

46  The provision of food was part of a nurse's role before the reforms of the late 19th century. During the Crimean War nurses took over the dietary needs of their soldier-patients. Anne Summers argues that in doing so, "female nurses entered an area which seemed to be simply more 'women's work'." Summers (2000), p. 35. Carol Helmstadter however argues that the exigencies of war meant the work became more than a mere domestic task. Helmstadter (2015). Jane Schultz points to the 'gentrification' of the patients' kitchen when it was taken over by middle-class ladies in the American Civil War. Schultz (2004), p. 35.

47  Vickers (1935), p. 124.

48  Caine (2001), p. 174.

49  Brock et al. (2015), loc592. See also Braybon/Summerfield (1987), p. 247.

50  For a useful discussion of the difficulties in recruiting nurses outside the famous, elite voluntary hospitals, especially those in London, see for example Bell (1991).

51  IWM, Documents.1274: Luker, Esther H.E., ARRC: Diaries from 1940–45, Preface, p. 5.

52  IWM, Documents.1274: Luker, Esther H.E., ARRC: Diaries from 1940–45, 5 November 1940.

53  IWM, Documents.1274: Luker, Esther H.E., ARRC: Diaries from 1940–45, 7 November 1940.

54  IWM, Documents.1274: Luker, Esther H.E., ARRC: Diaries from 1940–45, 16 December 1940.

would often have been performed by the medical staff, or at least supervised by them. Reflecting specifically on orthopaedic nursing, the text book, "Wartime Nurse", argued that the war "brought new and intensely interesting and vitally important duties",[55] many of which were willingly adopted by nurses of all specialities. Cynthia Toman cites one Canadian nursing sister, Pauline Lamont, "I did dressings and things I'd never seen before […] We were given trust. We were given responsibility."[56]

Toman argues, "It was gender, not nurses' abilities that constrained their work".[57] But it was also long-held attitudes towards the medical hegemony. Lamont may have performed complex dressings that in civilian life would have been a doctor's realm, but this work was handed to her by her medical colleagues who no longer had the time, or perhaps inclination to perform such tasks. This work was therefore contingent not only on the limited numbers of doctors and the geographic location of the hospital that created the necessity for nurses to take on additional and extended work, but also the doctors' willingness to relinquish such work. Clearly Col. W. was not prepared to do that and retained the medical prerogative to make decisions about what work he would extend to the nursing staff and what he would not. He thus retained the right to supervise the dressings-work of Luker and her colleague. This medical prerogative also extended to refusing to support nurses with patients. Behaviour that ensured the nurses knew that the doctor decided when they were professional colleagues, with professional accountability and responsibility and when they were subordinate workers, who should be supervised:

> We are just cleaning up after the transfusion when Pte Hughes, a gunshot wound of arm in plaster has a secondary haemorrhage. I have great difficulty in calling Capt. R and when he comes he's not very helpful. We give packets of morphine and pray hard. I go to Capt. R twice more, but he doesn't think fit to get up & help us, so I do what I think is best. But G + I are simply shaking with anxiety + there are lots of other ill patients as well.[58]

Sister Catherine Hutchinson also clashed with a medical officer over the boundaries between medical and nursing work. Hutchinson was sent to a ward where there was a patient who was suffering from Kala Azar, a debilitating tropical disease transmitted to human beings by the sand fly and which affects the liver and the spleen:

> Only recently (at that time) had a treatment been found, which was some metallic salt, highly injurious to tissues and therefore […] only to be given intravenously. The Consultant had ordered it, and it had arrived. Neither the Medical Officer nor the Sister had read the literature which stated categorically that the drug had to be given intravenously. The doctor therefore ordered it to be given intramuscularly, and the Sister so gave it – with disastrous results […] the MO [Medical Officer] put all the blame on the Sister,

---

55   Stirling of Keir (1940), p. 112.
56   Pauline Lamont, cited in Toman (2007), p. 124.
57   Toman (2007), p. 52.
58   IWM, Documents.1274: Luker, Esther H. E., ARRC: Diaries from 1940–45, 20 December 1940.

stressing that she had given the injection. In the rather apathetic state she was then in, she did not seek to avoid blame, which was rightly his.[59]

Harrison maintains that although military doctors admired the nursing sisters for their professionalism and technical skills, there was a level of friction between them.[60] Where nursing sisters had developed new ways of working to have their autonomy removed, caused them considerable irritation. Expectations that they would take the blame for mistakes made in the field, created a working environment that was not conducive to patient welfare and recovery. Hutchinson also recalled being angered and upset by doctors for taking patients to surgery even when the situation was hopeless and the nurses had fought hard for a more palliative manner of care.[61] Mary Morris wrote of her distress with the doctors' lack of sympathy for men with psychological war-damage, when she and her fellow nursing sisters believed that these men should be treated with kindness, compassion and sent home.[62] But angered as they were, there was little they could do.

Yet given the multiple points of potential conflict, clinical, professional and gendered, it is perhaps surprising that not more instances of difficulties have been located in the nurses' personal testimonies. Perhaps the reason for this is that nurses wished to make little of conflict and demonstrate collaboration with their medical colleagues, to show their increased autonomy and professional acumen. It may be that they were careful in their writings so as not to alert family, friends or the military authority to any problems that may have led to questions about their presence in war zones. It is also possible that there was an element of self-censorship in their letters home so that their friends and families believed that the military medical teams worked together for the war-effort.[63] Notwithstanding the impetus for nurses themselves to make much of inter-professional collaboration, evidence of such congenial relationships are found in doctors' and patients' testimonies too. Lieutenant-Colonel George Feggetter of the RAMC, was part of the medical contingent with Operation Torch that landed in Algiers in 1942. He wrote in his diary: "There is no doubt that the presence of female nurses on the day of the landing and for three or four weeks afterwards would have been a handicap".[64] Elsewhere however, he commends their work: "The efficiency of an operating theatre depended a great deal on the quality of the nursing staff and we were fortunate

59  IWM, Documents.11950: Hutchinson, Catherine A.: My war and welcome to it (2001), p. 112.
60  Harrison (2004), p. 32.
61  IWM, Documents.11950: Hutchinson, Catherine A.: My war and welcome to it (2001), p. 36.
62  IWM, Documents.4850: Morris, Mary: The diary of a wartime nurse, 28 June 1944, p. 116; Morris (2014), p. 100.
63  For a full and detailed discussion of the issue of censorship and self-censorship in the writings of Second World War nurses, see for example Brooks: Negotiating (2018), p. 12; Toman (2007), p. 72.
64  Wellcome Library, RAMC 1776: Feggetter, George: Diary of an R.A.M.C surgeon at war, 1942–1946, pp. 37–38.

in having excellent nurses, especially the sisters-in-charge."[65] RAMC Colonel J. R. McDonald's diary is replete with praise for individual nurses as well as their work more widely. Furthermore, the matron of his hospital attended the morning meeting with McDonald and the other senior medics.[66] Patients, including officer patients, also wrote of their praise for the nursing sisters, their work and the very positive effect their presence had on both the healthy and the ill and injured soldiers.[67] Indeed, it appears that nursing sisters were generally commended for their work, their clinical skills and their morale-boosting presence.

## Collaboration

*Socialising on active service: partying together*

In her diary for 20 February 1945, Sister Mary Morris wrote:

> Last night should have been my 'night off'. Bill [one of the medical officers] and Eric B came along to the Mess at 6 p.m. to collect me and Peggy. Eric invited us to the R.A.F. officers club in Brussels [...] They brought us back just after midnight and there was a message awaiting me to say that I must go on duty at once as a new convoy had come in.

> My bed never looked so inviting as I changed into my grey and scarlet uniform. There was absolute chaos in the ward. All the lights were on – stretchers on the floor and T.J. and Soeur Marie Anselma rushing around in circles. D. was trying to run both her ward and mine. Bill put on a white coat and joined me as we tried to bring some order to the situation and deal with the most seriously injured cases first.[68]

One of the significant differences between civilian hospital life and active service was the increased socialising between the nurses and medical staff. In most hospital training schools nursing students were disbarred from socialising with medical students and if caught could face dismissal.[69] There were occasional challenges to this prevailing ideology. Sister Penny Salter recalled her student nursing days at St. Mary's Hospital in London in which she identified both close friendships and romantic relationships between nurses and medical students. She wrote of her nursing colleagues and their medical student 'boyfriends' holding a joint party in one of the medical students' parents' home,[70] and remembered them all attending the theatre or sports events together.[71] According to medical historian Kevin Brown, the matron of St.

---

65  Wellcome Library, RAMC 1776: Feggetter, George: Diary of an R.A.M.C surgeon at war, 1942–1946, p. 66.
66  Wellcome Library, RAMC 944: McDonald, J.R.: A doctor goes to war, p. 206.
67  An officer (1944), p. 538.
68  IWM, Documents.4850: Morris, Mary: The diary of a wartime nurse, 20 February 1945.
69  UKCHN, Morris, Elizabeth: Personal correspondence with Jane Brooks, 14 August 2013.
70  IWM, Documents.17649: Salter, Muriel Kathleen (Penny): Long ago and far away: A distant memory: A diary, c. 1938–1970, pp. 31–32.
71  IWM, Documents.17649: Salter, Muriel Kathleen (Penny): Long ago and far away: A distant memory: A diary, c. 1938–1970, p. 7.

Mary's, Miss Milne herself decided that as there was a war on and the nurses and medical students needed to work together closely, they should be enabled to play together too.[72] It may be that the attitude did exist in other hospitals, but evidence of such ideas are scant. Nevertheless, Miss Milne's attitude worked in favour of improved relations on active service overseas. Salter was posted to Ramree Island in the Bay of Bengal. Because of the usual chaos of war, she did not reach the island until several weeks after she was expected, eventually arriving between Christmas and New Year 1944. When she did arrive therefore, there was a strong possibility that she would be reposted – her position having been filled by another nurse. However early contact with a naval officer who had been a medical student at St. Mary's and then meeting the Colonel who had also been at St. Mary's, precluded further posting and Salter stayed.[73]

On active service female nurses were often the only European women and specifically women officers of the British Army available for social engagements. In a realm in which, as Mary Morris recalled there could often be at least ten male officers to each female nurse,[74] the nurses held considerable social power. As I have argued elsewhere, nursing sisters were not blind to the social contract that could be made, in which they were able to marry someone from the officer class and the male officer gained a suitable partner in wartime and possibly a wife.[75] However, there were perhaps unseen ramifications for the nurses too. If the medical officers were used to seeing female nurses as their subordinates and 'servants' of the hospital, they would need to adjust these ideas in order to have access to these European women on active service. If they did not, the nurses would seek their partners elsewhere and frequently did.[76] Medical officers soon realised that if they wanted female company they would need to re-consider any hierarchical ideas about the nurse-doctor relationship and in the wake of any improved social relations, doctors learnt much about the nurses' abilities. Many of the nurses' personal testimonies point to a disregard for the normal rules of hospital work, etiquette and professional boundaries and identify a significant alteration in the attitudes of doctors to nurses, in which, "The medical officers were more than caring and loyal".[77]

When Salter was sent on well-earned leave in 1943, she took the night train to Banderwela in Sri Lanka, where there was a rest-house for officers. Arriving with a set of borrowed golf clubs, although she could not play, she was immediately requisitioned for a round of golf, by "Charles a Scottish doctor

---

72   Brown (2008), loc4295.
73   IWM, Documents.17649: Salter, Muriel Kathleen (Penny): Long ago and far away: A distant memory: A diary, c. 1938–1970, p. 131.
74   IWM, Documents.4850: Morris, Mary: The diary of a wartime nurse, 21 June 1944, p. 105; Morris (2014), p. 90.
75   Brooks: Negotiating (2018), p. 95.
76   Toman (2007), p. 99.
77   IWM, Documents.17649: Salter, Muriel Kathleen (Penny): Long ago and far away: A distant memory: A diary, c. 1938–1970, p. 109.

stationed with one of the Regiments of whom I had not previously met".[78] At Betty Parkin's desert hospital the sisters and medical officers erected a tent between their two messes, which they called the Bilharzia Arms – after one of the prevalent tropical diseases in Egypt – for socialising, listening to music and the occasional alcoholic drink.[79] Arriving in North Africa, unexpected and exhausted Sisters Geraldine Edge and Mary Johnston recalled the doctors and sisters sitting together in the lounge of the ship being served tea by the stewards.[80] One anonymous sister wrote to Dame Katharine Jones of the social activities organised in her CCS in Sicily in 1943. She detailed discussions organised by the colonel for all to attend, gramophone recitals organised by one of the other sisters and a unit newspaper for both staff and patients alike.[81] Sister Catherine Butland's unit in Tournai had a joint mess for medical and nursing staff.[82] Later with a unit in North Africa she wrote of, "a message was sent asking us to take tea with the Medical Officers […] a rather long affair."[83] The War Office Diaries for the QAs on 5 November 1939 stipulated that sisters were not to visit bars in France, or the officers' messes.[84] As the war progressed such rules were either completely disbanded or simply ignored.

The nurses' testimonies also demonstrate far more numerous occasions of collaboration and the removal of nurse-doctor hierarchies in the face of patient need, than points of conflict. Sister Jessie Wilson recalled the essential team work when she wrote, "it was obvious that it would take all the skill of both the Medical Officers and the nurses if those broken and smashed bodies were to get well."[85] It is this collegiality that belies the gendered and professional boundaries of the civilian hospital system. Hutchinson recalled one particular "high ranking consultant" arriving to do a ward round whilst her ward was in a state of chaos. Against all protocol: "We did the round together. He did not seem to mind that the MO in charge of the ward was absent but turned to me for any fresh information about each patient."[86] One anonymous Sister wrote to the Dame Katharine Jones, of their doctors who volunteered to stay up all night with the patients so that the nurses could get some sleep.[87]

78  IWM, Documents.17649: Salter, Muriel Kathleen (Penny): Long ago and far away: A distant memory: A diary, c. 1938–1970, p. 96.
79  Parkin (1990), p. 95.
80  Edge/Johnston (1945), p. 39.
81  MMM, Queen Alexandra's Royal Army Nursing Corps (QARANC) uncatalogued archive, Anonymous: Sicily, 58 Gen Hospital, 1943.
82  MMM, QARANC/PE/1/74/BUTL Box 8, Butland, Catherine M.: Army Sisters in Battledress or the Chosen Few or Follow Fate, p. 15.
83  MMM, QARANC/PE/1/74/BUTL Box 8, Butland, Catherine M.: Army Sisters in Battledress or the Chosen Few or Follow Fate, p. 35.
84  The National Archives, WO 177/14: Q. A. I. M. N. S. War diary: Volume III, 5 November 1939.
85  Private archive Jane Brooks, Wilson, Jessie Sarah Catherine: We also served, 1940 …, p. 50.
86  IWM, Documents.11950: Hutchinson, Catherine A.: My war and welcome to it (2001), p. 111.
87  A Sister QAIMNS (1944), p. 47.

On His Majesty's Hospital Carrier, "Leinster" on the Lake of Bizerta, an inland lagoon on the north-east tip of Tunisia, Sisters Geraldine Edge and Mary Johnston wrote of the dining saloon that was for the use of all, "'Abandon rank all ye who enter here' should have been written over the entrance, for all were equally welcome".[88] This abandonment of rank or at least altering the manner in which people of different ranks worked together became a necessary aspect of overseas medical services. The realisation that traditional hierarchical structures were not helpful and may indeed harm patients, became an important lesson in active service medical care. Sister Angela Bolton wrote in her autobiography: "The unquestioning obedience to doctors that had been instilled into us when we were training had changed to an easy comradeship that made life pleasanter and more productive of ideas for the patients' welfare."[89] Sometimes this relaxing of rank rules meant everyone, nurses, doctors and orderlies worked together but retained practice boundaries, other times it meant inter-changing work, but there is little doubt of the developing understanding that it was necessary to alter the manner in which patient care was performed.

*Relaxing professional hierarchies: working together*

Working at a hospital at Tobruk in 1942, one nursing sister wrote to Dame Katharine Jones:

> Every morning all patients, except those on the "Dangerously Ill" lists were taken from the wards and transferred to base hospitals, either by hospital ship or ambulance convoy. Fresh streams of stretchers began to arrive almost at once and the wards were soon as full as ever.

> During the night air-raids were now much fiercer [...] Sleep was a luxury. We began to feel we had been living like this all our lives, and the parties of a few weeks ago seemed like the fanciful dreams of some other existence.

> Under these conditions rank was barely recognised. Each had his [sic] task and set about it with a will. Medical Officers, Sisters and Orderlies fraternised completely only conscious of the particular job in hand [...] The orderlies were all well trained [...] The Medical Officers just worked and worked, unfalteringly, always cheerful and patient and giving every encouragement.[90]

This anonymous sister continued with a description of the organisation of the operating theatre in which six sisters worked at two operating tables. The roles therefore of nurse and surgeon were maintained in terms of clinical practice expertise, but the collaborative manner in which the roles were carried out were a far cry from civilian nursing practice. Sister Dorothy Bartlett in her

88   Edge/Johnston (1945), p. 45.
89   Bolton (1986), p. 195.
90   MMM, Queen Alexandra's Royal Army Nursing Corps (QARANC) uncatalogued archive, Anonymous: Middle East and the Hospital at Tobruk. December 1939 – October 1942, p. 8.

autobiography of her war-work described a working environment on a diph-
theria ward near Cairo, in which each had their particular tasks, the doctor administering serum "at any time he might be needed", the nursing sisters tend-
ing to the patients' diets and the orderlies supporting the sisters.[91] Sister Betty
Evans was posted to France with the 79 British General Hospital in 1944. In
her oral history she maintains that the nurses and doctors did separate jobs,
"we had the medical officers putting up the drips", but that "we worked in a
team of course."[92] Sister Laura Coward, on active duty in West Africa was
posted with a fellow nursing sister, a medical officer and two orderlies to care
for a patient suffering from blackwater fever. On arrival she described how the
doctors had performed the medical work of setting up intravenous fluids and
taking bloods before they arrived, suggesting a demarcation of work. Yet, she
and her fellow nurse then relieved the medical officers, so they could sleep,
suggesting some interchangeability of roles.[93]

As Emma Newlands argues, war offered opportunities of increased autonomy.[94] For the nurses, this meant they could make decisions on how they
organised their work and patients. But within these less hierarchical and
more collaborative relationships, doctoring work remained masculine scientific work and nursing female nurturing work.[95] If these interactions altered
the working relationships between nurses and doctors on active service, the
maintenance of work roles meant they were not particularly contentious. The
movement of nurses into what was considered to be scientific medical work
was more problematic. On the Home Front, nurses' engagement with work
such as anaesthetics gave rise to a series of hostile letters in the medical press.
One medical doctor, W. Stanley-Sykes wrote to the *British Medical Journal* that
nurse-anaesthetists were the, "bane of the second-rate American medical
school" and offered praise to the Canadians for outlawing the practice.[96]

The adoption of 'medical' tasks by nurses was not new. As Julie Fairman
and Patricia D'Antonio argue there have always been nurses who had little
use for the constraints of professional boundaries and were willing to undertake work in order to support their patients, even if that work was not considered the realm of nursing.[97] Where they saw a problem, they dealt with it.[98]
On active service overseas, the nursing sisters of the British Army were able

---

91   Bartlett (1961), p. 194.
92   Betty Evans, oral history interview 2014.
93   MMM, uncatalogued archive, Coward, Laura M.: A journey with the blackwater team in
     West Africa.
94   Newlands (2014), p. 9.
95   For a valuable discussion on the nature of medical and nursing work and the gender
     boundaries of each, see for example Dyhouse (1998), p. 125.
96   Stanley-Sykes (1941), p. 339. For a full and detailed discussion of the anger created by the
     move to enable nurses to given anaesthetics see Brooks: Negotiating (2018), pp. 148–149.
     It does appear that arguments surrounding the use and position of nurse-anaesthetists is
     on-going. See for example Aberese-Ako et al. (2015).
97   Fairman/D'Antonio (2008), p. 444.
98   Toman (2007), p. 64.

to re-negotiate the ideas of what could constitute nursing work and take on anaesthetics and even surgical interventions themselves with little opposition from their medical colleagues. When Sister Evelyn Cottrell was posted to Italy during the Battle of Monte Cassino, she was willing to perform minor surgery to salvage her soldier patients and support the medical officers who could then deal with more major surgical cases.[99] Sister Edith Stevenson administered anaesthesia during an amputation whilst island-hopping hiding from the Japanese and admits she and her nurse colleague would have probably done the amputation itself had they had the instruments.[100] Parkin, having been "waved away on several occasions [by the doctor]", became increasingly frustrated by one medical officer's inability to pass a naso-gastic tube on a patient with suspected poisoning: "swiftly I pinned it [the blanket] tight, shouted, 'Sit on his legs!' to the orderly and a nearby patient and got a firm grip on [the patient's] nose. A gasp, and the tube I had snatched from the MO went down. I left them to the messy job of the washout."[101]

It was not just in surgical work that nurses formed new areas of practice that they developed out of traditional medical roles. The care of malaria patients was a key nursing duty in the desert. In North Africa in 1943 malaria was responsible for eighty-three hospital admissions per thousand troops.[102] The ubiquity of the disease created levels of treatment regimens that could not be managed by the medical officers alone. As the war in the Middle-East and North Africa intensified, nurses developed their practice into the science of the diagnosis of malaria under a microscope. Sister Pat Moody described the interest she gained from learning to read slides, "I am learning bacteriology and spend a fair amount of my spare time peering down a microscope searching blood slides looking for malarial parasites."[103] According to Cynthia Toman, nurses soon became proficient at diagnosis and treatment.[104] In his 1943 edition of "Tropical Nursing", Arthur Leslie Gregg was stark in his assertion that the nurse on overseas service "should endeavour to make herself reasonably competent to recognise clinically all three types of malaria and, given the opportunity, an efficient nurse will soon learn to identify parasites under the microscope."[105] The recommendation that nurses should be proficient diagnosticians was a far cry from the belief she should be the deferent servant of the hospital that had been expected pre-war. But the requirement that nurses should be able to diagnose as well as administer nursing care was 'for the duration' only.

99   Evelyn Cottrell, oral history interview 1990.
100  IWM, LBY94/1636: Edith Stevenson: The Last Lap: Autobiography 1912–1986, pp. 14–15.
101  Parkin (1990), pp. 131–132.
102  Harrison (2004), p. 138.
103  Royal College of Nursing Archives, Moody, Patricia, Sister TANS: 76 General Hospital, BNAF. Letter to her mother. 24 July 1943.
104  Toman (2007), p. 134.
105  Gregg (1943), p. 99.

## Conclusion

Despite the occasional enlightened matron, most of the nurses who joined the QAs and went to war between 1939 and 1945 had trained in civilian hospitals that stymied their personal freedoms and demanded absolute obedience and deference to the system. Once in battle zones overseas, they and many of their medical officer colleagues realised that war service required a very different type of professional action, one grounded in professional collaboration, rather than the subservence of the nurse. This collaborative practice was understood as improving patient care and treatment regimens as nurses and doctors worked to heal men for the war effort. If the nursing sisters thought that these new modes of working would prevail at the end of the war, they were mistaken. In 1945, as the women of Britain were returned to the hearth and home, having supported the war effort 'for the duration', so demobilised nurses returned to find that hospitals wanted to re-establish pre-war models of work and practice boundaries. If nurses had hoped their war-time autonomy would remain, the power of the male and medical hegemony proved just how contingent nurses' wartime lives had been. Salter found her return to work in a British hospital, "boring".[106] Wilson was excited to organise her home posting with the matron for whom she had worked in the Middle East. She was however disappointed when she was warned she would have to "readjust" her ideas about nursing practices now she was back on home soil.[107] Even the Royal College of Nursing pamphlet, "The Re-Settlement of Nurses: Back to Civilian Life", published in December 1945, alerted demobilised nurses, "not [to] be disappointed if, because you have held a position of authority in the field, you do not step straight away into a similar position at home."[108]

On active service overseas, there was a clear demand for skilled care near the frontline to salvage men to return them to fight – nurses were vital to this service. At war's end with sufficient numbers of doctors in civilian practice to provide scientific treatment, the need for nurses to step outside the professional and gendered roles vanished. Unable to return to the stifling world of the civilian hospital, many simply left nursing and married. Of those who remained in the profession, public health work and overseas work with the colonial service became popular professional choices.[109] Professional arenas

---

106 IWM, Documents.17649: Salter, Muriel Kathleen (Penny): Long ago and far away: A distant memory: A diary, c. 1938–1970, p. 158.
107 Private archive Jane Brooks, Wilson, Jessie Sarah Catherine: We also served, 1940 …, p. 61.
108 Royal College of Nursing (1945), p. 1.
109 New research is showing that public health work was also the career of choice for many of the Jewish and Non-Aryan women who came to Britain as refugees in the 1930s fleeing Nazi Europe. Significantly for many of these women, medicine was their first choice of career, a profession that was not open to them in Britain at that time because of gender, language and financial reasons. That they should then choose the relative autonomy of community nursing and health visiting is perhaps testament to the less hierarchical nature of public health service.

that continued to provide autonomous and collaborative working conditions and enabled the demobilised nurses to use their considerable talents for patient benefit.

## Bibliography

*Oral histories (All held at the UKCHN, University of Manchester, unless otherwise stated)*

Anonymous, oral history interview of a nurse who trained at Booth Hall Hospital in Manchester between 1957 and 1960.
Cottrell, Evelyn Alma, Spears Unit, oral history interview by Lyn E. Smith on 9 July 1990 (Imperial War Museum Oral History Collection, Interview 12180).
Davies, Elsie, oral history interview by Jane Brooks at her home in Manchester, on 18 December 2012.
Evans, Betty, oral history interview by Jane Brooks via the telephone on 10 January 2014
'Frontline Females', BBC Radio 4 on 11 April 1998 & 18 April 1998[110] (British Library Sound Archive H9872/2 & H9890/2).
Hamilton, June (pseudonym), oral history interview by Jane Brooks at her home in the South of England on 19 October 2011.
Heaton, Roma, oral history interview by Jane Brooks, at her home in the North West on 18 September 2013.


*Archival sources*

### Museum of Military Medicine, Aldershot (MMM)

*QARANC/PE/1/74/BUTL Box 8*
Butland, Catherine M.: Army Sisters in Battledress or the Chosen Few or Follow Fate.

*Queen Alexandra's Royal Army Nursing Corps (QARANC) uncatalogued archive*
Anonymous: Middle East and the Hospital at Tobruk. December 1939-October 1942.
Anonymous: Sicily, 58 Gen Hospital, 1943

*uncatalogued archive*
Coward, Laura M.: A journey with the blackwater team in West Africa.

Of the informants for this research, Penny Salter joined the Medical and Nursing Service of Rhodesia (Zimbabwe), Betty Evans stayed in India until she married and returned with her husband to Britain. Catherine Hutchinson was the only nurse whose testimony has been used who it is known stayed in hospital nursing. She worked at East Grinstead Hospital which was the institution that performed much of the pioneering plastic surgery work and therefore was not typical.

110 In this programme Claire Rayner discussed their wartime nursing experiences with Monica Baly, Mary Bates, Glenys Branson, Constance Collingwood, Gertrude Cooper, Ursula Dowling, Brenda Fuller, Anne Gallimore, Monica Goulding, Daphne Ingram, Anita Kelly, Margaret Kneebone, Sylvia Mayo, Kay McCormack, Anne Moat, Phyllis Thoms and Margot Turner.

## Royal College of Nursing Archives, Edinburgh

Moody, Patricia, Sister TANS: 76 General Hospital, BNAF. Letter to her mother. 24 July 1943.

## Imperial War Museum, London (IWM)

Documents.1274: Luker, Esther H. E., ARRC: Diaries from 1940–45.
Documents.4850: Morris, Mary: The diary of a wartime nurse.
Documents.11950: Hutchinson, Catherine A.: My war and welcome to it (2001).
Documents.17649: Salter, Muriel Kathleen (Penny): Long ago and far away: A distant memory: A diary, c. 1938–1970.[111]
LBY94/1636: Edith Stevenson: The Last Lap: Autobiography 1912–1986.

## The National Archives, London

WO 177/14: Q. A. I. M. N. S. War diary: Volume III (1 to 30 November 1939).
Wellcome Library, London.
RAMC 944: McDonald, J. R.: A doctor goes to war.
RAMC 1776: Feggetter, George: Diary of an R. A. M. C surgeon at war, 1942–1946.
UK Centre for the History of Nursing, University of Manchester (UKCHN).
Collins, Barbara: Letters home from Sierra Leone, 1940–1941.[112]
Morris, Elizabeth: Personal correspondence with Jane Brooks, 14 August 2013.

## Private archive Jane Brooks

Foster, Susan (pseudonym): Personal correspondence with Jane Brooks, 8 September 2013.
Wilson, Jessie Sarah Catherine: We also served, 1940 ...[113]

## *Printed sources*

A Sister QAIMNS: An ambulance train in the evacuation from France, May 1940. In: Harrison, Ada (ed.): Grey and Scarlet: Letters from the War Areas by Army Sisters on Active Service. London 1944, pp. 40–49.

Aberese-Ako, Matilda et al.: 'I used to fight with them but now I have stopped!': conflict and doctor-nurse-anaesthetists' motivation in maternal and neonatal care provision in a specialist referral hospital. In: PLoS ONE 10 (2015), no. 8, pp. 1–20.

Abrams, Lynn: Oral History Theory. London 2010.

An officer: In Step with the QAs. 1.- An officer writes to his wife from the Anzio beachhead. In: Nursing Times (5 August 1944), p. 538.

Anderson, Julie: War, Disability and Rehabilitation in Britain: 'Soul of a Nation'. Manchester 2011.

Bartlett, Dorothy: Nurse in War. London 1961.

---

111  I am indebted to Penny's friends for providing me with full access to her diary and the various press reports of her wartime nursing experiences.

112  I am indebted to Rowena Quantrill, Barbara Collins' daughter for providing me with access to her mother's letters home during the war.

113  I am indebted to Jessie Wilson's family for providing me with access to this war memoir.

Beaumont, Caitriona: Citizens not feminists: the boundary negotiated between citizenship and feminism by mainstream women's organisations in England, 1928–39. In: Women's History Review 9 (2000), no. 2, pp. 411–429.

Beaumont, Caitriona: The women's movement, politics and citizenship, 1918–1950s. In: Zweiniger-Bargielowska, Ina (ed.): Women in Twentieth-Century Britain. Harlow 2001, pp. 262–277.

Bell, Liane: Shortages of nurses, 1928–1935: Was nursing going – or was nursing going on? In: History of Nursing Society Journal 3 (1991), no. 5, pp. 16–23.

Bevington, Sheila M.: Nursing Life and Discipline: A Study Based on Over Five Hundred Interviews. London 1943.

Bolton, Angela: The Maturing Sun: An Army Nurse in India 1942–45. London 1986.

Boschma, Geertje; Grypma, Sonya J.; Melchior, Florence: Reflections on researcher subjectivity and identity in nursing history. In: Lewenson, Sandra B.; Herrmann, Eleanor Krohn: Capturing Nursing History: A Guide to Historical methods in Research. New York 2008, pp. 99–121.

Boschma, Geertje et al.: Oral history research. In: Lewenson, Sandra B.; Herrmann, Eleanor Krohn: Capturing Nursing History: A Guide to Historical methods in Research. New York 2008, pp. 79–98.

Bourke, Joanna: The Second World War: A People's History. Oxford 2001.

Braybon, Gail; Summerfield, Penny: Out of the Cage: Women's Experiences in Two World Wars. London 1987.

Brock, Julia et al. (eds.): Beyond Rosie: A Documentary History of Women and World War II. Kindle ed. Fayetteville 2015.

Brooks, Jane: Negotiating Nursing: British Army Sisters and Soldiers in the Second World War. Manchester 2018.

Brooks, Jane: "Not Only with Thy Hands, But Also with Thy Minds": Salvaging Psychologically Damaged Soldiers in the Second World War. In: Nursing History Review 26 (2018) [article in press].

Brown, Kevin: Fighting Fit: Health, Medicine and War in the Twentieth Century. Kindle ed. Stroud 2008.

Caine, Barbara: English Feminism, 1780–1980. Oxford 2001.

Dickinson, Tommy: 'Curing Queers': Mental Nurses and their Patients, 1935–74. Manchester 2015.

Dyhouse, Carol: Women students and the London Medical Schools, 1914–39: The anatomy of a masculine culture. In: Gender & History 10 (1998), no. 1, pp. 110–132.

Edge, Geraldine; Johnston, Mary E.: Ships of Youth: The Experiences of Two Army Nursing Sisters on Board the Hospital Carrier Leinster. London 1945.

Fairman, Julie; D'Antonio, Patricia: Reimagining nursing's place in the history of clinical practice. In: Journal of the History of Medicine and Allied Health Sciences 63 (2008), no. 4, pp. 435–446.

Grayzel, Susan R.: At Home and Under Fire: Air Raids and culture in Britain from the Great War to the Blitz. Cambridge 2012.

Gregg, A[rthur] L[eslie]: Tropical Nursing. London 1943.

Hallett, Christine E.: Containing Trauma: Nursing Work in the First World War. Manchester 2009.

Hanson, Kathleen S.; Donahue, M. Patricia: The diary as historical evidence: The case of Sarah Gallop Gregg. In: Nursing History Review 4 (1996), pp. 169–186.

Harrison, Mark: Medicine and Victory: British Military Medicine in the Second World War. Oxford 2004.

Helmstadter, Carol: Class, gender and professional expertise: British military nursing in the Crimean War. In: Brooks, Jane; Hallett, Christine E. (eds.): One Hundred Years of Wartime Nursing Practices, 1854–1953. Manchester 2015, pp. 23–41.

Jones, Vera: A Time to Remember: A Record of Nursing Experiences, Impressions and Travels During World War II Contained in Letters Sent Home from The East. London 2005.

Keddy, Barbara et al.: The personal is political: a feminist analysis of the social control of rank-and-file nurses in Canada in the 1920s and 1930s. In: History of Nursing Society Journal 4 (1992–1993), no. 3, pp. 167–172.

Larson, Elaine: The impact of the physician-nurse interaction on patient care. In: Holistic Nursing Practice 13 (1999), no. 2, pp. 38–46.

Limbert, Paul M.: Discipline: A major problem in the nursing profession. In: Nursing Times (13 May 1933), pp. 462–465.

Marwick, Arthur: The New Nature of History: Knowledge, Evidence, Language. Basingstoke 2001.

Mayhew, Emily: The Reconstruction of Warriors: Archibald McIndoe, The Royal Air Force and the Guinea Pig Club. Kindle ed. Barnsley 2010.

McGann, Susan; Crowther, Anne; Dougall, Rona: A History of the Royal College of Nursing: A Voice for Nursing, 1916–90. Manchester 2009.

Morris, Mary: A Very Private Diary: A Nurse in Wartime. Ed. by Carol Acton. London 2014.

Newlands, Emma: Civilians into Soldiers: War, the Body and British Army Recruits, 1939–45. Manchester 2014.

Olson, Karen; Shopes, Linda: Crossing boundaries, building bridges: Doing oral history among working-class women and men. In: Gluck, Sherna Berger; Patai, Daphne: Women's Words: The Feminist Practice of Oral History. London 1991, pp. 189–204.

Parkin, Betty C.: Desert Nurse: A World War II Memoir. London 1990.

Rose, Sonya O.: Which People's War? National Identity and Citizenship in Britain, 1939–1945. Oxford 2003.

Royal College of Nursing (The Advisory Service): The Re-Settlement of Nurses: Back to Civilian Life. London 1945.

Schultz, Jane E.: Women at the Front: Hospital Workers in Civil War America. Chapel Hill, NC 2004.

Stanley-Sykes, W.: Nurse anaesthetists. In: British Medical Journal (1 March 1941), p. 339.

Starns, Penny: Nurses at War: Women on the Frontline, 1939–45. Stroud 2000.

Stein, Leonard I.: The doctor-nurse game. In: American Journal of Nursing 68 (1968), no. 1, pp. 101–105.

Stein, Leonard I.; Watts, David T.; Howell, Timothy: Sounding board: The doctor-nurse game revisited. In: The New England Journal of Medicine 322 (22 February 1990), pp. 546–549.

Stirling of Keir, The Hon. Mrs.: Orthopaedic nursing. I: The background of orthopaedic nursing. In: Mackintosh, J[ames] M[acalister]: War-time Nurse: An Anthology of Ideas about the Care and Nursing of War Casualties. Edinburgh 1940, pp. 101–112.

Summerfield, Penny: Reconstructing Women's Wartime Lives: Discourse and Subjectivity in Oral Histories of the Second World War. Manchester 1998.

Summers, Anne: Angels and Citizens: British Women as Military Nurses, 1854–1914. Newbury 2000.

Toman, Cynthia: An Officer and a Lady: Canadian Military Nursing and the Second World War. Vancouver 2007.

Vickers, M.B.: Tempting the invalid: A few hints on sick cookery. In: Nursing Times (9 February 1935), pp. 124–125.

Weaver, Roslyn: Games, civil war and mutiny: Metaphors of conflict for the nurse-doctor relationship in medical television programmes. In: Nursing Inquiry 20 (2013), no. 4, p. 280–292.

Wilks, Janet: Carbolic and Leeches. Ilfracombe 1991.

Wytenbroek, Lydia: Negotiating relationships of power in a maternal and child health centre: The experience of WHO nurse Margaret Campbell Jackson in Iran, 1954–1956. In: Nursing History Review 23 (2015), pp. 87–122.

# "Toothless Law": The Regulation (or 'Vaguelation') of Dentistry in Mandate Palestine[1]

*Eyal Katvan*

## Introduction

The requirement that practitioners of various professions (including dentistry) obtain a license (or register), as it existed in Mandate Palestine, dates back to 1918, with the British liberation of Palestine from Ottoman rule. In its 1926 Dentists Ordinance, the Mandate government established possession of a license as a precondition for practicing dentistry, with education and professional training as prerequisites for obtaining a license. Since that time, perhaps in contrast to the legislation regulating other professions, the Ordinance underwent frequent revisions, with amendments primarily in the areas of licensing and the activities in which those who do not meet the standards established by the Ordinance may engage. This study aims to demonstrate how the profession of dentistry developed within this "pressure cooker" of occupations centered on dental care – a "pressure cooker" with a safety valve of sorts[2] that allowed those who did not meet the licensing standards to practice nonetheless. That is, the British differentiated among various categories of practitioners so as not to deprive long-practicing professionals of their livelihood, on the one hand, without putting patients at risk of receiving unqualified care, on the other. The legislation in this area had to be amended repeatedly, primarily because new waves of immigrants led to new and varying demands for recognition as dental practitioners, alongside demands by qualified dentists, who insisted that unqualified individuals be prohibited from practicing.

I will argue that these mechanisms – which enabled qualified dentists to establish themselves and their profession by means of comparison with "others" – in fact also enabled the employment of those "others". The British faced pressure from various directions and demands from different types of parties who united their efforts through professional associations represented by lawyers. Within this context, as I will demonstrate, they took action by way of legislation that formed part of a professionalization (professional regulation) process. This legislation was deliberately vague, to ensure the authorities'

1    I wish to thank Dr. Tali Margalit, Prof. Aviva Halamish, Prof. Margalit Shilo, Prof. Zvi Triger, Prof. Assaf Likhovsky and the organizers and participants of the "Marketplace, Power, Prestige" workshop for their important comments and remarks. Special thanks to Dr. Moshe Kalman and Prof. Noah Lewin-Epstein for sharing important historical resources. This research is based on primary sources from various archives: Israel State Archives; Central Zionist Archives; The British National Archives; the League of Nations; Tel-Aviv Municipality Archives; Hadassah Archives; Lewin-Epstein's private Archive.
2    This idea is based on Waitzkin and Waterman's theses, claiming that the sick role in total institutions is an important factor and a tool to permit deviance for the sake of the inmate and the sake of the system. Waitzkin/Waterman (1974).

overriding objectives of protecting public health. At least in terms of its effect, the ambiguous nature of this legislation allowed practitioners to participate in the dental services marketplace, while also creating a system of stratification that enhanced the prestige of qualified practitioners and made it possible for others to claim a higher professional status. This "original sin" was intended to address the needs of professionally marginalized groups, but it also became the source of the stratification that exists today in the field of dentistry among dentists, dental technicians/mechanics, dental assistants/attendants, and hygienists.

The history of dentistry in Mandate Palestine generally, and that of the professionalization of dentistry specifically, has yet to be fully explored.[3] This study aims to fill that gap in terms of theory, adding a theoretical dimension by posing the question: What factors impeded or enabled the formation of this profession within such a multinational and multicultural setting? In particular, the study will examine the professional melting pot that served as a locus by drawing a range of professionals with varying degrees of education, certification, and training, all of whom claimed to belong to the mainstream of dentistry and sought to shape legislation to suit their own needs. I will show how, against this background of multidimensional pressure, the British regulating authority employed ambiguous legislation.

Two fascinating phenomena further enrich this discussion: First, what differentiated the regulatory process in Mandatory Palestine within the sphere of dentistry from the process vis-à-vis other professions was that it was "neutral" in terms of nationality. That is, most of the practitioners in this field were Jews who could afford to expose their interests and voice objection to professional "trespass" without being accused of sabotaging the enterprise of *aliyah* (Jewish immigration) and nation-building. The various requests for recognition as dentists reveal a range of underlying interests, some aimed at preventing others from entering the profession for narrow interests (thwarting competition), others driven by broader public interests (protection of service consumers). The absence of a national dimension allows us to expose internal professional rivalries as well as inherent tensions between the protection of public health and pursuit of professional interests.

The second phenomenon in this context is the correlation between the regulation of dentistry and that of another profession: Law.[4] As I will demonstrate, there are many parallels between the professionalization of the law and the professionalization of dentistry. We can therefore learn a great deal from the rich literature, including Israeli texts, regarding regulation of the legal profession as it relates to the regulation of dentistry: both are genuinely "free trades"[5] – in contrast, for example, to medicine, which became an organized profession perceived as a national interest; both apparently enjoyed only a

---

3    Cf. Katvan (2011); Katvan: Beginning (2010); De Vreis (2013).
4    On literature regarding the linkage between the legal and medical professions: Cf. Goold/Kelly (2009).
5    Cf. Miller (1986).

partial national commitment and as such had to struggle for their share of the market, mainly against "trespass" and "overcrowding" of the profession. There are, of course, differences among these professions, on which I shall elaborate below. Moreover, lawyers were involved in shaping the profession of dentistry through their representation of various professional associations, which in turn had an impact on legislative revision. As such, there is a strong relationship between the two professions and they provide mutual insights about one another.

The first part of this article reviews the current research and theoretical background relevant to these professions in terms of the elements of the profession and their regulation; the second part describes the regulatory process for dentistry in Mandatory Palestine until and slightly after the founding of the State of Israel; and the third part of the article addresses efforts to decipher the regulatory process and its implications in the context of the theoretical issues and compares it with the practice of law; the conclusions are presented in the summary.

## On Professions, Regulation, and Professional Competition

The legislative regulation of an occupation is one of the many aspects of what is customarily termed a "profession".[6] Another characteristic, for example, is extensive professional training on the basis of (academic) knowledge. An ethical code is another facet of a "profession", as is the existence of a professional association that acts to promote the status of these professionals and defend them from trespass and overcrowding of the profession.[7]

In effect, the legislative regulation of an occupation is often what makes it a profession. Such regulation often reflects the interests of these professionals through the unique rules of the profession, which (through registration or licensing requirements) permit only those who meet the standards of training and certification to practice, thus preventing competition for the same sector of the market.[8] Naturally, the legislator does not focus on protecting professional pressure groups solely for the benefit of the latter. One of the main rationales for such regulation stems from the authorities' interest in ensuring suitable quality services (such as healthcare) for its population or, perhaps, gathering information about the population.[9] This undoubtedly creates an economic and class advantage for those who hold the desired status, and in this context it is not surprising that many aspire to it – that is, claim to be members of the profession, at the exclusion of others.[10] Such competition for

6   Ellis (2012); Abbott (1988) in his research prefers to discuss wider theoretical questions instead of specific parameters; Macdonald (1995).
7   Cf. Katvan (2012).
8   Cf. Ogus (1994), p. 215.
9   Cf. Bartal/Katvan (2010).
10  Abel presents some of these parameters: "Thus the following elements are inseparably related: Differentiation and Standardization of professional services; formalization of the

professional hegemony is the source of attraction to regulated and protected occupations[11] as well as the source of professional stratification.

Hook and other researchers date the transformation of dentistry (which was known during ancient times as well)[12] into a profession to the 1940s (in the United States). According to Hook's research, three elements contributed to this transition: organization (the formation of an association of dental surgeons), education or professional training (the first dental school), and professionalized journals and literature.[13] All these, according to Hook, took place during 1839–1940, when dentistry was regarded as part of the medical practice.[14] Accordingly, specialized dentistry journals also contributed to professional segregation.[15] Likewise, with the establishment of the School of Dental Surgery in Baltimore in 1840, academic education began to replace education through mentoring. This transition, which took several decades[16], originated with legislation that made the completion of studies at a recognized institution a precondition for recognition as a dentist[17]. In England, too, uncertified practitioners were allowed to provide dental care as long as they did not present themselves as certified dentists[18], and the situation in Germany was similar[19]. In England, for example, the regulatory process commenced even before the adoption of the Dentists Act.[20] In fact, England's Apothecaries Act of 1815 distinguished between dentistry and other medical professions, thereby effectively defining the profession.[21] This is an example of the creation of a profession by means of segregation.

The practice of dentistry came to be legislatively regulated during the early days of the British Mandate in Palestine, first under the Public Health Ordinance (1918) and later, in 1926, with the enactment of a special ordinance for dentists. Elsewhere I have addressed certain aspects of the profession of dentistry[22] in Mandatory Palestine, including the question of knowl-

conditions for entry; persuasion of the public that they need services only professionals can provide; and state protection of the professional market against those who lack formal qualifications and against competing occupations. Educational institutions play a central role in attaining each of these goals." Abel (1979), pp. 82, 84.

11  Cf. Ziv (2017).
12  Cf. Haden/Machen/Valachovic (1998).
13  Cf. Hook (1985); Robinson (1940); Horner (1959).
14  Cf. Hook (1985), p. 349.
15  Cf. Hook (1985), p. 350.
16  Haden/Machen/Valachovic (1998) states that in 1865 only 15 percent of the 18,000 dentists in the US were medical schools' graduates. However, in 1920, less than 3 percent of the dental practitioners were trained through mentoring.
17  Cf. Haden/Machen/Valachovic (1998).
18  Morton (1912), pp. 71–78 presents also the Dentists Act, 1878, 41 & 42 Vict. c. 33, which forbid the unregistered to present himself as Dental Practitioner or as a Dentist.
19  Cf. Kuhlmann (2001), p. 445.
20  On regulation and professionalization in the UK see Langley/Newsome (2014); Gelbier (2005); Thorogood (2002); see also Forbes (1985); Richards (1968).
21  Cf. Bishop/Gelbier: Part 1 (2002); Bishop/Gelbier: Part 2 (2002).
22  On whether dentistry is a profession: Welie: Part 1 (2004); Welie: Part 2 (2004).

edge and the import of American scientific knowledge[23]. The development of dentistry in Mandatory Palestine was in fact shaped by American methods, imported by practitioners who soon became leading members of the profession, foremost among whom was Dr. Lewin-Epstein. Knowledge provided an important foundation for the consolidation of a professional identity and status. So too did the de-feminization of the profession – or, more precisely, the marginalization of women – which presumably enhanced the status and prestige of dentistry. At the same time, through their substantial volunteer activity, it was these women who upheld the social contract with the public.[24] This study aims to examine professional regulation through (usually primary) legislation[25] as a key element, in conjunction with the involvement of professional associations in this regulatory process, in the transformation of an occupation into a profession.

The Dentists' Association (*Histadrut Rof'ei HaShina'im*) was established in 1919. The very creation of the Association was a key element in the professionalization process[26], and the Association quickly set out to delineate and defend the boundaries of profession. Its founders approached the Zionist Commission (*Va'ad HaTzirim* – "Committee of Delegates" – the body responsible for liaising between the Jewish community and the British government), informed the latter of its own existence, and requested that henceforth any questions that arise regarding dentistry be referred to them. The draft bylaws of the Association, formulated in English, stipulated that only certified dentists could be admitted as members. The aims of the Association were framed as follows:

> Mutual scientific assistance, group subscriptions to periodicals, the establishment of a specialized library [...] public dissemination of accurate information regarding dental diseases and the rational systemization of this profession for the residents of the country, and the establishment of a professional association of dentists to explore issues of a professional nature.[27]

In time this association combined with other groups from various cities to create a dentists' union – *Histadrut Rof'ei HaShina'im*. Simultaneously there emerged several associations, each of which sought to maintain and promote the professional and regulatory status of its members: dental assistants, dental technicians/mechanics, and others.[28] As we shall see, there emerged in Palestine a sizable number of associations and organizations that did not belong to

---

23  Cf. Katvan: Beginning (2010); Picard (2009); Garant (2013).
24  Cf. Katvan (2011); Katvan (2019).
25  On legislation and professions see Bishop/Gelbier: Part 1 (2002); Bishop/Gelbier: Part 2 (2002).
26  Among others, due to the fact that these associations took part not only in the local arena, but in the international one as well, gaining recognition and prestige. Lewin-Epstein highlighted the international component: "The first milestone in the organization of the dental profession in this country was the dental conference in Tel Aviv in 1931, attended by 110 members of the profession." Lewin-Epstein (1939).
27  CZA, L4/483, Dentists' Association Regulation in Palestine.
28  Cf. Welie: Part 1 (2004), p. 531.

the same "mainstream" of dentists, but rather comprised practitioners whose aim was to enter the market despite the opposition of "conventional" dentists (who had been retroactively certified, at least to the satisfaction of the British legislator). Thus, as I will show, the efforts of associations in the legislative sphere were aimed at setting boundaries for the profession and preventing trespass. On the other side were unions working to secure authorization for their members to practice dentistry in Palestine, often through prominent lawyers. It is important to bear in mind, however, that had they not been united, they would not have been able to engage with the British authorities.[29] It was, as noted, an internal professional struggle.

The lawyers essentially mediated between the associations and the Mandate authorities (and later, the state institutions) that dealt with the legislative regulation of healthcare professions. The role of "mediation" on the part of lawyers in Palestine at that time was hardly a novelty; in fact this was the main role that lawyers, by virtue of their familiarity with the language or with the workings of government, took upon themselves.[30] In matters related to their representation of dentists, the extent of their involvement and prominence appears to have been exceptionally substantial. For these reasons, the legislative dynamics and the legal option of granting authorization to practice were, as noted, related to the involvement of various professional associations in the process. The latter were represented by the most prominent lawyers in Palestine at the time, a fact that, as we shall see, links the practice of dentistry with another profession taking shape simultaneously – namely, the legal profession.

It should be noted that the regulatory process in Mandate Palestine for dentistry was simpler than the process elsewhere or for other occupations because the legislation itself did not create the distinction between dentistry and other medical occupations. That is, it did not differentiate the practice of dentistry from the practice of medicine (a process that had long been underway in other countries)[31], because evidently there was a clear pre-existing distinction between these occupations (aside from the legal authorization for physicians to provide dental care for their patients, there was no link between the occupations)[32]. Regulation therefore focused primarily on setting standards that would determine who was qualified to engage in dental practice and who was not. Moreover, the Dentists Ordinance had been passed before the Medical Practitioners Ordinance, and the former in fact served as a model for the regulation of other professions[33], even though dentistry was less highly regarded and the Dentists' Association was less powerful than the Association of Physicians. Here too, developments paralleled the situation in England. Notably, however,

29  On the involvement of the dentists' association in the US regarding legislation: McCluggage (1959).
30  Cf. Likhovski (2006).
31  Cf. Haden/Machen/Valachovic (1998), p. 3.
32  CZA, J113/2699, Report of Subcommittee on Medical Education: Recommendation in Respect to Dental Education (ca. 1945).
33  Cf. PRO, CO 733/142/9.

physicians in Palestine were permitted to engage in dental practice.[34] As such, the practice of dentistry in Mandatory Palestine exemplifies a professional regulatory process that took place between and among practitioners with varying degrees of training and education – a process that informed the consolidation of the profession while also generating professional stratification.[35]

## The Legislative Regulation of Dentistry during the Mandate Period

### A Hybrid Law and the Role of Professional Associations

During the 1920s a variety of occupations in Mandate Palestine – including law, medicine, and midwifery, among others – underwent a process of regulation through legislation.[36] The Public Health Ordinance of 1918 made it a prerequisite to obtain a license in order to practice dentistry, medicine, or midwifery. The licensing standards specified three years of academic study at a recognized school of medicine or dentistry; a work permit was granted to those who could prove that they had practiced dentistry before May 16, 1918.[37] The licensing (and enforcement) standards apparently remained flexible, and even unqualified dentists began to practice. Presumably this explains why calls for the profession to be regulated legislatively – as the practice of pharmacy had been – began to surface as early as 1922.[38] There is no indication as to who initiated these calls, but from a letter written two years later it appears to have been the dentists of Mandate Palestine. A representative of the Dentists' Association in Jerusalem approached the director of the Department of Health and informed him that, since its establishment, the Association had been requesting a review of the issue of unqualified practitioners, and accordingly they were now appealing to him to clarify the matter.[39]

As noted, it was an organization formed on behalf of certified dentists that evidently launched the legislative process, which began with a proposal by the legal persona (the Attorney General) to the medical persona (the director of the Mandatory Department of Health) to regulate the practice of dentistry through legislation. The Attorney General was aware that Ottoman legislation

34  Cf. PRO, CO 533/440/12.
35  About the inter-professional struggles as shaping the profession: Adams (2004); Picard (2009), pp. 4–8.
36  On the regulation of health professions: Price (2002); on professionalization of medicine: Freidson (1988); for general background on the kinds of professional regulation: Adams (2009).
37  Cf. ISA, M-1554 (MG/27/3), Public Health Ordinance No. 7, Regulations governing the exercise of the Profession of Dentistry "in the public interest".
38  Annual report of the Department of Health, government of Palestine, for the year 1922: "A certain amount of unqualified dental practice exists and several requests have been made that an Ordinance similar to the Pharmacy Ordinance should be drawn up to regulate the practice of dentistry."
39  Cf. ISA, M-1554 (MG/27/3), Letter to the Director of Department of Health from Dr. I. B. George (Jerusalem's Dentist Association), 6/2/1924.

on the subject already existed, but he proposed new legislation based on English law. The law on which he wanted to draw had emerged under conditions
that would eventually arise in Palestine as well: disputes among the various associations in Britain, represented by lawyers; a temporary shortage of dentists
(especially during the two world wars); and solutions that included different
levels of licensing and the option for qualified dentists to employ uncertified
workers for "minor dental work". Apparently in 1916 – in response to the employment of uncertified practitioners in England, as well as the need to weigh
the shortage in dentists against concerns that preventing competition would
lead to higher rates – a commission was appointed to examine these issues.[40]
The very existence of the commission sparked controversy, as unregistered
dental practitioners were not represented.[41] Here too, lawyers represented the
unregistered practitioners, at the initiative of the commission itself, which preferred that lawyers speak for the issue rather than one of the unregistered dental care givers.[42] The commission's report, issued in 1919[43], sparked disagreement over the terminology used for various occupations. The controversy primarily surrounded use of the term "unregistered", in contrast to the original
1878 law, which had permitted use of the term "dental practitioners".[44] The
British were actually aware of the advantages of various colonies' legislation
over its own law, as evidenced by a memorandum from the president of the
Medical Council in England in 1916, stating that the legislation in England, as
interpreted by the court, was formulated to enable even unqualified practitioners to provide dental care. The author of the memorandum noted at the time
that the colonies' legislation was superior[45], and that even in states that did
not prohibit unqualified practitioners from engaging in dental care, they were
nonetheless prohibited from misleading the public through false representation of their qualifications[46].

The director of the Department of Health in Mandate Palestine was apparently well-versed in both the development of legislation in this field and the history of the profession in England, in contrast to the colonies, and was therefore
reluctant to rely on English law. In his view, because it focused primarily on
registration of rather than oversight over the profession, it did not protect the
public. The director's proposal is fascinating: he was aware of the differences

---

40  Cf. PRO, PC 119780. A similar committee will assemble in Palestine during WWII.
     See also PRO, PC 118389, Memorandum from Donald Macalister, the President of the
     Medical Council (July, 1916): "[...] to protect the public, and, *inter alia*, to enable persons
     requiring professional aid to distinguish qualified from unqualified practitioners [...] the
     *Dentists act*, as now interpreted, fails in both of these respects [...]". Emphases in original.
41  Cf. PRO, PC 119886. In Mandate Palestine as well, the British tend to prefer the quali-
     fied dentist's viewpoint.
42  Cf. PRO, PC120053; PRO, PC 120327.
43  Cf. PRO, MH 58/46; PRO, T1 12562.
44  PRO, PC 122377.
45  On the legislation in territories under the British regime see PRO, CO 323/1565/1; cf.
     Chiu/Davies (1998).
46  Cf. PRO, PC 118389, Memorandum from Donald Macalister (July, 1916).

as well as the correlation between public needs and the needs of the profession and of professionals. He proposed that the law in Palestine be more progressive than the law in England, where the problem of unqualified practitioners was on a much larger scale.[47] Yet the problem in Palestine, too, stemmed from the range and variety of certification standards and training methods in the countries from which practitioners of dentistry had immigrated:

> The Ottoman law allows no unqualified practice in any of the professions; it is much stricter than English law as regards medicine and pharmacy, and equally strict as regards dentistry and midwifery. The Central European countries from which the majority of the immigrants come, usually divide persons practising dentistry [...] into two grades. Thus, the dental surgeon (Zahnarzt) [...] grade I are fully qualified, while the Technical Dentist [...] Grade II, receive State recognition in their own countries and are allowed to practice [...] under certain restrictions [...] But on arrival in Palestine the [...] Technical Dentists find they have no recognised status at all [...] these semi-qualified persons feel therefore that they suffer a definite hardship [...] [It] is generally for the public good and it is not intended to modify the existing laws.[48]

Against this background, with "complete chaos in the area of dentistry, the Mandate government had to pass an ordinance in 1926".[49] The subsequent 1926 Dentists Ordinance established two ranks: dentists and dental practitioners (28 in total, a small minority of the registrants). These included anyone engaged in dental care before 1918 who, under the terms of the new Ordinance, would lose their employment (as they would no longer meet the licensing standards). At this point the Attorney General looked to the model adopted in Iraq, where anyone who had been practicing for a year prior to the new legislation could continue to do so.[50] Indeed, the new law seemingly combined the Iraqi ordinance with English law. It included a transition provision allowing dental care providers residing in Palestine in 1919 to continue practicing under the terms of the Turkish authorities' permit. They were regarded as "dental practitioners" rather than "dentists".[51] This system was also based on the 1921 English law[52] that aimed to prevent anyone who did not meet the standards from practicing, on the one hand, without undermining the rights of those already engaged in the profession, on the other[53] – in effect redefining and redrawing the boundaries of the profession while seeking to preserve certain rights for those already practicing, until they retire[54]. There is, however,

---

47  Cf. ISA, M-1554 (MG/27/3), letter from the Director of the Department of Health to the Attorney General (A. G.) (3/11/1923).
48  Annual report of the Department of Health, government of Palestine, for the year 1925.
49  ISA, G-5749/13; Lewin-Epstein (1939).
50  Cf. ISA, M-1554 (MG/27/3), a letter to the Director of the Department of Health from the A. G. (18/10/1923).
51  ISA, G-5749/13.
52  Cf. ISA, M-1554/1967 (Dentists Ordinance).
53  In other Ordinances, such as the Midwives Ordinance, the British allowed the unqualified midwives to practice, but within certain geographical boundaries. Cf. Bartal/Katvan (2010); Lewis (1945).
54  Cf. Personal Archive Katvan, Samuel Lewin-Epstein, "History of Dentistry in the Country" 1.

an alternative (or complementary) version of the rationale for the creation of this classification. Advocate Krongold, one of the prominent lawyers in Mandate Palestine and later Israel, attested that he and his colleague, Advocate Moshe Smoira (later the first president of the Supreme Court of the State of Israel), who represented the dental practitioners, had initiated the process because there was a shortage of dentists at the time and they were seeking British permission to recognize individuals working in the field as "dental practitioners".[55] In his view, the British evidently acquiesced but insisted on differentiating between a dentistry license and a temporary permit allowing practitioners to continue working.[56]

The law established yet another status: as in Britain, the ordinance allowed dentists and dental practitioners to employ assistants to perform "minor dental operations" under authorized supervision. The concept of "minor dental work" originated in the British law of 1921. As in Palestine, in England too the concept raised problematic questions of interpretation.[57] A historical assessment from 1925 reveals that during World War I there was a shortage of dentists, which made it necessary to employ women to provide dental care for schoolchildren. Various circumstances made their employment possible, and the permission became permanent with the 1921 legislation.[58] These women were known as "dental dressers" in England, and the definition of "minor dental work" was in fact designed to protect them. That provision, intended to address a specific problem in England, was "imported" to Palestine in 1926. In this sense the director of the Department of Health was correct in urging that the legislation, having created problems in this sphere in England, should be much stricter and clearer in Mandate Palestine. The provision was later to be "exploited" by dental mechanics.

According to Dr. Lewin-Epstein – among the first dentists in Mandate Palestine, who also imported American know-how and advised the authorities on the legislative process[59] – this provision was added at the request of dentists who themselves were unskilled in technical work. It is also conceivable that this is what Advocate Krongold had intended in his remarks. In any event, the provision was vague and therefore gave rise to disputes, especially during the 1930s[60], when new waves of immigrants, including dentists, arrived

55  ISA, K-27/21, Protocol of the sub-Committee of the Public Services regarding the amendments of the Dentists Ordinance (26/11/1950).
56  Cf. ISA, K-104/2, Protocol number 32/B of the sub-Committee of the Public Services (2/7/1957).
57  Cf. PRO, MH 58/45; see also CZA, J1/7657, Dr. Tzemach Report, p. 4.
58  Cf. PRO, MH 58/4, "Note on the history of dental dresser scheme"; see also PRO, NATS 1/554 (file 1918).
59  Samuel Lewin-Epstein, Dental Pioneer, dies at 76. Hadassah Archives, RG 2/HMO, 103d: "Throughout the Mandatory period, he was in constant call for professional counsel and in drafting of professional legislation by British authority"; Katvan: Beginning (2010).
60  Cf. ISA, M-323/1, Interview of the Chief Secretary with Lewin-Epstein and Glaszman (Dentists' Association), 5/1/1942.

from Germany[61], as did practitioners with other qualifications, such as dental technicians. Thus the ambiguous legislation, which was intended to address the needs of various pressure groups, created a professional stratification that correlated with the interests of all the parties involved.

### Difficulties in Implementation of the Ordinance
### (The Question of Recognized Institutions)

After issuing the ordinance, the British began to review requests from applicants claiming to have already been practicing as dentists before its adoption[62], as well as requests by applicants to be registered as dentists. They encountered problems stemming from the wide range of training and certification practices abroad.[63] At a certain point the High Commissioner called for the creation of a registry of "recognized institutions" of instruction in medicine and dentistry. It soon became apparent, however, that opinions differed, in particular between those who argued against discriminating among professionals from different countries and institutions (as this contravened Article 18 of the Ordinance)[64] and those who argued that this was precisely the role of the Mandate authorities: to protect public health through oversight over the professionals[65]. Moreover, the British were aware that those seeking to serve as professionals (in medicine, dentistry, and pharmacy) in Palestine had followed one of two professional training tracks in Europe: the first track included those who wished to practice the profession; the second track was primarily intended to draw foreign students seeking a diploma – one that, in fact, would not actually permit them to engage in that practice. The director of the Department of Health was concerned that, rather than complete a full course of studies, students would learn the profession during a brief stay in Europe at institutions where the standards were not particularly high. Therefore, in his view, no diploma should be accepted unless it permitted its holder to practice in the country that had actually granted the diploma.[66] Additional problems that arose in this context included the recognition of diplomas issued in Russia, where it was difficult to ascertain the type or validity of certifications.[67] Nor were the Russians always forthcoming about transmitting copies of diplomas, which made it difficult for petitioners to register in Palestine. Another prob-

---

61  Cf. Lavsky (2017).
62  Cf. ISA, M-1632/5190; ISA, M-322/7.
63  See also ISA, M-326/26, List of qualified dentistry schools (5/5/1931).
64  Cf. PRO, FO 371/18535.
65  Cf. PRO, CO 733/170/3.
66  Cf. PRO, CO 733/170/3, Letter from the Director of the Department of Health to the Chief Secretary (6/2/1929).
67  See for example CZA, J1/1711 (on recognition of Russian diplomas); compare with pharmacists licensing: CZA, S30/2131; PRO, FO 370/227 (file 1924–1926). See also High Court of Justice (H.C.) 37/38, Scharf v. Director of Medical Services. In: *Palestine Post* (11/7/1938), Law Reports.

lem related to the fact that various states whose institutions the British did not recognize also protested to the Mandate authorities.[68] The British were under pressure from many directions because of their commitments to the League of Nations and the writ of the Mandate, to other states and their varied accreditation processes, to the local residents and their health, and to practitioners in various fields, including – for our purposes – registered and qualified dentists as well as those who did not meet the prerequisites.[69]

## *Immigration from Germany, and Professional-National Questions*

In the mid-1930s a demographic shift took place among the professions of Mandate Palestine. The Nazi rise to power and Nuremberg laws resulted in the uprooting of many Jews, primarily from Germany (but Austria as well). A high proportion of Jews in Germany had worked in professions such as medicine[70] and law[71]. Some fled to Palestine and some sought refuge elsewhere. During this period, for example, Jewish dentists who had fled Germany to England were able to receive accreditation.[72] Indeed, they were seen as far more qualified than their British colleagues, according to a study by Louise London. Nevertheless, in England, local dentists opposed the granting of work permits to Jewish refugees.[73] Somewhat later, during 1937 and 1939, the British began to receive large numbers of petitions by Jewish physicians (and dentists) from Austria and Germany, and later from Italy as well[74], who were unable to practice in their own country because of racial laws[75]. They were primarily interested in receiving permission to practice in areas under British jurisdiction – namely, the various colonies of the British Empire. Professionals residing within those colonies, however, opposed such requests for fear of competition. They justified their opposition by arguing that they had been trained in England, or at least in accordance with British law, and should therefore be granted priority over those who had not undergone such an accreditation process.[76] The British, evasively, instructed the petitioners to approach the various colonies themselves and meet the relevant conditions for certification of each colony, as well as its relevant immigration conditions.[77]

---

68  Cf. PRO, FO 371/16930 (file 1933).
69  Cf. H.C. 81/35, Mazin v. Director of Medical Services. In: Law Reports of Palestine. London 1937, p. 435.
70  Cf. Niederland (1984).
71  Cf. Sela-Sheffy (2003).
72  Cf. PRO, CO 323/1564/7.
73  Cf. London (2001).
74  Cf. PRO, CO 323/1564/7; PRO, CO 323/1564/9.
75  Cf. PRO, CO 323/1462/3; PRO, CO 323/1462/6; PRO, CO 323/1564/7; PRO, CO 323/1564/8; Germany's New Aryan Legislation: Dentists Fall Before Nazi Axe. In: *Palestine Post* (18/3/1935), p. 3.
76  Cf. PRO, CO 323/1462/6, Copy of a report by Major Hallinan (11/2/1937).
77  Cf. PRO, CO 323/1565/1; PRO, CO 323/1565/2.

Only at a later stage – too late – did the British recognize the vast potential of bringing these experts to their various colonies[78], but still, they preferred the needs of those who met the British standards with those who did not which posed an obstacle that continued to bar the latter from the British colonies[79].

Some of the above-mentioned refugees arrived in Mandate Palestine, and their proportion of the professional population increased dramatically: between 1932 and 1934 the number of dentists tripled. The dentists themselves, alongside other professionals (physicians and lawyers) became targets of attack by the British and Arabs, and to some extent within the profession itself (in contrast to the situation in medicine). The latter were concerned about overcrowding of the profession (medicine, dentistry, and law). There were also concerns (or excuses) about uncontrolled immigration of practitioners who would later be unable to practice; furthermore, unchecked competition could have a negative impact on dentists already working in the country.[80] Perhaps above all else, though, the overriding British concern related to immigration by unqualified practitioners presenting themselves as dentists.[81] One of the problems the authorities faced in this regard was that dentists were able to immigrate under the laws that – until 1937 – permitted entry to anyone who could provide evidence of a specified amount of capital. The British were no less concerned about the vast discrepancy between Jews and Arabs across various professions.[82] This imbalance, in combination with their commitment to the parity principle, and their wish to halt the immigration, compelled the authorities to turn their attention to questions of legislative reform and legislative regulation of various professions.[83]

In 1934, Dr. Taufik Canaan, a physician and the first president of the Arab Medical Association in Palestine[84], requested that the British Department of Health place a limit on the number of ("regular") physicians granted a license annually. Canaan underscored that this was neither a political move

---

78  Cf. PRO, CO 323/1564/7, letter *Secretary* of State for the *Colonies to various colonies (30/9/1938)* suggesting to accept the Jewish physicians, whom are extremely qualified, and will probably strengthen the colonies.

79  PRO, CO 87/247/15; cf. Zamet (2009).

80  Cf. ISA, M-1170, letter (confidential) to the Chief Secretary from Director of the Department of Health (9/4/1932) – against the overcrowding of the professions which might harm those who already practice the professions in Palestine.

81  Cf. PRO, CO 733/261/11, Dentists (Amendment) Ordinance (1934), and Memorandum signed by the Attorney General. Explains that: "The dangers due to the overcrowding of the profession were reported to the Secretary of State [...]"; "[...] to restrict the grant of licences [...] to persons who are resident in Palestine and are Palestinian citizens or have entered Palestine as dentists in the appropriate category under the immigration law".

82  Cf. PRO, CO 733/261/11, letter from The High Commissioner for Palestine to The Secretary of State for the Colonies (17/3/1934), regarding the overcrowding of health and legal professions in Palestine, due to the immigration; ISA, M-1554/1973; ISA, M-1170 (IMM/4/2/7).

83  Compare with the struggle of women to become lawyers in Mandate Palestine, and the question of the parity principle: Halperin-Kaddari/Katvan (2009).

84  Cf. Shachar (2010).

nor an attempt to restrict or undermine Jewish immigration to Palestine, but
rather a professional concern about the negative impact on his own and his
colleagues' practices.[85] Right or wrong, he noted that long-practicing Jewish
dentists felt the same way but were not voicing their opposition for fear of
being accused of sabotaging *aliyah* (Jewish immigration).[86] The repercussions,
of course, included the prevention of immigration by those physicians who
lacked sufficient capital. As it turns out, the British conducted interviews with
various physicians across Palestine, government authorities, Jews and Arabs.[87]
The story that emerged from the interviews was consistent: the Arab physicians explained that no Jew would agree to the restrictions, as these would be
seen as restrictions on immigration rather than protection of the profession.
In the sphere of dentistry, the problems between the nationalities still existed,
but they took a different and far more moderate form because the two were
not actually in competition: there were very few Arab dentists in Mandate Palestine. The following graph illustrates the sharp rise in the number of dentists
between 1932 and 1933, with the percentage of non-Jewish dentists remaining
nearly constant.[88]

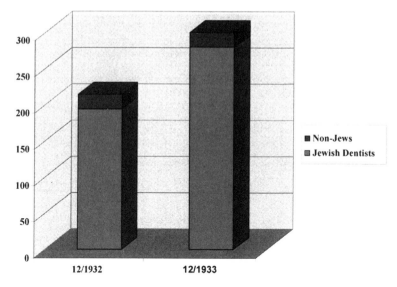

Graph 1: Jewish/Non-Jewish Dentists (1932/1933)

85   On using health and public health arguments in order to change patterns of immigration
     see Katvan: Landlord (2010).
86   Cf. PRO, CO 733/261/11, letter from Dr. T. Canaan to Dr. Harkness (25/7/1934).
87   Cf. PRO, CO 733/261/11, record of confidential conversations (Doctors).
88   369 More Doctors. In: *Palestine Post* (9/1/1934), p. 2.

One of the interviewees observed that, while the dental profession had not yet become "seriously overcrowded", he thought that Arab dentists "were suffering" as "there were a large number of dentists in the country of inferior professional standing. The influx of dentists had raised the standard of dental treatment amongst the Jewish section of the profession [...]."[89] In other words, even though Jewish immigration posed a potential threat to Arab dentists, as regards the profession of dentistry this interviewee saw the arrival of new dentists (especially from Germany) as a positive trend that would drive unqualified dentists out of the market. These perspectives posed a problem for the British: on the one hand, the immigrant dentists from Germany raised the local standards for dental services; on the other hand, Arab dentists could be negatively affected, even if not on the scale of the "competition" between "regular" Jewish and Arab doctors. Perhaps this is why the proposed amendment to the Dentists Ordinance of 1934 did not pass[90], and no legal restrictions were imposed on the immigration of dentists.

*Technicians and Dental Assistants*

Aside from minor protests by Arab dentists regarding professional overcrowding, there were objections on the part of the Dentists' Association, who claimed that unqualified dental practitioners were entering the country even though the legislation presumably prohibited this. The Association was primarily opposed to the entry of dental technicians and dental assistants. That is, in contrast to ("regular") physicians – who might have supported restrictions on the number of certified physicians but would never admit so publicly – the dentists acted, cautiously, in coordination with the Mandatory authorities. In 1935 the Dentists' Association wrote to the Mandatory Department of Health as follows: "Our societies have experienced [...] a strong and persistent competition on the part of the dental dressers, dental mechanics, and hygienists, who use all sorts of means and evasions to practice dentistry. Names of licensed dentists are purchased, misleading signboards."[91] In particular, representatives of the Association sought to rescind paragraph 2 (b) of the Dentists Ordinance, for fear that individuals coming from abroad would present a "certificate of practice" that in their view did not meet the legal standards for a license to practice dentistry.[92]

---

89  369 More Doctors. In: *Palestine Post* (9/1/1934), p. 2.
90  The Medical Practitioners Ordinance (Amendment) which meant to fix quotas did pass, especially due to Arab doctors pressures. LON, 6A/21184/668; PRO, CO 733/375/3. Several years later, the High Court of Justice ruled that the amendment is Ultra Vires. H.C. 15/38.
91  ISA, M-322/14, Letter to the Director of the Public Department of Health, from the representatives of the three (Jewish) Dental Societies (19/11/1935).
92  ISA, M-322/14, Letter to the Director of the Public Department of Health, from the representatives of the three (Jewish) Dental Societies (19/11/1935).

There was a context to their request: apparently some of the Association's more proficient dentists had been petitioning the authorities to rectify the situation for a while, but they were in the minority and their proposals had been rejected. In other words, the dentists had in effect been "tiptoeing through the tulips" because they were cognizant of the repercussions of acting against others within the profession. Yet as immigration increased, Lewin-Epstein recounted in retrospect, the number of dentists who themselves were trained in technical work also rose; eventually (in 1935) the Association voted to approach the Mandate authorities and request that it rescind the provision within the 1926 Ordinance permitting the employment of dental assistants engaged primarily in technical work under the supervision of a dentist. However, Lewin-Epstein added, the above-mentioned wave of immigration also included less qualified dentists who did not obtain a license but did exploit this provision in order to find employment. Rather than serve as dental assistants and work under the supervision of dentists, they purchased clinics where they employed dentists.[93] Thus the opening or leeway provided by the 1926 Ordinance, with its vague language, led to inter-professional problems a decade later, to the extent that dentists spoke out publicly against these "trespassers" who, in their view, posed a threat not only to the practice of dentistry but to the patient community as well.

The opposition to dental technicians in fact dated back to the early 1930s[94], as the 1926 Ordinance had not regulated their status. The British sought to ensure that the boundaries of the profession were maintained and that unqualified dental practitioners did not pose as dentists.[95] The debate around this issue was primarily semantic and focused on the question of how dental technicians may describe themselves and what phrasing they may use on the signposts of their laboratories. The dental technicians' union hired the services of Advocate Smoira (who, as noted, had represented the dental practitioners previously). Smoira unhesitatingly threatened to approach the High Court of Justice[96], and eventually a compromise was reached: dental technicians could refer to themselves solely as "dental mechanics"[97]. In 1938 the struggle intensified and the Association reiterated its request that dental mechanics be prevented from presenting themselves as dentists, especially on the signposts of their clinics.[98] In an appeal to the Chief Secretary, Association representatives even claimed that "given that the 1926 Dentists Ordinance speaks of 'healing practice', [...] one can surmise that dental services should

---

93  Cf. ISA, M-323/1, Interview of the Chief Secretary with Lewin-Epstein and Glaszman (Dentists' Association), 5/1/1942.
94  Already during the 1920s, the British examined applicants' diplomas: "in view of the large number of misrepresentations that we have discovered". CZA, S25/700, from Director of the Department of Health to Colonel Kisch (23/4/1923).
95  Cf. ISA, M-6601/30, letter from Director of the Department of Health to District Health Directors (22/1/1930).
96  Cf. ISA, M-6601/30, letter from Adv. Smoira to Senior Medical Officer (S. M. O.).
97  Compare with PRO, PC 101515.
98  Cf. ISA, M-322/14, letter dated 24/1/1938.

be viewed as a practice to be taught, even without a general or medical education. Apparently the legislator [regards] our country as undeveloped."[99]

The Dentists' Association's appeal to the authorities provoked resentment on the part of the Dentists' Assistants Association (founded in 1936). This union approached the Dentists' Association to voice its protest[100] while simultaneously its representatives sent a letter to the director of the Department of Health, explaining the three categories of practitioners in this field that existed in the country at the time:

> A. Certified/Qualified dentists with a certificate attesting to three years of study [...]
> B. Dental technicians/mechanics [...] who have no oral contact with the patient. C. Individuals who learned dental practice from dentists or at dental schools or institutions and completed an examination thereafter (private as well as state institutions), or during decades of practicing and specializing in the profession. [...] These are known abroad as 'dentists' and in countries such as Germany, Czechoslovakia, Romania, and others they legally use the title 'dentist' and are fully entitled to engage in private dental practice. This status and classification of dentists exists in many European countries, and in the main centers of Europe they constitute the majority of dental care providers. In our country there exists a third category [...] comparable to the classification of 'dentists' [...] who are entitled by law to provide dental services on an independent basis, and they are termed 'dental practitioner' [...] Since the adoption of the 1926 law, dentists of the type mentioned above have not been able to receive a license to practice independently as dental practitioners do, and in order to make a living we have been compelled to work as assistants under the supervision of a certified dentist.[101]

In other words, dental assistants could not obtain a license to work as "dental practitioners" – a classification whose original purpose was to enable continued employment by those who had been practicing before 1926. They therefore began working as dental assistants, but suddenly found themselves in competition with dental technicians. According to the dental assistants, the Association's request stemmed only from fear of competition and there was no reason why they should not be granted a license as dentists. The ambiguous legislation thus made it possible for them to work, but created an opening for dental technicians as well, which in turn triggered the opposition of qualified dentists when there was no longer a shortage of working hands.

Between 1938 and 1939, the Mandatory Department of Health and representatives of the Dentists' Association cooperated closely to promote legislative regulation (and to prevent dental technicians from being included in the law).[102] At the same time, the dental assistants were opposed to any amendment to the law that would result in their being regarded as "dental technicians".[103] Now too, as during the early days of the British Mandate, the problem lay in the difficulty of assessing the various accreditation methods and

---

99  ISA, M-322/14, letter dated 24/1/1938.
100 Cf. CZA, J1/2290, letter from Dentists' Assistants Association to Dentists' Association (28/6/1936).
101 CZA, J1/2290, Memorandum by the Dentists' Assistants Association (response to the Dentists' Association, 28/6/1936).
102 Cf. ISA, M-1554.
103 Cf. ISA, M-1554.

quality of professional training across different countries.[104] Evidently dental technicians who had provided dental services in their countries of origin continued to do so after arriving in Palestine as well, under the auspices of the 1926 Ordinance provision permitting them to carry out "minor dental work" under a dentist's supervision.[105] Association representatives believed that the legislative intent in relation to employment for the sake of "minor dental work" referred to dental assistants, not dental practitioners. But from that time the latter developed as an occupation, and in their view the court enabled this.[106] In light of the Association's protests, the Ordinance was amended to make it clear that dental assistants were prohibited from working as dental practitioners.

The dental assistants therefore sought to differentiate themselves from dental technicians – in contrast to the position of the dentists. The Dentists' Assistants Association approached the Department of Health, requesting that they not be identified with dental technicians but rather with dental practitioners (as distinct from "dentists"). In their view the 1926 Ordinance:

> provided the possibility of subsistence only to those who had been in the country working as dental practitioners for a certain period before the law entered into force. Therefore, others who had also been practicing in the country were excluded from the law, and in recent years their small number has grown with the addition of others who received first-class professional training in Europe [...] The above-mentioned union therefore represents dental practitioners who are prepared at any time to provide evidence and testimony of their perfect/complete professional qualification//that they are fully qualified professionals. Our members include professionals who were leaders in the field of dental healthcare/treatment/services [...] Our members have made their livelihood [...] under unique and difficult circumstances, working under the supervision of a licensed dentist. They are only permitted to provide minor dental work such as treating cavities, root canal work, extraction, and the like – that is, only the activities covered by Article 3 (2) (b) of the Dentists Ordinance may be performed by an assistant [...] Our members, upon arriving here, believed that they would be able to continue working independently as medical professionals, as they had in Europe. The members of our union/Association do not identify with the dental technicians, who also work in the field of dental practice, [but] without any prior professional training.[107]

During this period (1941–1942) most of the dental assistants were immigrants from Germany and Austria.[108] They appealed to various agencies for assistance, including the Jewish National Council (JNC, the main executive institution of the Jewish community in pre-state Israel) and the Central Office for the Settlement of German Jews in Palestine, among others.[109] The JNC took on the role of "mediator" between the dental assistants and the Dentists' Association, drawing criticism from the latter: "We object to your position, which supports the inequitable demands of a number of people, conflicts with the

104 Cf. ISA, M-1554, letter (undated) to S. M. O.
105 Cf. ISA, G-5749/13.
106 Cf. ISA, G-5749/13.
107 CZA, J1/6396, Dentists' Assistants Association to the Department of Health (24/3/1941).
108 Cf. CZA, J1/2290, list of dentists' assistants.
109 Cf. CZA, J1/2290.

interests of the dentists' community in the country, and endangers the health of the entire Yishuv [Jewish community in pre-state Israel]."[110] The Association's representatives were appealing to national sentiment as a basis for their claims. The dental assistants, who numbered approximately 30 at the time and feared that the amendments would apply retroactively, also approached the Mandatory Department of Health seeking recognition as dentists: "In the event that our above proposals are [...] accepted, we would willingly accept the revocation of Article 3 (2) (b) [...] in order to prevent those dental technicians/mechanics who are not professionally qualified from exploiting this law in the future."[111]

The 1940 amendment was intended to prevent unqualified practitioners from engaging in dentistry.[112] Smoira, representing the Dentists' Assistants Association[113], pointed out that approximately 30 individuals who were registered as "dental attendants" in Palestine had actually been trained in Europe, where they had served in senior positions. It was therefore imperative that these people be able to work legally and, in his view, just as such practice had been prohibited in 1918 and then enabled in 1926, the same measures should be taken in 1941; otherwise these individuals will lose their livelihood.[114] Advocate Volf, representing the dentists' union in Tel Aviv, argued that although the requirement for a diploma was welcome, the definition needed clarification as there were many graduates of various semi-academic institutes (in Germany, for example).[115] After the draft legislation was published, another lawyer, Goiten, representing about 200 dental mechanics, also submitted a petition opposing the amendment.[116] Each of the parties sought to reinforce its own standing by comparing itself against the other dental occupations.[117] At this stage the Attorney General became the address for appeals. He initially proposed an arrangement whereby dental technicians who had previously practiced could continue to engage in "minor dental work"[118], relying on the custom in the colonies, which guaranteed the rights of professionals who had previously been working to continue practicing[119].

110 CZA, J1/2290, letter from Dentists' Association to the "Vaad Leumi" (10/9/1941).
111 CZA, J1/6396, letter from the Dentists' Assistants Association to the Department of Health (24/3/1941).
112 Cf. ISA, M-5100/18, Dentists Ordinance, 1940 – Memorandum.
113 Cf. ISA, M-5100/18, letter from Adv. Smoira to the A.G. (21/4/1942). 12.000 dental surgeons-13.000 dental practitioners.
114 Cf. ISA, M-5100/18, letter from Adv. Smoira to the Legal Draftsman (21/7/1941).
115 Cf. ISA, M-5100/18, letter from Adv. Volf to A.G. and Director of the Department of Health.
116 Cf. ISA, M-5100/18, letter from Adv. Goiten to Chief Secretary; see also Dentatus, "Dentists and Dental Mechanics: Consequences of the New 'Dentists Bill'", in ISA, M-1554.
117 Cf. ISA, M-5100/18, document by Dr. Oigen Neumann (former Chair, Dentists' Association in Germany), describing the occupation of dental technicians in Europe.
118 ISA, M-5100/18, document by A.G.
119 Cf. ISA, M-5100/18, letter from Adv. Smoira to A.G. (21/4/1942), presents examples from other countries. Bellerby v. Heywoth (1910) A.C. 377. See also ISA, M-5100/18, regarding the South African legislation (1928).

In sum, opposition to the 1941 legislative proposal[120] came from multiple directions. The Dentists' Association objected to what they viewed as too much legal leeway[121]; dental assistants objected for fear that the ordinance would affect them negatively and identify them with dental technicians[122]; dental technicians argued that they were comparable to dental assistants who were permitted to carry out minor dental work; and some dentists also sought to prevent the exclusion of supervised dental technicians who carried out technical work because they themselves were not proficient in technical work[123]. The legislation was apparently delayed because there were so many interested parties opposing one another, or more precisely, claiming that they, rather than others, were qualified to practice dentistry. In addition, the Arab Dentists' Association had a response to the proposed legislation, on the condition that 40–50 individuals were affected. There were also a few Arab dentists for whom the amendment was necessary to enable their continued work.[124] At this stage the number of parties with an interest in the profession was quite large. Smoira explained in one of his letters that there were five categories of interested parties in the area of dental care/dental services:

Qualified dentists or dental surgeons;

Dental practitioners (temporarily authorized to practice);

Dental attendants (authorized to perform minor dental work under a dentist's supervision);

Dental attendants (not authorized to perform minor dental work);

Dental mechanics (not mentioned in the ordinance).[125]

Faced with this vast array of conflicting demands, the head of British medical services realized that the boundaries of dental practice were not clearly defined[126], and he decided to appoint a member of the Dentists' Association, Dr. Tzemach, to examine the issue[127]. During the subsequent investigation, anyone claiming to qualify as a dental practitioner who was not a dentist was called upon to register. A total of 95 dental assistants and 188 technicians then

120 Cf. ISA, M-323/1, Draft Ordinance (1941).
121 Cf. ISA, M-323/1, letter to the Director of Medical Services (D.M.S.) from Tel-Aviv Dentists' Association (8/7/1941).
122 Cf. ISA, M-323/1, letter to Chief Secretary from "Vaad Leumi" (7/10/1941), regarding the Draft Ordinance (1941).
123 Cf. ISA, M-323/1, letter to Chief Secretary from Dentists of Tel-Aviv (ca. 1941); Lewin-Epstein himself explained that the dentists who support them don't know the technical work.
124 Cf. ISA, M-1554/1967, Protocol of a meeting between Arab dentists' representatives and Government representatives (1/8/1943).
125 Cf. ISA, M-5100/18, letter from Adv. Smoira to A.G. (21/4/1942).
126 Cf. ISA, M-1554/1967, letter from Director of the Department of Health to Chief Secretary (11/9/1943): "Dentistry as a separate profession is younger than medicine, and its limits are not yet so clearly defined".
127 Cf. PRO, CO 859/62/15, letter from High Commissioner to Secretary of State to the Colonies (6/3/1942).

registered, and Dr. Tzemach visited each and every one of them.[128] About 40 met the requirements to practice dentistry, and the dentists agreed not to oppose their temporary licensing on the condition that a dental services section be established within the Department of Health, to ensure supervision of the dental technicians.[129] Interestingly, around this time a debate was taking place in England regarding the possibility of turning dentistry into an independent profession with its own board, separate from the physicians' medical board.[130] Quite possibly, the dentists were aware of this development, but in any event the very establishment of this section – a dentistry division within the Department of Health, led by Dr. Tzemach – provided another layer of reinforcement for dentistry as a profession.

*The Hygienists*

Few people know, but the practice of dentistry in Palestine during the late Ottoman period, and until the passage of the 1926 legislation, was primarily a women's occupation. These were mainly women from Central Europe and Russia who had undergone varying degrees of training and certification.[131] The matter was a source of concern for the British as well as leading professionals, and had served as an impetus for the 1926 legislation.

As observed above, this trend had come to a halt by the mid-1920s, and the proportion of women declined further during the 1930s, with a large wave of German immigrants that also had an impact on the size and composition of the dentists' community. In fact, however, during the first decade of the 20th century in Germany, about half the female dentists were Jewish women.[132] It should be noted in this context that women were involved in the professionalization process in Germany as well. At the same time, though, they were not regarded as experts but merely as qualified to practice, as Kuhlmann observes, "women were excluded from the official profession but as a result of the *Kurierfreiheit* of 1869 the vocational field was still open to them".[133] Thus women were able to integrate into the profession despite the objection of men.[134] In any event, there were far fewer women in the profession than in the United States or England[135], perhaps because they were prevented from

---

128 Cf. ISA, M-1554/1967, letter to Chief Secretary from Director of the Department of Health (11/9/1943); CZA, J1/7657, Dr. Tzemach Report (list of applicants).
129 Based on the South-African model, ISA, M-5100/21 (document 9/1944); PRO, CO 859/106.
130 Cf. PRO, MH 58/891 (1946).
131 Cf. Katvan (2011).
132 Cf. Kaplan (1994), pp. 144, 280, 289. Half of female dentists in Germany were Jewish (1908–1912). In 1907 were 165 female dentists in Germany: Clark (2008), pp. 216–217; cf. Schaeffer (1992), p. 48.
133 Kuhlmann (2001), pp. 442 (quotation), 446.
134 Cf. Kuhlmann (2001), p. 443.
135 Cf. Kuhlmann (2001), pp. 446 (3.3 percent female dentists in Germany in 1919), 451.

attending universities but could still practice the profession[136]. Those who wanted to study had to travel abroad.[137] Some of the women dentists who had been trained in Germany reached Palestine, and their numbers therefore grew, but their ratio relative to the number of male dentists declined.[138] Thus, if women comprised a majority of dentists in 1927 (71 percent), by 1952 they had become a minority (40 percent). There is no conclusive proof (although much circumstantial evidence) that the large proportion of women in the profession reduced its prestige. Outwardly the process was depicted as intended to ensure that those engaged in dentistry would be appropriately trained and qualified. In retrospect, however, it is apparent that the legislation resulted in the exclusion of women from dentistry.[139] At the same time, women began (not without resistance) to enter the lower ranks of dental care services. This process had its origins in a project that Dr. Segal attempted to launch shortly after the British arrival in Palestine: a pilot training course in dental hygiene for four female students. The initiative did not succeed.

In the mid-1930s, it was proposed that a course for "Hygienists" be opened (although the surrounding discussions make clear that the course was intended for "women hygienists"). While expressing support for the idea, Dr. Lewin-Epstein voiced concerns that

> the dentists' community would not agree to the proposed course. There was opposition to the profession of [female] hygienists on the part of the dentists' community in America as well, and now in Europe [...] Likewise one must clarify what the government position would be regarding such a course, given that the Department of Health regulations permit only those who hold a diploma in dentistry to provide oral treatment.[140]

The resistance lasted at least two more years, until it was proposed to regulate the work of dental nurses. In this instance as well, the Dentists' Association objected to regulatory legislation establishing a "new professional class" and thus triggering further competition.[141] The first graduating class of nurses completed its training in 1938. Representatives of Hadassah Medical Organization (HMO) then approached the dental clinic at "Beit HaBriyut" and the *clalit kupat holim* ("general sick fund"), requesting that they include nurses in the provision of dental hygiene services.[142] The response they received from the Dentists' Association in Tel Aviv was unequivocal:

> The above-mentioned school was founded in contravention of a decision by the National Council of the Dentists' Association, which was based on the reasoning that the gradu-

---

136 Cf. Kuhlmann (2001), p. 447.
137 Cf. Kuhlmann (2001), p. 450.
138 Compare with female doctors: Villiez (2009).
139 See Katvan (2011); Katvan (2019).
140 CZA, J113/7931, Hygienists Course meeting protocol (26/10/1936). On the history of this field see Motley (1976).
141 Cf. ISA, M-1554, note on a meeting of representatives of the Jewish Dentists' Association (21/4/1938).
142 Cf. TAMA, H4, M 1039, file 2109b, letter from Kliegler to HMO.

ates of this school, upon receiving a certificate, would undermine the livelihood of the country's dentists, whose situation is already quite difficult.[143]

In practice, there were women who worked as dental nurses, and we know of at least one who not only underwent training in Mandate Palestine but also completed an internship in the United States.[144]

## The Late Mandate Period

In 1944 a new draft amendment to the ordinance was issued.[145] It addressed the question of forming cooperatives for the provision of dental services. The Dentists' Association opposed this proposal as well.[146] Likewise, the dental assistants joined efforts and "with the assistance of skilled lawyers" managed to revise the proposal to include "dental practitioners".[147] The legislation, adopted in 1945, provided that until the designated date (March 1, 1946) one could apply for a permit to work as a "dental practitioner". In a special announcement, several members of the commission (including Lewin-Epstein) resigned in protest against the provision granting a license to dental practitioners who did not have at least 15 years of professional experience (here too, the British were accounting for professionals trained outside of the regular framework who had been practicing for years). Once again, the legislation had produced a toothless law, formulated in a way that left much room for interpretation and for the entry of unqualified practitioners into the profession. And once again the Association underscored the public interest:

> The Department of Health's original plan was altered, in complete contravention of the goodwill of the authorities, which aimed to provide quality dental care for the population by means of clearly formulated legislation […] The very existence of such a status [dental practitioners] poses a serious threat to public health.[148]

Soon thereafter, a new group, represented by Advocate Levitzki, also petitioned for accreditation. These were 25 unlicensed dental practitioners, mostly war refugees and experts in their field, who did not qualify for a license under Article 7 because they were not classified as residents (they had not been working as dentists in Palestine).[149] At this stage more requests began to sur-

---

143 TAMA, H4, M 1039, file 2109b, letter from Tel-Aviv Dentists' Association to the Director of Education Department, Tel-Aviv Municipality (1/8/1938).
144 See Unmoved by New York's Glamour: Ziona Carmi is Interested in Dentistry Only. In: *Palestine Post* (20/2/1934), p. 6.
145 Cf. ISA, M-5100/21, draft legislation (Dentists Ordinance), 1944.
146 Cf. ISA, M-5100/21, complaint by Adv. Friedman (Tel-Aviv Dentists' Association) to the Director of the Department of Health (25/12/1944). According to the complaint, a cooperative is not a "person", and therefore cannot practice. A similar discussion took place in the UK: PRO, PC 98841; PRO, MH 58/47, Dental Companies (Restrictions of Practice) Bill.
147 ISA, 5749/13.
148 ISA, 5749/13.
149 Cf. ISA, M-5100/21, letter from Adv. Levitzki to Chief Secretary (12/8/1946).

face, by way of lawyers, to amend the law so that it would not have a negative impact on war refugees, including those conscripted during the war.[150] In 1947 another draft ordinance was issued, this time focusing on oversight over recipients of a license to practice dentistry, and the possibility of license revocation. This too was a shift in the direction of more stringent oversight over practitioners.[151] And thus the Mandate era drew to a close.

## The Post-Mandate Era

The problems related to regulation of the profession continued after Israel attained statehood, as if in direct extension of the Mandate era. Issues that remained unresolved from the Mandate period – the problematic and vague legislation, discharged military dentists, and the immigration of new dentists – landed at the doorstep of the Israeli legislature. A few months after the founding of the state, Advocate Levitzki contacted the Ministry of Health on behalf of dental practitioners (dentists), explaining that they had requested but been unable to obtain a license from the Mandatory authorities because they were not residents of Palestine "for reasons of politics in general and of immigration", although the British nonetheless permitted them to work, and now they were seeking to regulate their status.[152] It appears that these were Jewish refugees who had arrived as illegal immigrants, and it was decided that their status would be addressed after the legality of their residence was resolved.[153] However, the Dentists' Association apparently opposed this arrangement with dental practitioners as well, and even refused to meet with representatives of the organization. Dr. Neumann, a representative of the Ministry of Health, was uncomfortable with this position and urged that "the Dentists' Association attribute less value to its opinion regarding dental practitioners if it turns out to have been critically influenced by economic considerations aimed solely at reducing the number of competitors".[154] At the same time, Advocate Krongold, on behalf of the dental practitioners who had received licenses during 1927 and 1928, petitioned for this group's status to be equated with that of dentists and provided evidence of their professionalism.[155] Once again we see how the various actors attempted to regulate their own status through comparison with

---

150 Cf. ISA, M-5100/21, letter from Adv. Parlas to Chief Secretary (23/11/1947), regarding the Ordinance's amendment; ISA, M-4986/5, regarding Dentists (Temporary Provisions) Ordinance, 1947; CZA, S21/4888 (licenses for discharged soldiers), a letter from Simon to Justice Frumkin (22/7/1946).
151 See also ISA, M-5100/21; PRO, CO 67/271/4; PRO, CO 859/31/10; PRO, CO 859/62/14.
152 Cf. ISA, G-187/4, letter from Adv. Levitzki to Department of Health (1/9/1948).
153 Cf. ISA, G-187/4, letter from Adv. Levitzki to the Ministry of Health (13/5/1949).
154 ISA, G-4287/10, Memorandum of a meeting between the representatives of Dentists' Association (16/6/1949).
155 Cf. ISA, G-187/4, letter from Adv. Krongold to Dr. Neumann (Ministry of Health), 16/8/1949.

dentists and differentiation from non-dentists. In this instance, those identified as long-standing "dental practitioners" (accredited before the original law of 1926) feared being identified as "dental practitioners" who had arrived in Palestine towards the end of the Mandate period. And, as happened during that period, all of these parties approached the state authorities en masse through lawyers.

In 1950 the Dentists' Association, now represented by Advocate Bernard Joseph, who was also a minister, appealed to the Attorney General, complaining that non-dentists were practicing dentistry.[156] At the same time it also published a proposed amendment to the Dentists Ordinance. The Association took advantage of the opportunity to propose revisions that would clarify the "vague" terms in the Mandatory legislation that establish who is entitled to practice and in what manner.[157] In an effort to clarify the wording of the legislation, the Hebrew Language Council proposed the term *shinan* for those who provide dental services as dental practitioners but are not qualified dentists.[158] An official statement of the Association asserted that the new proposed legislation (of 1950) was following the same approach as the laws of 1926 and 1945 in that it was permitting individuals without university training to practice – because of the need to integrate immigrants (European refugees) – when in fact there was no shortage of dentists (1:1,000, as opposed to 1:1,800 in the United States).[159] The Association raised two additional matters of principle: dental services are essential for the sake of public health, and dentistry is a branch of medicine in general.[160]

Once again, potential victims of the legislation sought to change it. Particularly notable were the new immigrants who had made their way to Palestine after being promised they would be able to earn a living as dental practitioners.[161] Veteran practitioners, too – those few who had been able to renew their work permit under the 1926 Ordinance (dental practitioners) – sought recognition as "dentists" rather than revocation of their status. Again they hired the services of Advocate Krongold, who had been handling their affairs for decades now.[162] Advocate Levitzki, for his part, argued that it was unreasonable to require unlicensed senior members of the Dental Practitioners' Association to take an examination.[163] Discussions within the Public Services

---

156 Cf. ISA, P-856/2, letter from Adv. Bernard Joseph to the Legal Advisor (31/7/1950); ISA, P-856/2, letter from Adv. Schwartz and Co.

157 Cf. ISA, P-856/2, Dentists proposal for amending Dentists Ordinance (1950).

158 Cf. ISA, K-27/18; ISA, G-187/7, memorandum of a meeting of Dentists' Association representatives and Dental Practitioners representatives in the Ministry of Health (15/1/1951).

159 Cf. ISA, P-856/2, Dentists' Association note (28/11/1950).

160 Cf. ISA, P-856/2, Dentists' Association note (28/11/1950).

161 Cf. ISA, K-27/18, letter from new immigrants committee – dental practitioners from abroad (13/7/1950).

162 Cf. ISA, K-27/18, letter from Adv. Krongold to the Minister of Justice (30/6/1950).

163 Cf. ISA, K-27/18, letter from Adv. Levitzki to the sub-committee of the Services Committee.

Committee regarding amendment of the Dentists Ordinance also highlight the efforts to set the boundaries of the profession, even at the risk of a negative impact on immigration and immigrants. Advocate Sheffer (on behalf of the Dentists' Association) opposed the amendment, although it was intended to assist in the absorption of immigrants, but he was willing to accept it on the condition that the age of those permitted to practice be raised (that is, only the older practitioners be entitled to work, as they would be unemployed otherwise). He argued that the approach of the 1945 law should not be followed, and that those who lack professional training should be prevented from practicing.[164]

## Discussion: 'Vaguelation'

It is evident that the legislative regulation of dentistry underwent frequent revisions. Regulation of the practice continued after Israel achieved independence as well. This was largely an extension of the legislative activity characteristic of the Mandate era. Shortly after the founding of the state its institutions began to collect information on dentists, to establish a base of knowledge for regulation of the practice.[165] There were two main drivers of regulatory revision: the two world wars, and the waves of immigration to Mandate Palestine (women dentists from Eastern Europe and Russia, dentists from Germany, Jewish refugees, and waves of immigrants who arrived after independence). In each case various pressure groups – the Dentists' Association as well as less qualified practitioners – tried to differentiate themselves from other groups, or to become associated with them, depending on circumstances. The British had to face these pressure groups, as well as the demands of Arab dentists to be counted as members of the profession or to have the immigration of Jews halted, the shortage or overcrowding of professionals, and the commitment of the British themselves to ensure public healthcare in Palestine in accordance with the writ of the Mandate. In other words, the British found themselves trapped among various pressure groups whose interests often shifted (for example, qualified dentists initially needed dental assistants but later did not), between Jews and Arabs, and between longtime practitioners and new arrivals. They were also under pressure to provide public health services (including for the British themselves) in accordance with the terms of the Mandate; as well as under the pressure of the parity principle and the anti-immigration policy that they enacted. For these reasons they adopted legislation that pre-

---

164 Cf. ISA, K-27/18, Protocol of the sub-committee of the Services Committee on amending the Dentists Ordinance (26/11/1950). These discussions continued in 1957. See ISA, K-104/2, Protocol number 35/b (18/6/1957).

165 Actually, the initial data has been collected by the "Vaad Leumi" in 1947. Soon after the establishment of the State of Israel further data has been gathered. ISA, G-4269/1; CZA, J1/7657; ISA, 4277/9, Report on preliminary dental survey of Israel made to the Medical and Dental Department of the South African (S. A.) Zionist Federation (1954).

served the old institutions (unqualified and women practitioners, for example) while allowing them to "fade away" and simultaneously cultivating new institutions (modeled on American methods).

Under these circumstances, the legislation adopted at each stage was formulated with ambiguity, as Lewin-Epstein describes: "This vague and ambiguous paragraph [minor dental work] was mainly responsible for all the forms of evasions practised by mechanics and other non-licensed persons".[166] This ambiguity was intended both to protect qualified dentists and to enable those who did not meet the qualification standards to continue or begin working, without causing qualified practitioners to feel the negative impact of professional trespass. Market needs, on the one hand, and pressure from professional associations, on the other, resulted in hesitant legislation whose ambiguity benefited new immigrants. This legislation was, however, intended to regulate the state of affairs at that particular time, when the British did not foresee how developments would unfold. In retrospect, it appears that those provisional "loopholes" created by the Mandatory legislator were unduly extended later, in the opinion of qualified dentists, and too narrow, in the view of those who did not qualify as dentists. The former cemented their standing in no small part by distinguishing themselves from the unqualified "others"; the latter (dental assistants, for example) sought to be classified with the higher ranks and distance themselves from any of the lower ranks (such as dental technicians). The result was professional (and gendered) stratification on a virtually unprecedented scale.

Hence, the original ordinance and subsequent amendments reinforced the distinction between dentists and other practitioners, which in turn enhanced the standing of dentists. Alongside this segregation, a hierarchy also emerged over the years as a result of the creation of "auxiliary professions" under the auspices of a dentist's supervision. This was comparable to the dynamics in the regulation of midwifery, when the practice of delivery was differentiated from the practice of medicine and midwives were subordinated to the supervisory authority of the (mainly male) medical establishment. Notably, the 1929 Midwives Ordinance was modeled after the Dentists Ordinance, to enable long-practicing traditional midwives (*dayas*) to continue working until the market could provide enough certified midwives. In other words, this model of balancing veteran and new (qualified) practitioners served other occupations as well, but in contrast to the Dentists Ordinance, the legislation on midwifery was unequivocal and not open to interpretation. Moreover, although the Midwives Ordinance was indeed a law that ostensibly "raised" the status of midwives to a profession, in fact this law of their own subordinated the midwives to physicians and resulted in a de-professionalization of their occupation.

The most appropriate comparison therefore, is to the legal profession, as I will explain. Neta Ziv, who has conducted extensive research on the regulation of the legal profession in Israel, describes three main approaches to the study of professions: the functionalist approach holds that "preliminary train-

166 A note in Lewin-Epstein's private Archive.

ing or study is a necessary condition for entering the profession, and the aim [of this prerequisite] is preservation of the public interest in the provision of legal services"[167]; the Weberian approach, in contrast, holds that "professional organization is driven by the self-interest [...] of maximizing the material profit, status, and symbolic gains of the profession's members"[168]; the third approach, ascribed to Abbott, asserts that knowledge is a central component of the inter-professional struggle[169]. Ziv proposes using all three approaches to decipher the dynamics of professional conduct.[170] I believe that this applies to the analysis of the regulatory process of dentistry as well, because there were many points of similarity between the two professions in those years. First, neither occupation apparently enjoyed much prestige during the Mandate era – at least not in the eyes of the Jewish community (*yishuv*). Ben-David, who researched the legal profession during the Mandate era, argues that the status of lawyers improved towards the end of this period, when members of the profession represented underground fighters (against the British).[171] Until that time they were seen as concerned primarily with their own narrow professional interests: the struggle against overcrowding and trespass. In my view this was also the situation in the case of qualified dentists. Like the legal profession, dentistry (in terms of Jewish engagement in the occupation) was not always seen as contributing to the Zionist enterprise. In contrast to "regular" healthcare, dental healthcare was not perceived – at least as represented in most of the relevant documentation – as part of the Zionist ethos. That is, the identification of physical health and body image with the Zionist ethos was one thing, but teeth were not necessarily part of this ethos.[172] Having said that, however, there were those who did invoke the terminology of national state-building, at least retrospectively[173]: "We shared with everyone else the feeling of pioneer responsibility and the faith that we were called upon to establish the basis for a strong and organized Jewish community, which was in the process of building its country. We believed that we would find our niche amongst the other professions."[174] Thus, dentists too strove to enhance their prestige by differentiating themselves from "others", and in so doing also indirectly advanced the professional interest of preventing competition. Over time, the Association's representatives increasingly used arguments based on "protection of the community of patients" (public health) to justify their demands. After the founding of the state, it probably became easier to prevent others from entering the profession: foreign rule, the prevention of *aliyah*, the

---

167 Ziv (2008), p. 448.
168 Ziv (2008), pp. 449–450. That is why lawyers create "social closure" according to Larson (1977).
169 Cf. Ziv (2008); on professions as based on knowledge, Macdonald (1995), p. 157.
170 Cf. Ziv (2008), p. 453.
171 Cf. Erez-Blum (2012).
172 Cf. CZA, J113/6144, letter from Dr. Segal to Dr. Szald (6/9/1920).
173 Cf. Ziv (2002/03).
174 Glasman (1971), p. 32.

dispute with Arabs, and questions of national identity were no longer factors. The situation was similar in the legal profession.

A second point of similarity was that during the Mandate era, lawyers were mainly focused on preventing professional overcrowding and trespass, two phenomena that still preoccupy the Israel Bar Association: With respect to trespass, this was primarily a struggle against a group known as "Petition Writers".[175] In the name of "public interest", lawyers endeavored to designate certain tasks solely to themselves, thereby barricading the legal marketplace and enhancing the uniqueness of the legal practice.[176]

With respect to the overcrowding of the profession[177]: The common assumption that there was not enough work for lawyers in Palestine was even more acute during the period of the British Mandate in Palestine (1917–1948). The British sought to limit immigration by limiting the entry of Jewish professionals seeking refuge primarily from Nazi Germany in the 1930s. The Chief Justices (British judges who headed in turn the judicial pyramid in Palestine) also complained about the overcrowding of lawyers. The fear of saturating the profession concerned both those already serving in the legal profession in Palestine and potential immigrants in the field. In 1926, given the economic crisis that afflicted the country, the argument of the overcrowding of the profession arose once again: "The crisis afflicting the country [...] caused serious harm to the legal profession. This has been particularly felt in light of the proliferation of lawyers and the great competition that developed as a result." Therefore, a noticeable decline of the profession was felt both in the spiritual sense ('every man does what is right in his own eyes') and in the material sense (given the lack of a tariff for the lawyer's fees).[178] Criticism regarding the overpopulation of lawyers appeared in the press as well. Nevertheless, professionals were cautious in their arguments about overcrowding of the profession because indirectly, such voices could be interpreted as opposition to the absorption of immigrants and cooperation with the British. The establishment of the State changed this position of the local jurists, making the opposition to the absorption of immigrant lawyers public. Apparently, this opposition was rooted in an ideology of concern for the public at large, which the lawyers representing this view were supposed to serve. By contrast, the foreign lawyers argued that the opposition was rooted exclusively in "fear of professional competition".[179]

As with dentists, even after Israel's founding there was resistance to the absorption of new immigrant jurists. The latter encountered opposition, or at least restrictions on their acceptance into the profession, in the form of exams and internships. The restrictions, which aimed to prevent competition

---

175 PRO, CO 733/413/12 (Petition Writers); PRO, CO 733/211/13. The matter was regulated in India during the 1930s as well: PRO, CO 535/101/7.
176 Cf. Ziv (2015).
177 Based on Katvan (2012).
178 Cf. Strassman)1984(.
179 CZA, S71/775, Newspaper cuts regarding immigrant lawyers' difficulties joining the profession (1940s–1950s).

and overcrowding of the profession, generated concerns about the presence of "unionism" among the country's lawyers.[180] Immigrant lawyers soon established their own organization to coordinate their struggle.[181]

Elsewhere, I showed how the claim of overcrowding actually united and galvanized the lawyers in a single cause, thus generating uniformity and unity as well as prestige in a market composed of very heterogeneous service providers. Throughout this process they relied on the "public interest" argument as a basis for preserving the unique contours of the profession.[182] In the case of dentistry, it was not concerns about overcrowding but rather opposition to the "other" that in fact united qualified dentists and enhanced their prestige, leading to professional stratification. Here too, they relied on the public health argument as a basis for granting the authority to practice solely to qualified dentists.[183] The rhetoric of opposition to the other was similar too. Both the lawyers and the dentists took measures to support the activities of uncertified practitioners or curtail overcrowding during the Mandate era as well, basing their arguments on the public good. Arguably the lawyers acted with greater caution, while the dentists, though not reckless, were less inhibited (in any case, the resistant to others did not harm the *aliyah*). The lawyers were operating within the framework of their own professional union, the Association of Lawyers, which created a sense of solidarity; the dentists and other variously qualified professionals, in contrast, operated under the auspices of several professional associations represented, for the most part, by lawyers (the same lawyers who defended the legal profession from trespass and overcrowding). After Israel attained statehood, the inhibitions dissipated, and the lawyers as well as the dentists openly set out to oppose the certification of new immigrants.

Moreover, as noted, a relationship formed between the two professions because leading lawyers served as representatives of the various associations, thus also playing a "mediating" role between the parties and the authorities. Unsurprisingly, lawyers were not seen as "struggling against" the Mandate authorities, as doing so would mean undermining the very essence of their practice and the positive relations they had cultivated in the corridors of power. These lawyers understood perfectly well the implications of professional overcrowding and competition, as exemplified above all by the Advocate Moshe Smoira, who in time came to represent the dental assistants. In a letter to his wife, Smoira, who immigrated in 1922, wrote that "there are already seven Jewish lawyers and the country doesn't need any more".[184]

In any event, we see how Ziv's three approaches to analyzing the dynamics of legal regulation also apply, in combination, to dentistry: training and education as a basis for protection of the public; preservation of self-interest;

---

180 Cf. CZA, S71/775, Newspaper cuts regarding immigrant lawyers' difficulties joining the profession (1940s–1950s).
181 Cf. ISA, G-4770/7, on the foundation of the organization of "Qualified Jurists" (1952).
182 Cf. Katvan (2012).
183 Cf. Katvan: Landlord (2010).
184 Smoira (2002), p. 12.

and the appropriation of knowledge as a core element. All these elements combine to provide us with a clear picture of the interests of dentists and their internal professional rivals.

## Summary

During the late Ottoman era the practice of dentistry began to undergo a process of professionalization: through Americanization, academization, de-feminization, self-organization and unionizing, and as noted, regulation through legislation – with a dispute between qualified and unqualified practitioners at the center of it all – each group and subgroup sought to establish its own identity by differentiating itself from the "other" with the lower degree of accreditation, and to be equated with those holding a higher degree of certification. The story of dentistry in Mandate Palestine is therefore also a story of cooperation and of efforts at segregation and identity formation. In this sense there is much similarity between the consolidation of this profession and the consolidation of the legal profession. In each case, prominent practitioners in the field cooperated with the British legislator to prevent professional trespass and overcrowding, that is, to provide a defense against the "other". Both were free trades that did not always rest on the national ethos and typically did not receive public funding. The outcome, however, was slightly different in each case: for the legal profession, the argument about overcrowding led to, or was intended to achieve, professional cohesion; for dentistry, the outcome was professional stratification, primarily because of inter-professional competition. As for dentistry, each party attached to the national feeling: for immigration or for public's health.

The situation in Mandate Palestine was unique: the model of legislation was mixed, based partly on the British code and partly on the Iraqi Ordinance (regarding those who practiced dentistry before British rule); the variety of professionals and semi-professionals from around the world, holding different kinds of diplomas made the process of professionalization and regulation through legislation even more complex.

Mandate Palestine therefore serves as a "laboratory" of sorts to examine the professionalization process in a multi-professional environment comprising practitioners from various parts of the world, representing a range of teaching methods, degrees of training, and certification. Each sought to build on the disadvantages of the other, employing pressure in various forms on the Mandate authorities, which for their part issued successive legislative measures that added consecutive layers to the professionalization process in a manner that benefited certified dentists: the legislation, ambiguous as it was, placed qualified dentists at the top of the pyramid. But the Mandatory legislator also granted uncertified practitioners the right to work, leaving leeway for inter-professional "ventilation". All of this took place against a background of struggles that turned professional status, prestige, and livelihood into matters of the highest priority for the parties involved, even at the expense of national issues (however – this vague legislation had its advantages: it enabled the immigration of less professional immigrants, and this is probably the reason the dentists, cautiously, promoted this legislation, knowing that it will not prevent immigrants to arrive in Palestine, even if they won't practice dentistry). And thus, as a result of this professional pressure pot, like a product of its British cooks, we inherited a multilayered system of professional stratification.

From 1957 through the early 1960s, there again arose practical problems regarding the licensing of immigrant dentists.[185] This time as well, the dental practitioners (dentists) accused the Dentists' Association of having disingenuous motives in seeking to prevent their licensing: "It is obvious to any thinking person that the dentists are concerned not with public health but with their own livelihood."[186] During the early 1970s disputes were still arising between the Ministry of Health and the Dentists' Association, and it was proposed that a department be created within the Ministry to advise the minister on dental healthcare. As noted, such a department had existed during the Mandate era. The Association has repeatedly demanded that health insurance for dental care also be regulated, and the question of immigrant dentists has resurfaced, as has a demand by the Association not to adopt the private laws proposed in this context for the granting of permits to new dentists.[187] This problem of balancing among level of training, protection of the country's own educational institutions, foreign graduates, and the influx of immigrant dentists continues to this day, and will presumably continue to affect the regulation of dentistry in the future as well.

"We are honored to honor the law", in the closing words of a letter from the dental services division of the Ministry of Health to "the community of experts in the fields of dentistry".[188] This somewhat archaic formulation obscures the fact that the letter was written in 2009. Yet the wording seems particularly appropriate and relevant in the context in which it was written: dentistry in Israel. The phrasing in effect tells a story of professional boundary delineation, the creation and regulation of a profession, and all of it by means of the law and with the assistance of jurists of the highest order.

---

185 Cf. ISA, N-14/51, letter from Dr. Meir (Ministry of Health) to the Dental Practitioners' Association (22/12/1960).
186 A Response to the Dentists' Association. In: *Davar* (30/12/1957), p. 6.
187 Cf. ISA, GL-12147/4, report on a meeting with the Minister of Health and the representatives of the Dentists' Association (11/12/1970); see also ISA, G-6524/21 (Russian Jewish immigrants, 1974).
188 http://www.health.gov.il/Download/pages/dent010409.pdf (last access: 25/07/2018).

# Bibliography

*Archives*

Israel State Archives, Jerusalem (ISA)

4277/9
5749/13
G-187/4
G-187/7
G-4269/1
G-4287/10
G-4770/7
G-5749/13
G-6524/21
GL-12147/4
K-27/18
K-27/21
K-104/2
M-322/7
M-322/14
M-323/1
M-326/26
M-1170
M-1170 (IMM/4/2/7)
M-1554
M-1554/1967
M-1554/1973
M-1554 (MG/27/3)
M-1632/5190
M-4986/5
M-5100/18
M-5100/21
M-6601/30
N-14/51
P-856/2

Central Zionist Archives, Jerusalem (CZA)

J1/1711
J1/2290
J1/6396
J1/7657
J113/2699
J113/6144
J113/7931
L4/483
S21/4888
S25/700
S30/2131
S71/775

## The British National Archives, London (PRO)

CO 67/271/4
CO 87/247/15
CO 323/1462/3
CO 323/1462/6
CO 323/1564/7
CO 323/1564/8
CO 323/1564/9
CO 323/1565/1
CO 323/1565/2
CO 533/440/12
CO 535/101/7
CO 733/142/9
CO 733/170/3
CO 733/211/13
CO 733/261/11
CO 733/375/3
CO 733/413/12
CO 859/31/10
CO 859/62/14
CO 859/62/15
CO 859/106
FO 370/227
FO 371/16930
FO 371/18535
MH 58/4
MH 58/45
MH 58/46
MH 58/47
MH 58/891
NATS 1/554
PC 98841
PC 101515
PC 118389
PC 119780
PC 119886
PC 120053
PC 120327
PC 122377
T1 12562


## The League of Nations, Geneva (LON)

6A/21184/668


## Tel-Aviv Municipality Archives (TAMA)

H4, M 1039

## Hadassah Archives, New York

RG 2/HMO, 103d

## Lewin-Epstein's private Archive

A note

## Personal Archive Katvan

Samuel Lewin-Epstein, "History of Dentistry in the Country" 1

## *Printed Sources*

Annual report of the Department of Health, government of Palestine, for the year 1922.
Annual report of the Department of Health, government of Palestine, for the year 1925.
369 More Doctors. In: Palestine Post (9/1/1934), p. 2.
Unmoved by New York's Glamour: Ziona Carmi is Interested in Dentistry Only. In: Palestine Post (20/2/1934), p. 6.
Germany's New Aryan Legislation: Dentists Fall Before Nazi Axe. In: Palestine Post (18/3/1935), p. 3.
H.C. 81/35, Mazin v. Director of Medical Services. In: Law Reports of Palestine. London 1937, p. 435.
H.C. 37/38, Scharf v. Director of Medical Services. In: Palestine Post (11/7/1938), Law Reports.
Lewin-Epstein, S[amuel]: Dental Health and Hygiene in Palestine. In: Palestine Post (9/5/1939), p. 12.

## *Literature*

Abbott, Andrew: The System of Professions. Chicago 1988.
Abel, Richard L.: The Rise of Professionalism. In: British Journal of Law and Society 6 (1979), pp. 82–98.
Adams, Tracey L.: Inter-Professional Conflict and Professionalization: Dentistry and Dental Hygiene in Ontario. In: Social Science and Medicine 58 (2004), pp. 2243–2252.
Adams, Tracey L.: The Changing Nature of Professional Regulation in Canada, 1867–1961. In: Social Science History 33 (2009), pp. 217–243.
Bartal, Nira; Katvan, Eyal: The Midwives Ordinance of Palestine, 1929: Historical Perspectives and Current Lessons. In: Nursing Inquiry 17 (2010), pp. 165–172.
Bishop, M[alcolm] G.H.; Gelbier, S[tanley]: Ethics: How the Apothecaries Act of 1815 Shaped the Dental Profession. Part 1. The Apothecaries and the Emergence of the Profession of Dentistry. In: British Dental Journal 193 (2002), pp. 627–631.
Bishop, M[alcolm] G.H.; Gelbier, S[tanley]: Ethics: How the Apothecaries Act of 1815 Shaped the Dental Profession. Part 2. The Chemist-Dentists and the Education of Dentists. In: British Dental Journal 193 (2002), pp. 683–686.
Chiu, G.K.; Davies, W.I.: The Historical Development of Dentistry in Hong Kong. In: Hong Kong Medicine Journal 4 (1998), pp. 73–76.

Clark, Linda L.: Women and Achievement in Nineteenth-Century Europe. Cambridge 2008.

De Vreis, David: From Porcelain to Plastic: Politics and Business in a Relocated False Teeth Company, 1880s–1950s. In: Enterprise & Society 14 (2013), pp. 144–181.

Ellis, Uri: What do you mean when you say: "Profession". In: Analiza Irgunit [Organizational Analysis] 17 (2012), p. 12.

Erez-Blum, Shimon: The "juridical underground": the involvement of Jewish lawyers in the Zionist struggle in 1938–1947 in mandatory Palestine. PhD diss. Tel Aviv Univ. 2012.

Forbes, Eric G.: The Professionalization of Dentistry in the United Kingdom. In: Medical History 29 (1985), pp. 169–181.

Freidson, Eliot: Profession of Medicine. Chicago 1988.

Garant, Philias Roy: The Long Climb. From barber-surgeons to doctors of dental surgery. Batavia, IL 2013.

Gelbier, Stanley: 125 Years of Developments in Dentistry, 1880–2005. Part 2: Law and the Dental Profession. In: British Dental Journal 199 (2005), pp. 470–473.

Glasman, Mirta: The History of Dentistry in Israel – Part I. In: Israel Journal of Dental Medicine. Journal of the Israel Dental Association 20 (1971), pp. 31–34.

Goold, Imogen; Kelly, Catherine (eds.): Lawyers' Medicine. Oxford 2009.

Haden, Karl N.; Machen, Bernard J.; Valachovic, Richard W.: The Value of the Dental School to the University, 75th Anniversary Summit Conference. Washington, D.C. 1998, available at: http://www.dns.adea.org/publications/Documents/1valachovic.pdf (last accessed: 08/11/2018).

Halperin-Kaddari, Ruth; Katvan, Eyal: The Feminist Proposal is really Ridiculous. Women's Battle to Become Advocates in Pre-State Israel. In: Mechkarey Mishpat [Law Studies] (2009), pp. 237–284.

Hook, Sara Anne: Early Dental Journalism: A Mirror of the Development of Dentistry as a Profession. In: Bulletin of the Medical Library Association 73 (1985), pp. 345–351.

Horner, Harlan H.: The Association and Dental Education. Part I: 1840–1938. In: The Journal of the American Dental Association 58 (1959), pp. 123–130.

Kaplan, Marion A.: The Making of the Jewish Middle Class. Oxford 1994.

Katvan, Eyal: That was the Beginning: Professionalization and Americanization of Dentistry in (Pre-State) Israel. In: Journal of the History of Dentistry 58 (2010), pp. 147–156.

Katvan, Eyal: Who is the Landlord? Quarantine and Medical Examinations for Immigrants at the Gates of Eretz-Israel (1918–1929). In: Korot 20 (2010), pp. 37–71.

Katvan, Eyal: The History of Dentistry in pre-State Israel: The De-Feminization Process. In: HaMishpat 16 (2011), pp. 173–208.

Katvan, Eyal: The "overcrowding the profession" argument and the professional melting pot. In: International Journal of the Legal Profession 19 (2012), pp. 301–319.

Katvan, Eyal: Women Entering the Professions in Mandatory Palestine. In: NASHIM (forthcoming, 2019).

Kuhlmann, Ellen: The Rise of German Dental Professionalism as a Gendered Project: How Scientific Progress and Health Policy Evoked Change in Gender Relations, c. 1850–1919. In: Medical History 45 (2001), pp. 441–460.

Langley, P[hilip] P.; Newsome, P[hilip] R.H.: Professionalism, then and now. In: British Dental Journal 216 (2014), pp. 497–502.

Larson, Sarfati Magali: The Rise of Professionalism: A Sociological Analysis. Berkeley 1977.

Lavsky, Hagit: The Creation of the German-Jewish Diaspora. Berlin 2017.

Lewis, Lilly: Restrictive Legislation and its Concomitants. In: The Accounting Review 20 (1945), pp. 198–200.

Likhovski, Assaf: Law and Identity in Mandate Palestine. Chapel Hill, NC 2006.

London, Louise: Whitehall and the Jews, 1933–1948. Cambridge 2001.

Macdonald, Keith M.: The Sociology of the Professions. London 1995.

McCluggage, Robert W.: A History of American Dental Association. Chicago 1959.

Miller, Arie L.: The Doctor's Legal Status. In: Mishpatim 17 (1986), pp. 510–529.

Morton, John N.: The Law Relating to Medical Practitioners and Dentists in Great Britain. London; Edinburgh 1912.

Motley, Wilma E.: Ethics, Jurisprudence and History for the Dental Hygienist. 2nd ed. Philadelphia 1976.

Niederland, Doron: The Influence of Immigrant Medical Doctors from Germany on the Evolution of Medicine in Eretz-Israel. In: Cathedra 30 (1984), pp. 111–160.

Ogus, Anthony I.: Regulation – Legal Form and Economic Theory. Oxford 1994.

Picard, Alyssa: Making the American Mouth. Dentists and Public Health in the Twentieth Century. New Brunswick, NJ 2009.

Price, David: Legal Aspects of the Regulation of the Health Professions. In: Allsop, Judith; Saks, Mike (eds.): Regulating the Health Professions. London 2002, pp. 47–61.

Richards, N. David: Dentistry in England in the 1840s: the first indications of a movement towards professionalization. In: Medical History 12 (1968), pp. 137–152.

Robinson, J. Ben: The Foundations of Professional Dentistry. Baltimore 1940.

Schaeffer, Conroy Mary: Women Pharmacists in Russia Before World War I: Women's Emancipation, Feminism, Professionalization, Nationalism, and Class Conflict. In: Edmondson, Linda (ed.): Women and Society in Russia and the Soviet Union. Cambridge 1992, pp. 48–76.

Sela-Sheffy, Rakefet: The Jekes in the Legal Field and Bourgeois Culture in Pre-Israel British Palestine. In: Iyunim bi Tequmat Yisrael 13 (2003), pp. 295–322.

Shachar, Yoram: Taufik Canaan Article – An Introduction. In: Halperin-Kaddari, Ruth; Katvan, Eyal; Shilo, Margalit (eds.): One Law for Man and Woman: Women, Rights and Law in Mandatory Palestine. Ramat Gan 2010, pp. 515–519.

Smoira, Esther: Hebrew Zionist Women. Tel Aviv 2002.

Strassman, Gabriel: The Robed: History of the Legal Profession in the Land of Israel. Tel Aviv 1984.

Thorogood, Nicki: Regulating Dentistry. In: Allsop, Judith; Saks, Mike (eds.): Regulating the Health Professions. London 2002, pp. 108–119.

Villiez, Anna von: The Emigration of Women Doctors from Germany under National Socialism. In: Social History of Medicine 22 (2009), pp. 553–567.

Waitzkin, Howard B.; Waterman, Barbara: The Exploitation of Illness in Capitalist Society. Indianapolis 1974.

Welie, Jos V. M.: Is Dentistry a Profession? Part 1. Professionalism Defined. In: Journal of the Canadian Dental Association 70 (2004), pp. 529–532.

Welie, Jos V. M.: Is Dentistry a Profession? Part 2. The Hallmarks of Professionalism. In: Journal of the Canadian Dental Association 70 (2004), pp. 599–602.

Zamet, John: The Anschluss and the Problem of Refugee Stomatologists. In: Social History of Medicine 22 (2009), pp. 471–488.

Ziv, Neta: Combining Professionalism, Nation Building and Public Service: The Professional Project of the Israeli Bar 1928–2002. In: Fordham Law Review 71 (2002/03), p. 1621.

Ziv, Neta: Who Moved my Gown? On Unauthorized Practice of Law in Israel. In: Bar-Ilan Law Studies (2008), pp. 439–489.

Ziv, Neta: Who Will Guard the Guardians of Law? Lawyers in Israel between the State, Market and Civil Society. Ramat Gan 2015.

Ziv, Neta: Unauthorized practice of law and the production of lawyers. In: Katvan, Eyal; Silver, Carole; Ziv, Neta (eds.): Too Many Lawyers. London 2017, pp. 175–192.

*Internet*

http://www.health.gov.il/Download/pages/dent010409.pdf (last access: 25/07/2018)

# Counselling Diabetics – The Hampered Development of Educational Programmes for Patients with Diabetes in Germany[1]

*Aaron Pfaff*

## Introduction

In Germany, more than six million people suffer from diabetes mellitus, costing the country approximately 35 billion Euros per annum.[2] Hence, diabetes is one of the most common and for the health system most burdensome disease. In order to minimise symptoms and to avoid long-term consequences, it is important that patients are thoroughly informed about their disease and are able to perform most therapeutic measures by themselves. In comparison to the immense costs for medication and medical technology, training the patients had long been neglected. As a consequence, there have been numerous avoidable problems and conflicts in the interaction between patients and medical staff.[3] A particular persistent complaint by the patients is that doctors only take little time to explain treatment-related issues[4] and that they use a language too complicated for the patients (too many technical terms)[5]. A possible result of this is the patients' reduced therapy compliance. It is one of the tasks of the Association of Diabetes Counselling and Training Professions in Germany ("Verband der Diabetes-Beratungs- und Schulungsberufe in Deutschland e. V.", VDBD) to address this conflict by providing a link between doctor and patient by serving as a mediator. While suggestions for informing patients better were already made in the 19th century[6] and were subsequently demanded with increasing urgency by experts, for a long time it seemed unimaginable to have structured training sessions with dedicated expert staff. Due to the lack of access to experts on diabetes whose number was at all times low given the social-medical significance of the clinical

---

1   This article is based on the German article in the collection by Pfütsch and Hähner-Rombach: Pfaff (2018).

2   German health report by the "Deutsche Diabetes Gesellschaft" (DDG) and the "Deutsche Diabetes Hilfe" (diabetesDE) from 16/11/2016: https://www.diabetesde.org/system/files/documents/gesundheitsbericht_2017.pdf (last accessed: 31/10/2018).

3   In the German original the author mainly used the female versions of the nouns when referring to the tutors in diabetes training as they were mainly women during the time under investigation.

4   A meta-analysis published in 2017 showed that the doctor-patient contact in Germany lasted on average barely seven minutes. Especially in comparison to Scandinavian countries but also to the US, Germany scored lower in this area. Cf. Irving et al. (2017), p. 6.

5   The *Diabetes-Journal* also includes numerous reports from patients who complained that doctors hardly took any time to explain things to them and didn't use patient-friendly language. For instance in: Schöller (1981) and *Diabetes-Journal* (1985), no. 3, p. 98.

6   Cf. Bouchardat (1875), p. 188.

picture, the majority of patients relied mostly on their general practitioners (GPs). Dependent on the GP's subject knowledge and didactic skills as well as his or her time available, the care for the patients could vary significantly. With a very complex and in everyday-life very present chronic disease such as diabetes, there is also the risk that patients are overwhelmed with their disease when they have not received sufficient help and training. This results in some patients resisting the allopathic treatments altogether and looking for alternative, allegedly simpler solutions. In particular the promises of being completely healed from diabetes contribute to patients moving away from academic medicine and insulin therapy.

> I hear of course what secret "miracle drugs" are used. Especially popular at the moment, particularly in Baden-Wuerttemberg, are green coffee beans with a spread of garlic on top that have to be chewed on an empty stomach. [...] Also very common in our country is the "sugar bracelet", a metal bracelet to cure diabetes mellitus that has be worn day and night.[7]

These are only two examples from a report by the "diabetes counsellor"[8] Marianne Romeick about alternative treatments that she had to face during her work. The report was written in 1980 in the context of receiving the "Gerhardt-Katsch-Medaille", an honour for individuals who made outstanding contributions to the training of diabetes patients. This award must alternately go to doctors and medical laypeople. With Romeick, a freelancer was honoured[9], which illustrates the great need for advice on diabetes. Simultaneously, it is an indication for the numerous internal and external problems in the diabetology of the 1970s and 1980s, which had hindered educating patients with diabetes until then. At the time, Romeick had been a diabetic herself for 25 years already and she was one of the first who fought for intensive training for patients suffering from diabetes mellitus. Even at the beginning of the 1980s, the goal of a patient-oriented, individually adjustable training (i. e., adapted according to age, gender, type of disease and manifestation, living situation etc.) seemed far off. This was the case despite the fact that training from dedicated expert staff had been demanded since the 1920s.

While the American diabetologist[10] Elliot Proctor Joslin (1869–1962) had already recognised in the 1920s that informing the patients was necessary, more than half a century passed in West Germany until the development of a health profession for the training of and caring for patients with diabetes was initiated in the late 1970s. A few more decades were required to achieve a fully differentiated occupational profile with different levels of qualification

---

7    Romeick (1980), p. 245.
8    Romeick called herself a "diabetes counsellor", anticipating the later term. Cf. Romeick (1980), p. 245.
9    N. N. (1980), p. 242.
10   Only since 2003, Germany has introduced the occupational profile of a diabetologist, which can be obtained by completing additional training (specifying that he or she has to work for at least 18 months in this field to receive the title "Consultant of Diabetology") in the subjects of internal medicine and endocrinology. In the following I will refer to doctors who had worked in the area of diabetology before 2003 as diabetologists.

even though to this day (2017) there is no state recognition of the profession in the Federal Republic of Germany, which is the ultimate goal. Even in 2017 a profession specifically designed to match this disease and to serve as an interface between doctor and patient is still rare.

The stagnation or decline of diabetology as a department[11] makes the counselling professions for diabetes gain even more significance as they have to bear the major load of caring for these patients. In the context of the growing social-medical significance of diabetes this is particularly important.

In the following I will analyse the formation of this health profession from its beginnings with committed female diabetics to the independent occupational profile of diabetes counsellors and diabetes assistants with its increasing professionalisation, including an independent professional organisation. I focus on the specific mechanisms and areas of conflict that went along with the professionalisation and differentiation, and also include the various interests and co-operations of the individual agents.

My corpus of sources consists of files from the company archives of the Bayer AG and Merck KGaA, publications by the professional organisation, the German Diabetes Society ("Deutsche Diabetes Gesellschaft", DDG) and association of non-professionals, the German Diabetes Association ("Deutscher Diabetiker Bund", DDB), in particular the journal of the association, the *Diabetes-Journal*[12], files and foundation documents of the VDBD, informational literature from the time, medical studies, normative texts and interviews[13] with contemporary witnesses, including initiators and participants, of the first training courses.

To integrate the formation of the counselling professions for diabetes better into the evolution of modern diabetes therapy after 1922, I will begin with a brief summary of the development until 1950.

## Development until 1950 – changes of the disease and therapy

When diabetes changed from being a fatal disease to a chronic condition due to the invention of insulin in 1922, fundamental changes in diabetes therapy became necessary. Until then the most common therapy was a hunger therapy that countered the diabetic coma. Nonetheless the patients died usually

11 One of the reasons for the disappearance of many expert clinics is the mainly outpatient treatment of diabetes patients through GPs (90 per cent). Often, the patients are only referred to consultants in case of severe complications and subsequent diseases. Cf. Diabetes-Ratgeber (Diabetes Guide). Situation of diabetology: https://www.diabetes-ratgeber.net/Diabetes/Stirbt-die-Diabetologie-524591.html (last accessed: 31/10/2018).
12 Until March 1971, the journal was published as *der diabetiker*, from April 1971 onwards it had the title *Diabetes-Journal*. Subsequently, for reasons of simplicity I will only refer to the *Diabetes-Journal*.
13 I would like to give my special thanks here to Dr. Anja Waller who conducted and transcribed the interviews with Marlies Neese, Anne Lütke Twenhöven, Klaus Funke, Gisela Müller, and Bettina Brandner.

within a few years. After the introduction of insulin in 1922 completely new therapeutic problems became central. Which principles were supposed to be applied in treating this chronic disease? Questions about diet, frequency and dosing of the insulin, and everyday factors such as family, job, or placement in society demanded answers.

While some therapeutic approaches worked in theory they were difficult to implement in everyday practice. For a long time, therapies commenced during a two-week hospital stay often failed because the inpatient schedule of treatments could not be applied to everyday life outside. A daily schedule that was planned by the minute could help to get diabetes "under control" and to prevent metabolic lapses, but few could fulfil such requirements in every-day life. The job, holidays, a disease, or simple social engagements such as a family party could disturb the metabolism.

In addition, not many of the treating doctors knew enough about the disease during the first decades as there were few sources of information on extended routine treatment of diabetes mellitus. Before 1922 only type 1 diabetes[14] was known and, because of the fatal outcome, the number of patients remained very low. Only very few doctors had to deal with diabetes. Elliot Joslin's demand that each patient with diabetes had to be his or her own doctor is thus understandable. He argued for a therapy that was adapted to the real-life situation of each individual patient. While this seemed a straightforward approach, the few diabetologists available could not teach the patients the required information. According to Joslin, this task should have been taken on by qualified "teaching nurses".[15]

In the German-speaking countries, this development remained initially without effect, and the prevailing ideal was to find the right dose of insulin for the patient during a hospital stay. Since there were only few hospitals with the necessary qualified staff, new institutions were needed to remedy this situation. For instance, in 1930 Gerhardt Katsch (1887–1961) founded a home for diabetics in Garz on Rügen, which was the beginning of the Central Institute[16] for Diabetes in Karlsburg. According to his therapeutic model, patients with diabetes should spend a longer period of time in the home to learn everything that they needed to know for their own everyday life. They were supposed to work and prove their productivity and performance during this "occupational therapy".[17] Katsch constructed diabetes as what he called "con-

---

14  Type 1 diabetes is an autoimmune disorder in which the insulin-producing cells are destroyed. The body no longer produces its own insulin and hence an insulin therapy is always necessary. Type 2 diabetes is far more common (90 per cent). Initially, insulin is still being produced, however, its effectiveness (insulin resistance) is reduced and without intervention this also affects the insulin release in the long term. Risk factors are foremost being overweight and lack of movement.

15  Nassauer/Petzoldt (1991), p. 64.

16  The institute was the leading institution for research and treatment of diabetes in East Germany. In 1994, it was taken over by a private hospital group. See also Bruns (2014).

17  Grote (1951), p. 51.

ditional health"[18] that one could achieve when complying with the therapy requirements. The plan was to build more hospitals with similar therapeutic models or therapies that drew on this model.

Yet, we must not assume that the doctor's requirements were guided by an idealistic partner relationship between doctor and patient. We can read in the contemporary guide books how the information was to be provided, and it increasingly served to aid both the doctor and the patient. For instance, in the guide for diabetics "ABC für Zuckerkranke" ("Diabetics from A-Z") by the diabetologist Ferdinand Bertram we read the following: "1. Do not tell anyone that you are suffering from diabetes! 2. Always stick to your diet – be careful when injecting insulin – strengthen your body with regular muscle training!"[19]

Following the style of the Ten Commandments there were another eight rules that were all also written in the imperative. Similar to the religious model Bertram's rules were not to be questioned. The patient with diabetes was regarded as a receiver of commands. The reason for this style was mainly the fear of many prevalent wrong ideas about the disease and the "well-meaning" suggestions of the people around the patient.

It was the task of the treating physician and increasingly also GPs to communicate these commands. These doctors themselves had received their knowledge from similar guide books such as the one by Bertram.[20] The early complaints after being released from hospital from both doctors and patients illustrate that many things were either forgotten at home or mistakes slipped in. While the one side criticised the bad treatment and unclear communication, the other side was horrified that the patients did not comply with the orders so that metabolic lapses occurred quite frequently.

Since there was no institutionally organised diabetics care in 1930, the foundation of the German Diabetes Association in 1931 was supposed to provide a possibility for diabetics to organise and have a single point of contact. Through the journal *Wir Zuckerkranken* (We Patients with Diabetes), the predecessor of today's *Diabetes-Journal*, the members of this organisation for non-professionals could become informed and new members attracted. In the co-opting of the health care system during National Socialism and the resignation of the first president, the German Diabetes Association was integrated into the German Health Association ("Deutscher Gesundheitsbund"). During the war, the activities of the German Diabetes Association seem to have been slowly discontinued and the journal was last mentioned in 1943.[21]

---

18  Cf. Katsch (1958).
19  Bertram (1947), p. 50.
20  Bertram published both a guide for patients and one for doctors and medical students.
21  Cf. Roth (1993), pp. 2–8.

## Reorganisation – association of non-professionals and everyday problems

In 1951, the journalist Robert Beining re-founded the DDB alongside the publication of the new journal of the association, *der diabetiker* (the diabetic). The articles still mainly had a didactic character: the majority were educational articles, then there was a section with questions and answers, and finally there were articles on numerous social problems that emerged with the disease. Yet, it quickly turned out that only a vanishingly small proportion of patients with diabetes could be reached this way.[22] Other methods of training patients gained attention.

While at least an organisation for non-professionals existed again from 1951 onwards, it took many more years before a medical association for experts was founded. Since many diabetes experts had emigrated during the NS time, German diabetology suffered from a massive brain drain and undertook huge efforts to re-connect with the international research community. Due to the low number of diabetes patients[23], which was also an effect of the war, at this point in time diabetes was a disease that few experts studied. Only in 1965, the expert association DDG came into existence. Until then it was very difficult to ensure a consistent approach and depending on the medical infrastructure, the therapy could vary greatly for patients. In particular there are dramatic descriptions of the differences in care between cities and the countryside.[24]

First pilot projects that studied a more intensive training for diabetes patients were started in the middle of the 1950s. There were different opinions on who was supposed to teach the patients and some doctors critically questioned their own role. "The diabetes doctor takes on the role of a teacher and trainer which is in fact a task that is very alien to his actual work."[25]

In times of general social change, the role of the doctor also changed, and the credibility of the doctor as a model and "health educator" began to unravel.[26] This development had its own conflicts. While conflicts with the treating doctor had long been under-represented[27] in the *Diabetes-Journal*, from the middle of the 1970s onwards this was more intensively discussed. Yet even the new generation of diabetologists with new didactic approaches could not train the numerous patients and additional suggestions on training patients were shared in the journal. One idea was to use nurses with the appropriate

---

22   By the mid-70s the editions reached 28,000 copies per month. *Diabetes-Journal* (1973), no. 12, p. 434.
23   For instance, in the American occupation zone approximately 13,000 diabetes patients were counted during a survey on the insulin provision for diabetics. HStA Stgt, EA 1/014 Bü 493/1, Letter 25/05/1948.
24   Cf. Petrides (1962), pp. 295–297.
25   Banse (1959), p. 60.
26   Cf. Halhuber (1978), p. 507.
27   It only appears sporadically to distinguish between physicians and diabetologists.

additional training, yet there were already dietitians in place[28], and finally there was the option that the patients should teach each other. The argument was that the patients would know best what their problems were and what uncertainties they had to face every day. It was believed that they would have the necessary empathy to gain the trust and the co-operation of other patients.[29] The doctor was of course to remain in charge to monitor the training and to prescribe further therapies. This structure was not new.

Similar to the diabetes centre in Berlin[30], diabetes counselling offices opened from the 1950s onwards in larger cities, for instance in Heidelberg and Hamburg. However, often these had to deal more with existential questions rather than disease-specific training. Many patients with diabetes lost their jobs or had huge problems to find a new one, or they struggled with having children; often the advice was to refrain from getting pregnant altogether and health insurances often refused to accept patients with diabetes.[31]

In these circumstances it seemed to be progress that there were centres at all that patients with diabetes could visit to get answers to their questions. With respect to the treatment and management of the disease, all that was on offer were published training materials[32]; the "ABC für Zuckerkranke" thus reached 14 editions by 1970. The publications differed depending on the author's view and attitude and it was not always a given that the author was a doctor. The area of diabetes treatment often was also the area for personalities with questionable expertise, including people who promised a cure and shady therapies. The experts warned of such false promises and emphasised the necessity to have one's dose established while staying at the hospital.[33]

Letters by readers reveal how dangerous the environment could be for diabetes patients when they talked about the tips and pieces of advice they had received from acquaintances. "And when we came home we were really bombarded with good advice from the relatives, neighbours and friends – but these were tips that sounded so very different than what the doctor had said. One or the other person might have thought at the time: 'What should I stick to now?'"[34]

The spectrum of advice for healing diabetes was wide: There was everything from the bracelet mentioned above and tea for diabetics, South-American roots and electrical devices. Patients who lived in the countryside were perceived as being in particular danger because it was difficult to get information to them or to train them. To help this situation, diabetes counsellors were supposed to visit them at home – at least in an ideal world,

---

28  Dietary schools had been in existence since 1928. Pannhorst (1972) and also see: Thoms (2004).
29  Cf. Romeick (1963), p. 89.
30  The centre was founded in 1935 as the first counselling centre. Cf. Bernhard (1954) and Kloss (1956), p. 53 and Romeick (1954), p. 29 and Bertram (1953).
31  Cf. DDB Orts- und Landesverband Hamburg (1961), p. 29 and Himstedt (1962), p. 7.
32  *Diabetes-Journal* (1968), no. 12, p. 496.
33  Cf. Dennig (1954), p. 213.
34  Romeick (1955), p. 172.

as Romeick and many doctors during the 1950s proposed.[35] Many doctors
were stretched to their limits in this alien role of a teacher. From a didactic
point of view, they were criticised for their lack of empathy.[36]

Many training articles in the *Diabetes-Journal* had been written very much
in the sense of a doctor-patient hierarchy that was built on discipline and military obedience. Thus we read in 1960 in an article titled "Die Zuckerkrankheit
als Schicksal und Verpflichtung" ("Diabetes as a destiny and commitment"):

> Those people who join the d i a b e t e s   b a t a i l l o n when they receive their diagno-
> sis of diabetes must visit a  r e c r u i t m e n t   s c h o o l like any member of the army.
> In this school he must learn the basics of metabolism and diet; he must learn to calculate
> using the food tables, to weigh the food in practice and also gain a sense of proportion,
> he must learn to determine the sugar in urine, the dosing of insulin; and he must learn to
> use the "c a r a b i n e r": the insulin syringe.[37]

It is understandable that particularly young patients had problems with the
language of this kind. Another common analogy for the diabetes treatment
was that of a driver, even though for a long time diabetes patients had significant problems to get a driver's license, independent of the quality of their
metabolic adjustment. "The diabetic as an 'u n l e a r n e d   d r i v e r' – and
in addition with a faulty, (metabolism) machine that requires particular skills –
is as  d a n g e r o u s  as an untrained driver of a car [...]."[38]

The situation in East Germany was similar at the time even though the
political opinion becomes more obvious in many statements. The journal
*Heilberufe* wrote in 1959: "Each patient with diabetes must acknowledge the
large help he receives from the state and must not abuse it. That means he
must comply with all orders he receives. He contributes to building socialism
that will bring him and all future generations a better life."[39]

Independent of the political or military tint, it emerges that psychologically negative motivational elements were heavily used. Especially the sword
of Damocles with respect to possible long-term effects (blindness, amputation)
was often evoked.[40]

Yet, also on the side of the patients a lot of resistance had to be addressed.
Injecting insulin made many patients feel uncomfortable. In addition to
non-diabetes specific worries, such as a fear of needles or injections, there
were also concerns about the drug itself as emerges in a letter from 1958 that
worried parents had sent to the journal: "Is a **cure possible here? I am worried that the insulin treatment will make the disease worse over time.**"[41]
Another educational article reports that a patient said something along the
lines "I'd rather shoot myself than injecting a needle".[42]

35   Cf. Romeick (1955), p. 173.
36   Cf. Petrides (1962), p. 296.
37   Brückner (1960), p. 150. Emphases in original.
38   Brückner (1960), p. 150. Emphases in original.
39   Cited after: Jörgens (2001), p. 46.
40   Cf. Dennig (1954).
41   *Diabetes-Journal* (1958), no. 8, p. 210. Emphasis in original.
42   Rottenhöfer (1954), p. 149.

In this context, diabetes counsellor Marianne Romeick tried as one of the first to close the gaps in patient training in a practice-oriented way. Since she was a patient herself, many doctors regarded her as particularly qualified for this role. Yet Romeick learned quickly that you cannot assume any knowledge in a layperson.[43]

She worked in the care centre for diabetics in Heidelberg. Here, first steps were taken, at least on a local level, to offer counselling that was adapted to the needs of the patients. Romeick thought about pedagogical approaches and asked to what extent patients with diabetes could feel patronised by the term "social care".[44] Yet she called herself a "diabetes social carer" ("Fürsorge-rin").[45] The counselling included the whole spectrum from medical questions to social or legal issues. After one year, already 170 patients with diabetes of all ages were looked after.[46] Romeick saw her main task as being an "inter-preter between doctor and patient".[47] In delineation to dietitians, this care for diabetics focused more on disease-specific and psychological problems.

In any case, the area of nutrition was increasingly taken on by the die-titian. This development did not stop at diabetology, as the article "Diet is the major chance – a profession for women turns into a career: dietitian" promoted this job. In 1960, there were approximately 700 dietitians in West Germany. Yet, there was a much bigger need and the 30 official training facil-ities were overcrowded. To be accepted into the programmes, the women had to attend a domestic science school at least for a year and complete an intern-ship in a kitchen for another year.[48] The training lasted two years, due to their medical knowledge for nurses the time was reduced to one year. An essential reason for the attractiveness of the job was the official state recognition of the occupational profile. This included the payment classification into band A for employees ("Tarifordnung A", TO.A) and later the collective agreement for civil servants on a contractual basis ("Bundes-Angestelltentarifvertrag", BAT). The protection of the name of the profession and the duration of the training (two years) in all federal states of Germany were determined by the Act for Dietitians ("Diätassistentengesetz", DiätAssG) in 1974.[49]

Another advantage for the development of the profession was the creation of professional associations. In 1960, there were two. Even at this point in time, there was a tendency for further professionalisation: After three years of profes-sional experience, dietitians could apply for jobs as nutritional advisers. One of

---

43  Cf. Romeick (1987), p. 95.
44  Romeick (1954), p. 29.
45  Romeick (1963), p. 85.
46  Cf. Romeick (1955), p. 172.
47  Romeick (1963), p. 85.
48  Cf. Heimann (1960), p. 242.
49  After 1945 the length of the training had initially been subject to the individual states and lasted between two and four years (including a probationary year). Cf. Verband der Diätassistenten (Association of Dietitians). Berufsgeschichte (History of the Profession): https://www.vdd.de/diaetassistenten/berufsgeschichtederdiaetassistenten/ (last accessed: 31/10/2018).

the central schools for further education was the Institute for Nutrition Advice and Diets ("Institut für Ernährungsberatung und Diätetik") in Dusseldorf.[50]

This competition was a problem for the development of counselling professions in diabetes because nutrition and diet were in the hands of a different professional group that had its own organisation. Other possible areas such as training in self-management, were still the responsibility of the treating physician. The missing link was a personal training that was specifically adapted to the problems of patients with diabetes. While this area could also include issues of diet, according to Romeick, it was mainly supposed to provide support in managing everyday life. Personal visits with patients were a central point for her.[51] Only at home the counsellor could recognise the specifics of the patient and the problems with the therapy. Furthermore, an evaluation had shown that only eight per cent of all diabetes patients were informed about their diet.[52] There were for instance misunderstandings like "carbohydrates ["Kohlenhydrate"] were not the same as cabbage ["Kohl"] [...]", which have phonetic similarity in German or that butter had to be included when calculating the amount of calories.[53] Only during a home visit a counsellor could find out whether the patient merely complied with the therapy immediately before a visit at the doctor's office, the commonly observed behaviour. Another problem was that while the patients additionally received all information from the counselling session in writing, they did not always understand the teaching materials. For that reason, Romeick regarded an initial counselling always as advisable and suggested, if necessary, a follow-up later on. Already at the end of the 1950s, it emerged that working in small groups was the best method. The diabetes carer was in Romeick's mind more of an independent counsellor than a doctor's assistant because she often addressed issues that went beyond the purely medical context.[54]

## New pathways – hospitalisation or outpatient dose finding

An important step in the following development of diabetes treatment happened after the foundation of the medical expert association in 1965, mentioned above. Furthermore, the increasing significance of diabetes resulted in new approaches in the public management of the disease. Investigations had shown that the number of patients with diabetes who had not been discovered was much higher than expected and that the feared long-term effects could be mitigated through an early recognition.[55]

50   Cf. Heimann (1960), p. 242.
51   Cf. Romeick (1963), p. 85.
52   Cf. Romeick (1955), p. 173.
53   Cf. Romeick (1963), p. 85.
54   Cf. Romeick (1963), pp. 86–88.
55   Reliable numbers were hard to come by at the end of the 1950s, but estimates varied from one-tenth of a per cent to one per cent. Cf. Banse (1955), p. 46.

Following the model of the investigations the diabetologist Volker Schliack had conducted in East Germany in 1952[56] in 1967 the largest so-called "early detection campaign" was conducted in Munich. To get more reliable data with respect to the prevalence, distribution of age and gender, and connections to being overweight or other cases in the family, each person in Munich received a letter with a urine sugar test strip (glukotest) per post. The people were asked to send it back to the Medical Association after completing the test.[57] This data resulted in previous estimates of diabetes in West Germany being revised upwards.

With the discovery of new oral diabetic medications[58], from the middle of the 1950s onwards there was now also a third treatment option in addition to diet and insulin substitution. This meant that there was even more material for the doctors to explain. Naturally, patients found a treatment with pills far more attractive than insulin injections.[59] Since this therapy was not an option in insulin-dependent cases (diabetes type 1 or advanced type 2), a lot of explaining and persuading was necessary in these cases to explain to patients why they had to administer injections. This was not only true for the patients, as even some of the doctors needed some extra lessons here.[60]

Altogether these factors resulted in an increasing need for education and communication of information that could neither be satisfied by the doctors nor the expert association DDG nor the self-help organisation DDB.

With the increasing prevalence of diabetes, the cities and communal hospitals also felt the need to act. For instance, the 57th meeting of the Health Select Committee of the German Association of Cities and Towns discussed in collaboration with the 43rd meeting of the working group "Communal Hospital Sector" ("Kommunales Krankenhauswesen") on 27th/28th June 1968 in Stuttgart the recommendation for diabetes care. A draft on improving the care for patients with diabetes planned the hiring of "social workers with special prior training". The spectrum of tasks was defined as follows: "To support doctors in the care for patients with diabetes special carers/social workers are necessary. They should be trained so that they can advise the patients in all questions of diet and nutrition, show him or her how to administer injections and provide support with all social questions."[61]

The necessity of special care for patients with diabetes was not questioned at the meeting of the German Association of Cities and Towns. Yet, neither the cities nor their public health offices were to be put in charge because the legal concerns were too big. There were too many issues unresolved, especially with respect to who would be responsible at either the council or the

---

56  Cf. Banse (1955), p. 47.
57  Cf. N. N. (1971).
58  Before there had also been some oral anti-diabetic drugs, for instance diguanidin (synthalin A), that had to be taken off the market because of their toxicity. Cf. Beyer (1978).
59  Cf. Lübken (1972).
60  Cf. Interview on 19/01/2015 with Marlies Neese (transcription at the Institute for the History of Medicine of the Robert Bosch Stiftung, Stuttgart).
61  StA Stgt, 19/1 Bü 748, Draft 28/12/1967.

towns, so that finally the recommendation was to delegate the responsibility for hiring staff to the DDB without, however, resolving the cost regulation.[62] Hence there was no binding regulation agreed on in 1968 because the participants agreed that the recommendations of the Association of Cities and Towns could only provide a framework and that the implementation had to be adapted to the local situation.[63] The biggest problem, however, were the requirements in this area of work as the health office criticised:

> It will be difficult to attract suitable staff who can fulfil all the separate demands. A social carer would not have the required knowledge in the area of diet advice, a dietitian likewise would not know about social care. To monitor the technique of administering injections is still task of the treating doctor [...].[64]

This is a brief summary of the dilemma that training in diabetes faced at the end of the 1960s.

There has been no non-medical profession in nursing or health care that needs to cover such a broad spectrum of work areas. Drawing on the US, other options were also discussed that at least questioned the necessity of human training staff. There, training with electronic devices was tested. So-called teaching machines of the type "auto-tutor" were supposed to take over the large quantities of training.[65] Yet, these succeeded neither in the US nor in West Germany because "nobody seriously expects that automatic teaching machines can replace the persona of the doctor while training and informing patients".[66]

Despite all of these signals a concrete solution was nowhere in sight, neither at the communal nor the state level, and only intentions were shared. The committee "social medicine" ("Sozialmedizin") that had been founded together with the foundation of the DDG in 1965 concluded:

> The fantastic experiences that other countries (England, Switzerland, US, among others) have made with trained diabetes carers and that could be confirmed in Germany mainly by Marianne Romeick in Heidelberg and Duisburg have caused us to consider this issue with special attention. Unfortunately, the success of the previous efforts has only been meagre so far.[67]

Yet, the welcome speech at the opening of the third conference of the expert association DDG reveals that training was increasingly at the centre of attention. The president at the time, Werner Creutzfeldt, said that German diabetology "in general has caught up with international research".[68] He meant that effects of the brain drain that had followed the time of National Socialism had been overcome. He continued that diabetology would include "the training

---

62  StA Stgt, 19/1 Bü 748, Letter 25/06/1968 and early report from 06/06/1968.
63  StA Stgt, 19/1 Bü 748, Letter 10/11/1967.
64  StA Stgt, 19/1 Bü 748, Letter 10/11/1967. Emphasis in original.
65  Cf. Schweisheimer (1966).
66  Schweisheimer (1966), p. 14.
67  Petrides (1966), p. 191.
68  Creutzfeldt (1969), p. 185.

and guiding of patients more than in any other field within medicine".[69] The cooperation between organisations for non-professionals and expert associations was also increased. Their relationship had been somewhat problematic until the end of the 1960s. Creutzfeldt commented on this in his speech as follows: "Due to its hard work the earlier, a rather peculiar advocacy group [he means the DDB, A. P.] has evolved into an organisation that is looking with us for opportunities to enable patients with diabetes to live with the often-cited 'conditional health'."[70]

An improvement of the relationship was particularly important with regards to the training courses that the regional chapters of the DDB organised themselves (in 1968 this happened in 70 regional chapters). On the side of the DDG the diabetologists Karl Schöffling and Hellmut Mehnert among others were working on an educational programme for patients.[71] Numerous articles in the *Diabetes-Journal* illustrate that international comparisons became increasingly important. The US especially was portrayed in every regard as a leader and one prominent topic was the self-management which had been established there to a much larger extent. Simultaneously, such comparisons were often used to criticise the people who were involved at home. This becomes notable with respect to the often-postulated differences in mentality such as: "For the European observer, it is extremely impressive to observe that patients who come from all social demographics are so eager to learn."[72]

While hardly any concrete measures had been decided on by the end of the 1960s, there emerged a re-examination of training focussed on the particular needs of individual patients. Finding the right dosage for the patients while they were in hospital and without a connection to their everyday life had not proved to be successful. Similarly, it became clear that the physicians were unable to take care of all aspects of the diabetes therapy due to the increasing work load. While in many hospitals the dietitians had taken on the role of teaching the patients about dietary aspects, social issues and questions of frequent follow-ups had to be handled by somebody else. The idea was to transfer the responsibility to both the patient and non-medical assistants; the latter did not yet exist in the form that was required.

An important area of work was the gradually increasing significance of self-managing one's metabolism. While this had been recommended already at the end of the 1960s the implementation in a large scale was still far away. With the emergence of new opportunities for glycaemic control this responsibility progressively shifted to the patients. Yet, without appropriate training on the handling of devices, documenting the blood sugar values and having information on additional measures, the patients' monitoring their metabolism was still not adequate. With the enormous potential market of patient training, this area also became interesting for another agent in the field of diabetes

69   Creutzfeldt (1969), p. 186.
70   Creutzfeldt (1969), p. 186.
71   Creutzfeldt (1969), p. 186.
72   *Diabetes-Journal* (1963), no. 2, p. 52.

therapy: the pharmaceutical and medical device industry. The target group included approximately 30,000 physicians.[73] While there were approximately 250,000 potential users among patients with diabetes type 1[74], the market potential in the area of type 2 diabetes was massive. A financially strong and influential agent like the industry could provide further impulses with regard to patient training.


## Training and industry – support or exertion of influence?

Similar to the US, diabetology in West Germany had a factional debate on what constituted an adequate metabolic management. In the US, the discussion focussed on the question of whether the management should be strict or loose.[75] The debate in West Germany could not be as sharply delineated but the German speaking diabetologists equally disagreed on how the patient's self-monitoring was supposed to work. At the beginning of the 1970s, means for self-monitoring were indeed available. For the simpler version, i.e., checking the urine, there were commercial tests in different versions available, e.g., tablets (clinitest), test strips (clinistix, glukotest), optical instruments (polarimeter), and reagent solution (glycurator). For the glycaemic self-management, the first test strips entered the market during the 1960s (dextrostix, haemogluko-test).[76]

Self-testing one's metabolism was a big issue for training foremost because it required huge (educational) efforts. Not only the hands-on requirements such as a thorough and correct completion of the tests had to be taught, but the patients also needed to be informed about the underlying knowledge about the metabolic processes. This included basic subjects such as the measured parameters and the rough categorisation of the results. During the 1960s most of the experts still agreed though that only in absolutely exceptional cases the patients should be allowed to adjust the therapy (dose, diet) after interpreting the values by themselves.[77]

With respect to the problems many patients had with measuring parameters, such as bread units and a correct calculation of the total amount of calories in their diet, new measuring units such as mg/dl, mg% or mmol/l posed an additional burden and hence were a source for errors.[78] While the industry initially focussed on the doctors, it recognised that the target group of the pa-

---

73  BAL, Compur 1979 Vol. 2 Bayer Diagnostika-Entwicklung für das Compur-Mini-Photometer-System, p. 49.
74  SMA Erlangen, 2/513 MDS Laufende Bedarfsstudie zum Projekt "Mikrodosierung von Insulin" (Ongoing demand study for the project "Micro-dosing of insulin"), with a determination of the future development, p. 10.
75  Cf. Mauck (2010), pp. 245–304.
76  For instance in: BAL, 386/55 Bayer Diagnostics, Progress in Diabetes Management Through Innovation.
77  Cf. Mascher et al. (1969) and Dehmel (1969).
78  Cf. Chefredaktion (1978), p. 197.

tients had the bigger market potential long-term. The argument was that the best opportunity to dispel concerns of many diabetologists regarding a good self-management of one's metabolism were well-trained patients.

This also influenced Romeick's later career path. From January 1970 on-wards, she began to hold independent educational presentations both for doc-tors and patients. In her annual reports she informed the Ministry of Health in Stuttgart about her work. Using economics in her argumentation, she had succeeded at times to persuade the health insurances to pay for her talks. Romeick reported that she had to negotiate her pay with each local health insurance individually. By contrast, pharmaceutical companies were far more open. During larger events such as conferences of the International Diabetes Federation (IDF), the DDG, or the DDB, it had become tradition for the industry to attend and showcase itself. Now, the companies increasingly also presented themselves at local events.[79] While the associations and conferences critically regarded the business interests of the industry, they depended on its support.

In the US, the companies had already much more influence in the area of patient training. Under the leadership of the company branch Ames, since 1962 every quarter the journal *Diabetes in the News* was published that informed about new developments in therapy and reported especially on success stories of patients with well-controlled diabetes. While in 1973 the journal published 100,000 copies, ten years later the number was already 700,000. When in 1973 the "American Association of Diabetes Educators" was founded, Ames was involved with this association from the very beginning. In collaboration with the British Diabetic Association, from 1977 onwards the cartoon "Rupert the Bear" was published that was supposed to explain diabetes to children.[80] In the US, there had been radio shows such as "Quiz Kids", "One Man's Fam-ily", or "Barn Dance" that were sponsored by Miles with which the company ensured a strong presence in the public eye for a longer period of time.[81]

In Germany such efforts were more modest. At the end of the 1960s, Boehringer Mannheim had started to publish records for patients with dia-betes and donate or fund guide books and training materials.[82] While the marketing for a good publicity was far away from American dimensions the development headed into a similar direction.[83]

This became particularly evident during presentations that were meant to satisfy the significantly increased need for information due to the gradual implementation of self-tests of one's metabolism. This resulted in pharmaceu-tical companies appointing speakers to introduce the latest innovations and to

79  HStA Stgt, EA 8/601 Bü 387, Report of the experiences of the year 1979.
80  Cf. Cray (1984), pp. 86–87.
81  Cf. Gardner (2013).
82  Popular materials were, e.g., fake food made of plastic to estimate portion sizes and/or the nutritional values. Kurow (1972), p. 405.
83  N.N. (1967), p. 61.

explain the self-management using the companies' products.[84] Romeick also worked as a speaker and gave presentations to doctors collaborating with the companies Novo and Boehringer Mannheim. At times the doctors were really surprised about the low level at which patients (non-professionals) needed to be informed. The discrepancy between the doctors' expert knowledge and the ability to appropriately teach became again evident during these talks.[85]

Romeick stated that she gave nearly 2,000 presentations in ten years (1970–1980). For instance, in 1977 she gave 179 talks to 8,234 listeners. Since both the presentations for doctors and the presentations for patients became very popular and received positive feedback, another target group within diabetes therapy was considered: nurses and doctors' assistants. Next to the treating physician, these had been responsible until then for routine tasks, often without any deeper specific knowledge on diabetes. In collaboration with the insurance company AOK in Rhineland-Palatinate and Baden-Wuerttemberg, from the middle of the 1970s onwards advanced training courses were organised for the assistants.[86]

## Appropriations – experiences abroad and new committees

By now, Romeick was no longer the only person working in this area. While the training programmes of the DDB and DDG were always distributed in written form[87], this did not result in informing the majority of the patients with diabetes. A group of largely younger diabetologists pursued this goal. Because of their experiences abroad these doctors introduced additional ideas and approaches into German diabetology.

Due to the international recognition of the Joslin Hospital in Boston, many European diabetologists went there for internships and returned with new inspirations. Among them were for instance Hellmut Mehnert (Munich), Michael Berger (Dusseldorf), and Jean-Philippe Assal (Geneva). The latter had attracted type 1 diabetes himself while he had been working on his dissertation.[88] After his return he was appointed at the university hospital in Geneva and worked on making the therapy more patient-friendly. The patients were to receive simple rules, and for managing their metabolism this meant, for instance, a pattern of "if-then" decision rules.[89]

In 1977, in addition to Viktor Jörgens, the doctor in residence Michael Berger stayed at Geneva as well. Subsequently, first studies on new methods for training patients were conducted at the German diabetes centre in Dussel-

---

84   HStA Stgt, EA 8/602 Bü 64/2, Letter 27/02/1987.
85   HStA Stgt, EA 8/601 Bü 387, Report of the experiences of the year 1979.
86   HStA Stgt, EA 8/601 Bü 387, Reports of the experiences from the years 1977 to 1980.
87   Ständer (1968), p. 496.
88   Cf. Interview on 15/12/2015 with Viktor Jörgens (recording private archive Pfaff).
89   Private archive Pfaff, documents Viktor Jörgens.

dorf.[90] These included self-managing one's metabolism and a meeting with the pharmaceutical representative Katharina Wasser. Mrs. Wasser was persuaded to collaborate on patient training and her employer Miles released her from her work and even bore the costs for the first three years of her employment in Dusseldorf.[91] This model of assistants who the pharmaceutical companies paid for was adopted by, for instance, Boehringer Mannheim or Hoechst.[92] Just as in the US the link between medical staff and pharmaceutical industry was early established in the training of the patients. Yet, these few counsellors could not cover the demand. According to a calculation of the diabetologist Karl Schöffling at the end of the 1970s, approximately 3,000 assistants would have been necessary for the counselling on diet and diabetes.[93] He regarded them by all means as mediators that were to relieve the doctor as the primary educator.

Besides, at this time an increasingly critical debate had begun on the strongly hierarchical and formal training used over the previous decades. In articles such as: "On mistakes during the training of patients"[94], doctors were denounced because of their elitist behaviour and their inability to defer to the patients and explain the facts in an understandable language[95]. The image of the doctor as the only "health educator"[96] had also become obsolete in the context of the social changes after 1968 and the doctor's authority was questioned particularly in social matters. The biggest barriers were noticed here between patients and chief consultants. Diabetes counsellors who were closer to the everyday reality of the patients were supposed to bridge this gap. Training sessions in groups that had been demanded before and were supposed to be regularly repeated should prevent patients from returning to their old everyday routines. For instance, Carola Halhuber points out that

> the public health education and individual educators must influence reference groups and reference norms more. If the patient cannot find such a group after completing his health training, he or she will be socially isolated or will fall back to old habits.[97]

A "pre-study for the creation of a training concept for chronically ill patients" that had been conducted as part of a doctoral dissertation concluded that 72 per cent of the responding patients wanted to use every opportunity to get informed. However, they were very passive in this endeavour: only 38 per cent knew a journal for non-professionals and less than 10 per cent had a subscription or other access to such a publication. The goal of the new training

---

90   Cf. Berger et al. (1983).
91   Cf. Interview on 15/12/2015 with Viktor Jörgens (recording private archive Pfaff).
92   Cf. Interview on 23/07/2015 with Hellmut Mehnert (recording private archive Pfaff).
93   Cf. Janka (1979), p. 395.
94   Halhuber (1978), p. 504.
95   In a patient survey (n=512), 91 per cent criticised that the doctor would not listen enough and 89 complained about the usage of too many technical terms. Cf. Scholz (1988), p. 43.
96   Halhuber (1978), p. 505.
97   Halhuber (1978), p. 506.

was thus to overcome such passivity, in particular as most of the questioned patients (86 per cent) assumed that their knowledge about diabetes was sufficient. Every second patient relied however on one or more household remedies that were used in addition to the therapy.[98]

Studies from Austria concluded furthermore that patients with diabetes were willing to go to training sessions as long as they took place in their immediate neighbourhood. With a distance of four to five kilometres the willingness to attend significantly fell.[99] Counselling had to be brought to the patient and not vice versa. Policy-makers were thus informed and advised. Experience had shown that they were most open to economic arguments. For that reason, the success of diet counselling was supposed to be presented in a cost-benefit calculation. Likewise, this was later the case for diabetes counselling. Hiring a dietitian, including expenses for teaching materials, transport etc. in 1978 cost approximately 26,000 German marks per annum. With an estimated number of 1,200 diabetes patients per counsellor per year and a federal counselling system for all diabetes patients who were overweight, for oral anti-diabetic drugs alone more than 130 million German marks were supposed to be saved per year.[100] The validity of such calculations must be questioned though because they only take individual factors into account. Yet, they illustrate that the arguments in the debate were increasingly socio-economical. Support came in many cases from the pharmaceutical industry that funded additional counsellors from the end of the 1970s.[101] The companies bore the costs for a certain period of time, in most cases three to five years, after this time was up, the costs had to be covered by other sources. Since shutting down the services that had been provided until then would have hardly been explainable, most institutions bowed to the "power of facts"[102], accepted the inevitable and paid the costs in the future. This was also the case in the diabetes centres in Dusseldorf and Munich. Thus, the industry played a considerable role in creating the first offices for diabetes-specific counselling.

This was also the time period during which the DDG held internal discussions that led to the foundation of the committee "Non-professional Work" in 1978. The *Diabetes-Journal* says on its foundation:

> The foundation of this committee reveals that the German Diabetes Society wants to increasingly address the problems that patients with diabetes face. One of the committee's tasks is to organise the training and advance the education of patients with diabetes in collaboration with the German Diabetes Association, i. e., the association of non-professionals.[103]

---

98  Cf. Janka (1979), p. 394.
99  Cf. Sulzer (1992).
100 Cf. Petzoldt (1978).
101 Cf. Petzoldt (1978).
102 Interview on 23/07/2015 with Hellmut Mehnert (recording private archive Pfaff).
103 N.N. (1978), p. 449.

In this way the research and professionally oriented direction of the DDG was broadened through the aspect of patient training.[104]

The training methods that Assal used in Geneva caught on quickly in Dusseldorf and a team at the German diabetes centre, led by Michael Berger, started a series of public lectures all over North Rhine-Westphalia at the beginning of 1980. Due to the large interest, at times these lectures were held every two weeks. In addition to the heads of the team consisting of the doctors Michael Berger, Viktor Jörgens, and other doctors from the German Diabetes Centre, the team included dietitians and also Katharina Wasser. The latter is mentioned with the title "diabetes training nurse (new type of profession)" in the *Diabetes-Journal*.[105] The formerly typical form of teacher-centred presentation was replaced with working in small groups. After an introductory presentation, the participants were supposed to discuss different subjects in their groups and introduce these afterwards to the other groups. Explanations were not to be given by the experts but by the diabetes patients themselves.[106] The idea was to counter the common previous complaint that the training had been too complicated and theory heavy because of the terminology.[107] The statistical surveys revealed that action was required. It was assumed that barely 100,000 to 200,000 of the roughly two million patients with diabetes in West Germany received the opportunity to attend appropriate training. The main reason for that was supposedly the lack of qualified staff.[108]

In 1980, the members of the committee "Non-professional Work" also began to develop a curriculum to train future diabetes counsellors.[109]

A problem was here to agree what the minimal qualification of a future counsellor was supposed to be. First brainstorming included only those nurses, dietitians, and doctors' assistants who had had at least a year of experience dealing with diabetes patients. Later drafts provided the opportunity to gain such practical experience after the training at a diabetes centre was completed. The theoretical part of this additional training was supposed to be three months long and end with an exam before a committee of the expert association DDG before the participants received their certificate. In this way the DDG tried to standardise the diabetes therapy through certificates issued by the association and simultaneously stabilise the status of the expert society. An obligatory annually continued education was supposed to provide a quality that could keep pace with the continuously changing requirements of a modern diabetes therapy.[110] A first curriculum was agreed on in 1981

---

104 In the meantime the diabetologist Jean-Philippe Assal from Geneva had advanced the training also at the European level. Within the European Association for the Study of Diabetes (EASD) he led a study that investigated further opportunities for educating patients. Cf. Chefredaktion (1980), p. 436.

105 Cf. DDB (1981), no. 1, p. 28, and no. 3, p. 113.

106 Cf. DDB (1981), no. 1, p. 28.

107 Cf. Lange (1981), p. 106.

108 Cf. Chefredaktion (1981), p. 241.

109 Cf. Willms (1981), p. 409.

110 Willms (1981), p. 409.

and afterwards the planning for the first course of a continued education programme began. Now, for the first time binding criteria for a future professional profile of a diabetes counsellor had been created.

The first course began in 1983 at the diabetes centre in Dusseldorf and
ran for eight weeks in total (320 hours)[111] that were divided into two sections
of four weeks each[112]. In addition to medical basics the lesson planning and
video training on self-monitoring and behavioural training were taught.[113]
The participants regarded the planning of lessons as particularly difficult.[114]
At the end there was a final exam before a committee of diabetologists, the
president of the DDB and a state-certified educator who served both as committee member and minute taker.[115] After the first training course, 25 diabetes counsellors received their certificate, 22 of which were women and three
were men.[116] Of these 25, 13 were dietitians, nine were female nurses, and
three were male nurses. In the following two courses in Munich and Mainz,
51 participants were enrolled of which only one was a man. The age of the
participants ranged from 25 to 39 years.[117]

Even though the methods had changed, the goal of the training remained
clearly defined. "The goal of training patients with diabetes is to achieve and
maintain compliance with the therapy."[118]

## The first diabetes counsellors

In the future, this goal no longer had to be achieved by the physician but by
the diabetes counsellors as became also evident in the educational articles in
the *Diabetes-Journal*. Until the beginning of the 1980s such articles had nearly
exclusively been written by doctors (especially senior physicians at the diabetes centres). Now, this increasingly shifted to the newly created training teams.
Notably, the first teams in Dusseldorf and Schwabing published numerous
articles and took on an annual series of articles in the *Diabetes-Journal*. With
the shift from doctor to training staff, the style of the articles also changed.
Linguistically, the new articles were written in a much clearer language, technical terms were increasingly reduced to a minimum and the suggestions were
kept short and to the point. In contrast to the early "commandments" that
had been written in the imperative, now the advice was formulated in the
subjunctive, i.e., as a recommendation. For instance, in the series of articles
titled "Mrs Oppler is diabetic" the most important aspects from self-managing

---

111 To compare this to the training of nurses, see Hähner-Rombach (2018).
112 Cf. Scholz (1988), p. 64.
113 Cf. Scholz (1988), pp. 71–72.
114 Cf. Scholz (1988), pp. 96–97.
115 Cf. N.N.: Beruf (1984), p. 234.
116 Cf. N.N.: Hurra (1984), p. 275.
117 Cf. Scholz (1988), p. 169.
118 Böninger (1984), p. 317.

one's metabolism to going on holiday were covered using a case example and a practically relevant language without technical terms.[119]

With regard to achieving encompassing educational efforts these teams that mainly worked locally were not enough. In addition to the few hospitals/ doctor's offices that specialised in diabetes treatments another way had to be found, namely a more decentralised type of training.

A similar need had become evident in the nutritional counselling; here the trend had shifted towards counselling at the doctor's office that was decentralised. In a pilot project in Berlin, within two and a half years a dietary adviser had taught 4,365 patients with diabetes in 75 doctor's offices. In some cases, she had seen the patients up to seven times.[120] The need for such qualified staff was huge and not only for diabetes training. Each relevant journal contained job offers.

Since nutritional training had previously been the field of the dietitians, their professional association tried to include dietary counselling into the diabetes training but covered by specially trained dietary experts so that the area of diet and nutrition would not have to be covered by the diabetes counsellors.[121] The ideal construction of a triple team consisting of doctor, dietary adviser, and diabetes counsellor must hence be understood as a product of a health political debate that focussed on prevention and defining the roles of competing health professions.

Without their own advocacy group, the diabetes counsellors could hardly make themselves heard. Their resentment grew when the expert society DDG recommended that they should join the self-help organisation DDB.[122] If they had followed this advice, diabetes counsellors would have been grouped with the organisation for non-professionals in the long term, i. e., they would have hardly been able to influence decisions regarding their field of expertise.

Yet, first attempts to found their own association in 1984 were not successful due to internal conflicts.[123] The diabetes counsellors received very little support from the DDG, some of their members expressly opposed the foundation of an independent association of diabetes counsellors. Their opinion was that diabetes counsellors could join the DDG at least as associate members and use their influence in this way. Thus, in 1990 two diabetes counsellors joined the committee "Non-professional Work" of the DDG.

For further intra-professional communications, the annual obligatory training courses were used. During the work meetings between 1989 and 1991 nothing more happened than discussing steps to return to the goal of founding an association. Another focus was to standardise the advanced training

---

119 For instance: Toeller/Schuhmacher (1983).
120 Cf. Kurow (1972), p. 405.
121 Cf. N. N. (1976), p. 135 and Chefredaktion (1983), p. 200.
122 Cf. Interview on 25/02/2015 with Bettina Brandner (transcription at the Institute for the History of Medicine of the Robert Bosch Stiftung, Stuttgart).
123 The treasurer at the time disappeared with the funds. Cf. Interview on 25/02/2015 with Bettina Brandner (transcription at the Institute for the History of Medicine of the Robert Bosch Stiftung, Stuttgart).

courses everywhere. Until then, each centre for diabetes had implemented the
guidelines of the DDG differently, and at times the annual training courses for
the counsellors were subject to significant changes.[124] As a result, the training
courses were the topic of several conferences that had the goal to ensure the
standardisation of the programmes, in particular after it had become possible
to invoice the training. This happened after 1 July 1991 when the National
Association of Statutory Health Insurance ("Kassenärztliche Bundesvereini-
gung", KBV) and the supplementary insurance funds concluded the diabetes agreement.[125] With this recognition of the importance of training patients
with diabetes, the goal to found an independent association of diabetes counsellors was even more vehemently pursued. Finally, on 13 November 1992 the
successful foundation was reported. During the fourth conference of diabetes
counsellors in Bad Hersfeld, the 71 members present agreed on the foundation of the association.[126] Among them were many diabetes counsellors of the
first two training sessions in 1983/1984 and 1985/1986.[127] In the following
years, numerous unresolved questions had to be answered. While on the one
hand efforts were made to gain state recognition of the profession of diabetes
counsellor, on the other hand the unification of Germany had raised the question of care for the patients with diabetes in the newly added East-German
states.[128]

## Differentiation and new educational programmes –
## the diabetes assistant

Considering the very different health systems in West and East Germany,
namely the federalist one in the West and the centralist outpatient system in
the East, there was, of course, a need to address the fact that both staff and
patients had been educated differently than in the West.

Initially the outpatient clinics had simply continued in the polyclinics as
before. Then, the Minister for Labour, Social Affairs, Health, Women and
Family Affairs in Brandenburg at the time, Regine Hildebrandt, initiated a pilot project. Drawing on the West German system, specially trained staff were
supposed to take on the care of patients with diabetes in dedicated doctor's

---

124  History of the VDBD, cf. https://www.vdbd.de/Templates/main.php?SID=131 (last ac-
     cessed: 31/10/2018).
125  Cf. Chefredaktion (1991), p. 2 and Chefredaktion (1992), p. 2.
126  Minutes of the foundation of the VDBD, cf. https://www.vdbd.de/Downloads/VDBD_
     Gruendungs-Protokoll_13111992.pdf (last accessed: 31/10/2018).
127  Cf. Interview on 19/01/2015 with Anne Lütke Twenhöven (transcription at the Institute
     for the History of Medicine of the Robert Bosch Stiftung, Stuttgart).
128  History of the VDBD, cf. https://www.vdbd.de/Templates/main.php?SID=131 (last ac-
     cessed: 31/10/2018).

surgeries. The required staff was supposed to be trained in specially created advanced education programmes.[129]

The first agreement on the billing for the care and training of diabetes patients between the insurance AOK Potsdam and the Association of Statutory Health Insurance Brandenburg provided for hiring a diabetes counsellor in every dedicated surgery.[130] Yet, the doctors rejected this idea because of the long training time and new concepts had to be developed. After creating multiple concepts that were all rejected for various reasons, the model of the diabetes assistant was adopted. The diabetologist Klaus Funke in collaboration with the DDG and the Central Institute in Karlsburg were crucial for this development.

Similar to the outpatient clinics, the diabetes assistant was supposed to primarily work in the outpatient area. Revised requirements for advanced training were supposed to result in less centralised courses in the continued professional development of diabetes counsellors.

The programme was supposed to consist of two parts, each lasting 14 days with an oral examination before an examination board at the end. 25 and 22 nurses, respectively, participated in the first two courses.[131]

The VDBD was critical of this development and focussed particularly on additional qualifications and quality assurance, because it did not want to have to put up with a qualitative step backwards in its efforts for professionalisation.[132]

A few years later, the additional qualification of diabetes assistants to become diabetes counsellors became possible.[133] Again, Klaus Funke worked on a concept in collaboration with the committee "Education and Additional Training". The first attempt to equalise the status of assistants and counsellors at the beginning of 1997 failed because of the resistance of the VDBD. However, opening up towards other professions that dealt with therapies for diabetes were considered.

The conflicts between assistants and counsellors that I sketched out here were not so much a part of fundamental problems within diabetes therapy but rather a part of negotiating the professionalisation process. Hence, the groups came closer together because, on the level of the various associations, a unified procedure to implement long-term goals was inevitable. In the year 2000, the VDBD was renamed into Association of Diabetes Counselling and Training Professions in Germany. Thus, counsellors and assistants were joined

---

129 Cf. Interview on 02/02/2015 with Klaus Funke and Gisela Müller (transcription at the Institute for the History of Medicine of the Robert Bosch Stiftung, Stuttgart).

130 Die ersten 10 Jahre VDBD (The first ten years of the VDBD), cf. https://www.vdbd.de/Downloads/VDBD_Historie_erste_10_Jahre.pdf (last accessed: 31/10/2018).

131 Cf. Interview on 02/02/2015 with Klaus Funke and Gisela Müller (transcription at the Institute for the History of Medicine of the Robert Bosch Stiftung, Stuttgart).

132 Die ersten 10 Jahre VDBD (The first ten years of the VDBD), cf. https://www.vdbd.de/Downloads/VDBD_Historie_erste_10_Jahre.pdf (last accessed: 31/10/2018).

133 Cf. Interview on 02/02/2015 with Klaus Funke and Gisela Müller (transcription at the Institute for the History of Medicine of the Robert Bosch Stiftung, Stuttgart).

in one organisation even though both career paths continued to exist. This was also a reason for the growth of the number of VDBD members from 71 (1992) to 1,765 (2001).[134]

## Conclusion and further development

While the need to train patients was already evident in the 1920s, it took more than half a century until the first approaches for a structured education programme had been developed. Until far into the 1950s it was solely the task of physicians to inform their patients, yet often these were GPs without specialisation in diabetology. Hence, often the patients had to stay in special hospitals or sanatoriums to acquire the necessary knowledge about their disease. Yet it became apparent that, despite the foundation of a self-help organisation and first counselling offices for diabetes, no appropriate training was truly available. Doctors had poor didactic and pedagogical skills, leading to a lack of treatment compliance and a higher tendency to listen and adhere to advice from non-professionals. At this problematic interface the professionally trained expert was supposed to come in. On the one hand she was supposed to teach the patients the necessary knowledge without the burden of technical language and the doctor's authority that was regarded as a hindrance in the basic training. On the other hand, she was supposed to advise on treatments only in coordination with the physician. Considering the many open questions with regard to the training, funding, and positioning within the health system there were numerous conflicts between diabetologists and diabetes counsellors who began to get organised, especially in the first years after the introduction of the first advanced educational courses. These conflicts erupted in various ways; for instance, for a long time doctors preferred to add the term assistant or training nurse as an addition to the title of the emerging profession to ensure that the subordinate role under the doctor was also linguistically apparent.

Common to all these professions are their constant adaptation to internal and external influences to legitimise themselves with respect to competing professions and associations. In the health system there are numerous agents with diverging interests. For the diabetes counselling and training professions, this means they have had to continuously expand and adapt their educational content, for instance with topics like hypertension and diabetic foot.[135] With the implementation of additional advanced training, as for instance podology DDG, consultant psychologist DDG, wound assistant DDG or the two diabetes nurses (hospital/long-term), there is now even further differentiation taking

---

134 Die ersten 10 Jahre VDBD (The first ten years of the VDBD), cf. https://www.vdbd.de/ Downloads/VDBD_Historie_erste_10_Jahre.pdf (last accessed: 31/10/2018).

135 Diabetic foot is a disease that results from diabetes mellitus because a poor circulation and damage to the nerves (neuropathy) result in a poor healing of wounds. The main cause is a badly controlled blood sugar.

place. New conflicts of professionalisation seem to be unavoidable because the working areas often overlap and additional associations outside of either diabetology or the DDG (e.g., podologists) strongly represent the interest of their members.

A hindrance is that state recognition has not been achieved in the entire country because of the resistance in the various states.[136] The only exception is Rhineland-Palatinate that has had a law in this regard since 2009.[137] Some other states (Thuringia) also show progress but a breakthrough is not yet in sight.[138]

The states argue for instance with the existing freedom of occupation and the goals to reduce bureaucracy and regulations. In addition, laws and regulations on further education are missing which poses additional problems. Adding 200 hours to the current curriculum and expanding it thus to 720 hours seems inevitable in order to comply with the minimum requirements of further education that is imposed by the federal government. Yet, in doing so the DDG would also have to comply with the federal framework with all its advantages and disadvantages for the funding body. Hence the efforts that are put in are rather restrained. Yet, while a limited interest is evident and the need for counsellors is undisputed, not everyone regards a stronger treatment team of doctor-counsellor-patient as desirable.[139] From the very beginning there was resistance within the DDG regarding binding regulations for further education and examinations that have only been slowly eliminated.

With various working groups on topics such as quality assurance, increase of performance, public relations and professional profile, further professionalisation will be pursued in the future. In 2017 the VDBD had already 3,800 members.[140]

---

136 State recognition VDBD, cf. https://www.vdbd.de/Templates/main.php?SID=163 (last accessed: 31/10/2018).

137 State regulations concerning the implementation of state laws on the further education in health professions ("Landesverordnung zur Durchführung des Landesgesetzes über die Weiterbildung in den Gesundheitsfachberufen", GFBWBGDVO) from 13/02/1998, cf. http://landesrecht.rlp.de/jportal/portal/page/bsrlpprod.psml?pid=Dokumentanzeige& showdoccase=1&js_peid=Trefferliste&documentnumber=1&numberofresults=1&from doctodoc=yes&doc.id=jlr-GFBWBGDVRPrahmen&doc.part=X&doc.price=0.0 (last accessed: 31/10/2018).

138 State recognition. Diabetologie-Online, cf. https://www.diabetologie-online.de/a/staat liche-anerkennung-der-stand-der-dinge-1692600 (last accessed: 31/10/2018).

139 Cf. Interview on 02/02/2015 with Klaus Funke and Gisela Müller (transcription at the Institute for the History of Medicine of the Robert Bosch Stiftung, Stuttgart).

140 VDBD Overview, cf. https://www.vdbd.de/Downloads/170709_Faltblatt_VDBD_auf_ einen_Blic.pdf (last accessed: 31/10/2018).

# Bibliography

*Archives*

Bayer Archiv Leverkusen (BAL)

386/55 Bayer Diagnostics
Compur 1979 Vol. 2 Bayer Diagnostika-Entwicklung


Stadtarchiv Stuttgart (StA Stgt)

19/1 Bü 748


Siemens MedArchiv Erlangen (SMA Erlangen)

2/513 MDS Laufende Bedarfsstudie zum Projekt "Mikrodosierung von Insulin"


Hauptstaatsarchiv Stuttgart (HStA Stgt)

EA 1/014 Bü 493/1
EA 8/601 Bü 387
EA 8/602 Bü 64/2


Private archive Pfaff

Documents Hellmut Mehnert
Documents Viktor Jörgens


*Literature*

Banse, Hans Joachim: Zuckerkrankheit – ein soziales Problem unserer Zeit. In: Diabetes-Journal (1955), no. 3, pp. 45–49.
Banse, Hans Joachim: Schulung und Information von Zuckerkranken. In: Diabetes-Journal (1959), no. 3, pp. 60–62.
Berger, Michael et al.: Bicentric Evaluation of a Teaching and Treatment Programme for Type 1 (Insulin-Dependent) Diabetic Patients: Improvement of Metabolic Control and other Measures of Diabetes Care for up to 22 Months. In: Diabetologia 25 (1983), pp. 470–476.
Bernhard, Hella: Deutsche Diabetiker-Betreuungsstellen. 16. Die Diabetes-Zentrale der Krankenversicherungsanstalt Berlin. In: Diabetes-Journal (1954), no. 8, pp. 140–141.
Bertram, Ferdinand: ABC für Zuckerkranke. Ein Ratgeber für den Kranken. 3rd ed. Stuttgart 1947.
Bertram, Ferdinand: Deutsche Diabetiker-Betreuungsstellen. 6. Diabetiker-Klinik im Allgemeinen Krankenhaus Ochsenzoll (früher A.K. Langenhorn). In: Diabetes-Journal (1953), no. 11, pp. 165–166.
Beyer, Jürgen: 20 Jahre Diabetestherapie mit Tabletten. In: Diabetes-Journal (1978), no. 10, pp. 394–397.

Böninger, Ch.: Diabetiker-"Schulung". Anregungen zur besseren Verwirklichung ihrer Ziele. In: Diabetes-Journal (1984), no. 7/8, pp. 314–317.

Bouchardat, Apollinaire: De la Glycosurie sucré son traitement hygiénique. Paris 1875.

Brückner, R.: Die Zuckerkrankheit als Schicksal und Verpflichtung. In: Diabetes-Journal (1960), no. 6, pp. 150–152.

Bruns, Waldemar: Die Geschichte der Diabetologie in der DDR. In: Deutsche Diabetes Gesellschaft (ed.): 50 Jahre Deutsche Diabetes Gesellschaft. Berlin 2014, pp. 68–79.

Chefredaktion: Alles neu macht der Mai? Oder Blutzucker in mmol/l? In: Diabetes-Journal (1978), no. 5, p. 197.

Chefredaktion: Europäischer Diabeteskongreß in Athen. In: Diabetes-Journal (1980), no. 11, p. 436.

Chefredaktion: Woran liegt's? In: Diabetes-Journal (1981), no. 6, p. 241.

Chefredaktion: Weiterbildung zum Diabetesberater. In: Diabetes-Journal (1983), no. 5, p. 200.

Chefredaktion: Ein Meilenstein in der Schulung. In: Diabetes-Journal (1991), no. 7, p. 2.

Chefredaktion: Schulung auf dem Prüfstand. In: Diabetes-Journal (1992), no. 4, p. 2.

Cray, William C.: Miles 1884–1984. A Centennial History. Englewood Cliffs, NJ 1984.

Creutzfeldt, Werner: Hauptaufgabe. Schulung der Diabetiker. In: Diabetes-Journal (1969), no. 5, pp. 185–186.

DDB (ed.): Der Deutsche Diabetiker-Bund informiert. In: Diabetes-Journal (1981), no. 1, p. 28; no. 3, p. 113.

DDB Orts- und Landesverband Hamburg. In: Diabetes-Journal (1961), no. 2, pp. 29–32.

Dehmel, K. H.: Diabetikerschulung. In: Diabetes-Journal (1969), no. 6, pp. 220–222.

Dennig, Helmut: Erfahrungen eines Krankenhausarztes mit Zuckerkranken. In: Diabetes-Journal (1954), no. 12, pp. 212–214.

Gardner, Martin A.: Quiz Kids. The Radio Program with the smartest Children in America 1940–1953. Jefferson, NC 2013.

Grote, Louis R.: Diätetische und Insulintherapie des Diabetes mellitus. In: Diabetes-Journal (1951), no. 10, p. 51.

Hähner-Rombach, Sylvelyn: Aus- und Weiterbildung in der Krankenpflege in der Bundesrepublik Deutschland nach 1945. In: Pfütsch, Pierre; Hähner-Rombach, Sylvelyn (eds.): Entwicklungen in der Krankenpflege und in anderen Gesundheitsberufen nach 1945. Frankfurt/Main 2018, pp. 146–194.

Halhuber, Carola: Über Fehler bei der Schulung von Patienten. In: Diabetes-Journal (1978), no. 12, pp. 504–507.

Heimann, Wilhelm: Diät ist die große Chance. Ein Frauenberuf macht Karriere. Diätassistentin. In: Diabetes-Journal (1960), no. 9, p. 242.

Himstedt, Monika: Soziale Probleme der Diabetiker. Unter besonderer Berücksichtigung der jugendlichen Diabetiker. In: Diabetes-Journal (1962), no. 1, pp. 7–9.

Irving, Greg et al.: International variations in primary care physician consultation time. A systematic review of 67 countries. In: BMJ Open 7 (2017), no. 10, pp. 1–15.

Janka, Hans-Uwe: Möglichkeiten und Grenzen der Diabetikerschulung. In: Diabetes-Journal (1979), no. 10, pp. 394–395.

Jörgens, Viktor: Von der "Schulung" zum "Training". In: Diabetes-Journal (2001), no. 12, pp. 43–48.

Katsch, Gerhardt: Zur bedingten Gesundheit des Diabetikers. In: Diabetes-Journal (1958), no. 9, pp. 225–234.

Kloss, Anton: 31 Jahre Insulin. In: Diabetes-Journal (1956), no. 3, pp. 51–54.

Kurow, Günther: Ambulante Diätberatung in Gruppen. In: Diabetes-Journal (1972), no. 11, pp. 404–405.

Lange, Heike: Zum Thema Schulung … In: Diabetes-Journal (1981), no. 3, pp. 104–106.

Lübken, W.: Kann ich nicht Tabletten nehmen? In: Diabetes-Journal (1972), no. 7, pp. 255–256.

Mascher, E. et al.: Ausnahmsweise. Anpassende Insulinbehandlung bei "labilem" Diabetes. In: Diabetes-Journal (1969), no. 6, pp. 205–210.

Mauck, Aaron: Managing Care. The History of Diabetes Management in Twentieth Century America. PhD diss. Harvard Univ. 2010.

N. N.: Schallplatten. Als Diabetiker gesund leben. In: Diabetes-Journal (1967), no. 2, p. 61.

N. N.: Lehren aus der Münchner Diabetes-Aktion. Nach einem Bericht der Bayrischen Landesärztekammer. In: Diabetes-Journal (1971), no. 9, pp. 322–325.

N. N.: Tagungsprogramm der 11. Jahrestagung der DDG. In: Diabetes-Journal (1976), no. 4, p. 135.

N. N.: Ausschuß für "Laienarbeit" von der Deutschen Diabetes-Gesellschaft gegründet. In: Diabetes-Journal (1978), no. 11, p. 449.

N. N.: Verleihung der Gerhard [sic] Katsch-Gedächtnis-Medaille. In: Diabetes-Journal (1980), no. 6, p. 242.

N. N.: Hurra – Wir haben's geschafft! Die ersten 25 von der Deutschen Diabetes-Gesellschaft ausgebildeten Diabetesberater möchten sich vorstellen. In: Diabetes-Journal (1984), no. 6, p. 275.

N. N.: Neuer Beruf: Diabetes-Berater/in. In: Diabetes-Journal (1984), no. 5, p. 234.

Nassauer, Luise; Petzoldt, Rüdiger: Grundlagen der Diabetesdiät. Viel Theorie und wenig Praxis. In: Diabetes-Journal (1991), special issue "40 Jahre Diabetes-Journal", pp. 64–69.

Pannhorst, Rudolf: Fast zwanzig Jahre DGE. In: Diabetes-Journal (1972), no. 12, pp. 439–441.

Petrides, Platon: Irrwege und Fehler in der Behandlung des Diabetes. In: Diabetes-Journal (1962), no. 10, pp. 295–300.

Petrides, Platon: Aktuelle sozialmedizinische Diabetes-Probleme. In: Diabetes-Journal (1966), no. 6, pp. 191–193.

Petzoldt, Rüdiger: Kosten und Nutzen der Diätberatung. In: Diabetes-Journal (1978), no. 2, pp. 54–57.

Pfaff, Aaron: "Man darf keine Kenntnisse beim Laien voraussetzen!" – Die Genese der Diabetes-Beratungs- und -Schulungsberufe. In: Pfütsch, Pierre; Hähner-Rombach, Sylvelyn (eds.): Entwicklungen in der Krankenpflege und in anderen Gesundheitsberufen nach 1945. Frankfurt/Main 2018, pp. 383–422.

Romeick, Marianne: Deutsche Diabetiker-Betreuungsstellen. 5 (a). Diabetikerfürsorge in Heidelberg. In: Diabetes-Journal (1954), no. 2, p. 29.

Romeick, Marianne: Hausbetreuung der Diabetiker. In: Diabetes-Journal (1955), no. 9, pp. 172–174.

Romeick, Marianne: Aufgaben einer Diabetes-Fürsorgerin. In: Diabetes-Journal (1963), no. 3, pp. 85–89.

Romeick, Marianne: Dolmetscherin zwischen Arzt und Patient. In: Diabetes-Journal (1980), no. 6, pp. 244–246.

Romeick, Marianne: Schulungserfahrung. In: Diabetes-Journal (1987), no. 2, p. 95.

Roth, Sabine: Entwicklung und Aufgaben des Deutschen Diabetiker-Bundes. Med. diss. Univ. Düsseldorf 1993.

Rottenhöfer, Helmuth: Diabetiker-Schulung. 9. Die Behandlung der Zuckerkrankheit. In: Diabetes-Journal (1954), no. 9, p. 149.

Schöller, Alex: Meine Krankenhauserfahrungen. In: Diabetes-Journal (1981), no. 12, pp. 478–479.

Scholz, Vera: Weiterbildungslehrgang zum Diabetesberater. Entwicklung und Evaluation eines Kurses zur Ausbildung von medizinischem Assistenzpersonal zur Schulung von Patienten mit Diabetes mellitus. Med. diss. Univ. Düsseldorf 1988.

Schweisheimer, W.: Lehrmaschinen bei Patienten mit Diabetes. In: Diabetes-Journal (1966), no. 1, pp. 13–14.

Ständer, Heinz: Der DDB berichtet. An die Mitglieder, Freunde und Förderer unseres Bundes. In: Diabetes-Journal (1968), no. 12, pp. 496–498.

Sulzer, Michael: Diabetikerbetreuung auf dem Land. In: Diabetes-Journal (1992), no. 5, pp. 4–5.

Thoms, Ulrike: Zwischen Kochtopf und Krankenbett. Diätassistentinnen in Deutschland 1890–1980. In: Medizin, Gesellschaft und Geschichte 23 (2004), pp. 133–162.

Toeller, Monika; Schuhmacher, Waltraud: Frau Oppler hat Diabetes. Harnzucker und Blutzucker kann man selbst messen. In: Diabetes-Journal (1983), no. 12, pp. 524–528.

Willms, Berend: "Laienarbeit". Aus der Arbeit des Ausschusses "Laienarbeit" der Deutschen Diabetes-Gesellschaft. In: Diabetes-Journal (1981), no. 10, pp. 408–409.

*Internet*

Diabetes-Ratgeber. Situation of diabetology: https://www.diabetes-ratgeber.net/Diabetes/Stirbt-die-Diabetologie-524591.html (last accessed: 31/10/2018).

Landesverordnung zur Durchführung des Landesgesetzes über die Weiterbildung in den Gesundheitsfachberufen (GFBWBGDVO), 13. Februar 1998: http://landesrecht.rlp.de/jportal/portal/page/bsrlpprod.psml?pid=Dokumentanzeige&showdoccase=1&js_peid=Trefferliste&documentnumber=1&numberofresults=1&fromdoctodoc=yes&doc.id=jlr-GFBWBGDVRPrahmen&doc.part=X&doc.price=0.0 (last accessed: 31/10/2018).

Deutscher Gesundheitsbericht der Deutschen Diabetes Gesellschaft (DDG) und der Deutschen Diabetes Hilfe (diabetesDE) as of 16/11/2016: https://www.diabetesde.org/system/files/documents/gesundheitsbericht_2017.pdf (last accessed: 31/10/2018).

State recognition. Diabetologie-Online: https://www.diabetologie-online.de/a/staatliche-anerkennung-der-stand-der-dinge-1692600 (last accessed: 31/10/2018).

VDBD Overview: https://www.vdbd.de/Downloads/170709_Faltblatt_VDBD_auf_einen_Blic.pdf (last accessed: 31/10/2018).

Minutes of the foundation of the VDBD: https://www.vdbd.de/Downloads/VDBD_Gruendungs-Protokoll_13111992.pdf (last accessed: 31/10/2018).

The first ten years of the VDBD: https://www.vdbd.de/Downloads/VDBD_Historie_erste_10_Jahre.pdf (last accessed: 31/10/2018).

VDBD History: https://www.vdbd.de/Templates/main.php?SID=131 (last accessed: 31/10/2018).

State recognition VDBD: https://www.vdbd.de/Templates/main.php?SID=163 (last accessed: 31/10/2018).

Verband der Diätassistenten. Berufsgeschichte: https://www.vdd.de/diaetassistenten/berufsgeschichtederdiaetassistenten/ (last accessed: 31/10/2018).

*Interviews*

Interview on 19/01/2015 with Marlies Neese (transcription at the Institute for the History of Medicine of the Robert Bosch Stiftung, Stuttgart).

Interview on 19/01/2015 with Anne Lütke Twenhöven (transcription at the Institute for the History of Medicine of the Robert Bosch Stiftung, Stuttgart).

Interview on 02/02/2015 with Klaus Funke and Gisela Müller (transcription at the Institute for the History of Medicine of the Robert Bosch Stiftung, Stuttgart).

Interview on 25/02/2015 with Bettina Brandner (transcription at the Institute for the History of Medicine of the Robert Bosch Stiftung, Stuttgart).

Interview on 23/07/2015 with Hellmut Mehnert (recording private archive Pfaff).

Interview on 15/12/2015 with Viktor Jörgens (recording private archive Pfaff).

# List of Authors

**Geertje Boschma, PhD, RN, Professor**
School of Nursing
University of British Columbia
T201–2211 Wesbrook Mall, Vancouver BC V6T 2B5
geertje.boschma@ubc.ca

**Jane Brooks, PhD, RN, Senior Lecturer**
Division of Nursing, Midwifery and Social Work
University of Manchester
Oxford Road, Manchester, M13 9PL, UK
jane.brooks@manchester.ac.uk

**Eyal Katvan, Dr., Dr., Senior Lecturer**
College of Law & Business
26 Ben-Gurion St., Ramat Gan, Israel
drkatvan@gmail.com

**Karen Nolte, Prof. Dr.**
Institut für Geschichte und Ethik der Medizin
Ruprecht-Karls-Universität Heidelberg
Im Neuenheimer Feld 327
D-69120 Heidelberg
karen.nolte@histmed.uni-heidelberg.de

**Aaron Pfaff, M. A.**
Institut für Geschichte der Medizin der Robert Bosch Stiftung
Straußweg 17
D-70184 Stuttgart
aaron.pfaff@igm-bosch.de

**Pierre Pfütsch, Dr.**
Institut für Geschichte der Medizin der Robert Bosch Stiftung
Straußweg 17
D-70184 Stuttgart
pierre.pfuetsch@igm-bosch.de

**Christoph Schwamm, Dr.**
Institut für Geschichte der Medizin der Robert Bosch Stiftung
Straußweg 17
D-70184 Stuttgart
christoph.schwamm@igm-bosch.de

**Eileen Thrower, APRN, CNM, Assistant Professor**
Frontier Nursing University Carrollton, Georgia
195 School St., Hyden, KY 41749, USA
eileen.thrower@frontier.edu